This book is a study of schizophrenia in a modern psychiatric hospital. Its purpose is to develop a contextual understanding of schizophrenia by studying the clinical setting in which this disorder is experienced, diagnosed, and treated. It arises from an anthropological investigation of the day-to-day work of clinical staff: admitting patients, writing in their case records, and talking about them at case conferences.

The author, who is both a psychiatrist and an anthropologist, focuses on three core professions — psychiatry, psychiatric nursing, and social work— examining the relationships among them in terms of team work and professional autonomy. He offers a penetrating analysis of the language used by hospital staff as they write and talk about their patients and the way in which this practice both reflects and defines the attributes of schizophrenia.

The book traces the evolution of the concept of schizophrenia, showing how contemporary theoretical constructs are applied by clinical staff. It shows how the organizational features of a modern psychiatric hospital have fundamental consequences for the way in which schizophrenia is constituted as a diagnostic category and a moral state, with broader implications for how we understand the person.

In its analysis of the schizophrenia team and of those experiencing the disorder, this book reveals to mental health professionals many of the unspoken assumptions of their role. It also confirms to social scientists and clinicians the power of the ethnographic approach in psychiatric research.

The Psychiatric Team and the Social Definition of Schizophrenia

STUDIES IN SOCIAL AND COMMUNITY PSYCHIATRY

Volumes in this series examine the social dimensions of mental illness as they affect diagnosis and management, and address a range of fundamental issues in the development of community-based mental health services.

Series editor
PETER J. TYRER
Professor of Community Psychiatry, St Mary's Hospital Medical School, London

Also in this series

The Psychiatric Team and the Social Definition of Schizophrenia

An Anthropological Study of Person and Illness

ROBERT J. BARRETT

University of Adelaide
Adelaide, South Australia

Foreword by BYRON J. GOOD

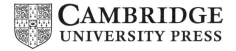
CAMBRIDGE
UNIVERSITY PRESS

Published by the Press Syndicate of the University of Cambridge
The Pitt Building, Trumpington Street, Cambridge CB2 1RP
40 West 20th Street, New York, NY 10011-4211, USA
10 Stamford Road, Oakleigh, Melbourne 3166, Australia

First published 1996

Printed in the United States of America

A catalog record for this book is available from the British Library

Library of congress cataloging-in-publication data

Barrett, Robert J.
    The psychiatric team and the social definition of schizophrenia /
Robert J. Barrett.
        p.   cm. — (Studies in social and community psychiatry)
    Includes bibliographical references and index.
    ISBN 0-521-41653-1 (hc)
    1. Schizophrenics—Rehabilitation—Social aspects.   2. Mental
health care teams.   3. Psychiatric hospitals—Sociological aspects.
4. Schizophrenia—Treatment—Social aspects.   5. Social
epistemology.   6. Social control.   I. Title.   II. Series.
RC514.B3666   1996
362.2′6—dc20   95-43459   CIP

ISBN 0-521-41653-1 Hardback

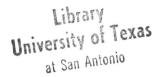

To Mitra

Contents

Foreword

Bearing a deceptively modest title, *The Psychiatric Team and the Social Definition of Schizophrenia*, this book provides a remarkable analysis of psychiatric knowledge and practice in a late twentieth century asylum.

'Ridgehaven Hospital' is a state institution in Australia undergoing transformations easily recognizable to any who have observed or worked in large psychiatric hospitals in North America or Europe. Once a total institution in Goffman's sense, a place where chronically mentally ill men and women lived out their lives, at the time of Dr. Barrett's research Ridgehaven was progressively reducing the number of its beds, discharging former patients into the community, and exploring new approaches to care. It had come to emphasize relatively brief hospital stays to stabilize the acutely ill, to provide them initial medical and pharmaceutical treatments, and to begin their rehabilitative services. In place of long term hospitalization, most patients were being sent back into the community where they face far less centralized surveillance and care than that provided under the old regime. This book thus provides a report on the status of the asylum and the practices it houses as the era of the 'Great Confinement' draws to a close after more than 300 years.

Barrett's book joins Sue Estroff's *Making It Crazy* and Lorna Rhodes' *Emptying Beds: The Work of an Emergency Psychiatric Unit* in analyzing a central component of the mental health system that is emerging as 'deinstitutionalization' moves forward. In conversation with the work of Michel Foucault, all three writers demonstrate that institutional powers and surveillance, though diffused, are pervasive in the lives of the mentally ill in the new regime as they were in the old. Barrett's primary interest, however, is not in the asylum as an institution of repression or in "schizophrenia" as a category justifying disciplinary procedures—one line of critical theory stimulated by Foucault's writing. Instead, this work starts from an assumption that institutionalized power is a "productive force which generates categories of knowledge and practice" and undertakes a detailed examination of everyday speaking practices through which 'schizophrenia', 'the schizophrenic', and 'the person with schizophrenia' are constituted as objects of medical practice and a domain of highly specialized knowledge in the contemporary hospital. It is in this context that psychiatric "teams"—psychiatrists, nurses, and social workers joined together to form an "Acute Team," a "Rehabilitation Team," and a "Schizophrenia Team"—are shown to be far more than incidental organizational groupings for providing care. They are formally assembled professionals who reconstitute individual patients as multidimensional "cases," evaluated in broad 'biopsychosocial' terms and treated accordingly.

By taking on the role of ethnographer, Barrett—a psychiatrist as well as anthropologist—submits the "taken for granted ideas and practices," the common-sense language of everyday psychiatric work, and the organization of time, space, and people at Ridgehaven to sustained 'archaeological' analysis. He moves from the surface of professional groupings and their claims to authorized knowledge, to a less visible, procedural level of speaking and writing practices, to a set of deep historical formations that exert their influence on the everyday contours of psychiatric knowledge. Layer by layer, a set of key discursive forms that serve as the building blocks of this knowledge are uncovered, allowing a number of conclusions to be drawn that have relevance well beyond Ridgehaven.

First, whatever the fate of totalizing institutions in this postmodern era, and whatever the limits of the psychiatric armamentarium, Barrett shows that the metanarrative of "progress" remains as powerful in psychiatry as in the rest of medicine. It is apparent in the organization of space at Ridgehaven: "progressive" forms of care are provided in the newest buildings in the front of the complex, while remnants of the old institution, the locked wards in which custodial care is provided for chronic patients, are hidden away in the buildings at the rear of the institution, an embarrassing reminder of psychiatry's ancient history. Space and time are thus joined by a common historical narrative, and confinement is "transposed to the past and depicted as having been rendered unnecessary by humane care . . . and modern medicine." This image of progressive care requires a category of patients susceptible to diagnosis and worthy of therapeutic investment. Not surprisingly, those patients most resistant to treatment and return to the community are excluded from this trajectory and end up in the care of nurses rather than the multidisciplinary Schizophrenia Team. Claims that psychiatric knowledge and therapeutics are advancing—along with neurobiology—are thus preserved, and patients, treatment forms, and bureaucratic practices are all submitted to moralizing judgements rendered in the language of progressive history.

Subtly embedded in assumptions about social and scientific progress is the counterimage of "degeneracy." Barrett's historical archaeology traces the distinction between chronic, degenerative mental illness, which is almost always incurable, and circular or periodic forms, which are curable, back through the writings of Emile Kraepelin to the institutional settings for psychiatric knowledge production in the nineteenth century asylum. These asylums provided a gathering of patients and a set of techniques that facilitated the development of a *Klinisches Bild*, a "clinical picture" of insanity, through a layering of case descriptions mapping out course and prognosis of illness. When linked to colonialist and evolutionary theorizing about non-progressive or degenerate races, and to concerns about moral degeneracy associated with the urban industrial poor, the image of insanity as degeneracy which is rooted in heredity provided a powerful model for observation and interpretation and a justification for eugenics as a social project. While we now know that long term confinement produced much of the chronicity that came to be seen as a hallmark of schizophrenia, it is remarkable how persistent in psychiatry is the distinction between chronic, degenerative disorders and circular or periodic disorders. Several decades of longitudinal studies have shown that schizophrenic illnesses are often periodic, while "bipolar" illnesses are often chronic and degenerative; nonetheless, the historic image of *dementia praecox* as the classic degenerative disorder is subtly present in contemporary psychiatric practice as it was in the old asylum.

The image of the disintegrated self is also unearthed as a part of everyday clinical lore in Ridgehaven, as well as in popular talk about schizophrenia. Rooted in the romantic ideal of the coherent and unitary self, an ideal associated with nineteenth century nationalists' efforts to resurrect a whole from a fragmented people, the counterimage of the dissociated, fragmented, or split person persists in the popular imagination and everyday psychiatric knowledge.

While these images are potent symbolic resources with enormous subterranean force, Barrett's most powerful analyses are of everyday practices rather than symbols and semantics. In two central chapters of the book, Barrett provides an ethnographic account of the most mundane practice through which the work of psychiatry is accomplished: writing and speaking. Data about every patient who enters Ridgehaven are recorded in a chart. Writing in the chart, providing a record of intake interviews and evaluations, is part of the everyday routine of members of the psychiatric team. However, as Barrett's careful comparisons of tape-recorded interview texts and written notes in patients' charts make clear, writing is no simple copy of the patient's verbal accounts. Writing is the central act in the construction of a 'case' of schizophrenia. It is a professional account that documents the presence of symptoms necessary for a diagnosis; more than that, it is an account that characterizes the illness as an active agent in control of an ultimately passive patient. The first act of incorporating a patient into the clinical world is thus an act of writing that defines him or her as a case.

Barrett shows, however, that this is only the first step in situating the patient within a therapeutic trajectory. Such a trajectory is a movement through time—from the origins of the illness to potential and hoped for outcomes. It is a passage through space—through the physical spaces of the hospital and back into the community, as well as through metaphoric spaces of being out of one's mind before returning to reality.

And it is a moral trajectory from a case of schizophrenia to a person who can be held responsible for his or her actions. Barrett argues that facilitating or enacting this trajectory, transforming the patient from case of schizophrenia to moral agent, is the central objective of treatment at Ridgehaven. And contrary to all expectations, Barrett discovered in his research that the most "unprofessional" forms of talk by members of the psychiatric team—off-hand comments about whether a patient was 'acting' in order to gain admission to the hospital, whether he was playing up to the staff or manipulating the physicians, for example—were crucial to the reestablishment of the patient as moral agent. Such talk was informal, judgmental, and explicitly subjective; staff at Ridgehaven, as elsewhere, were embarrassed to be heard using such language by any outsiders. However, rather than simply signifying disrespect for the patient or relieving tensions among the staff, Barrett argues, such talk is central to the therapeutic work of the team, to monitoring the patient's 'progress' and effecting the transformation of a case into a moral actor.

These findings, as well as the analytic methods from which they are derived, have significance for some of the most difficult problems facing mental health workers and consumers in the current era. How can psychiatric patients be 'empowered' in the context of emerging institutional arrangements? How can agency be restored to those suffering from severe and sometimes debilitating mental illnesses? How can schizophrenia be refigured, represented in new and less constraining ways, given the over-determined nature of symbolic resources we inherit for talking about this disorder? How are we to understand and value those writing and speaking practices associated with clinical work, and how might the subversive resources of everyday speech be employed in 'psychoeducational' efforts employed with families and sufferers? If social response and cultural interpretations are important for explaining course and outcome of schizophrenic illness, as recent research suggests, refiguring mental illness may be essential to the emergence of more positive therapeutic trajectories for those who are ill. And if the historical record is to be a guide, the progress of biological psychiatry is likely to be achieved in a cultural medium that reproduces many of the most disempowering contradictions of Euroamerican psychologies.

Tucked away in the conclusion of this book is one of Barrett's most provocative suggestions. "When we gather together a group of people with schizophrenia in order to study this illness," he suggests,

> it must be recognized that we are categorizing them on the basis of cultural principles which first began to form in eighteenth century Europe, which crystallized in the nineteenth century, and which have become consolidated and transformed in this century. It would be astonishing indeed were we to identify a singular biochemical process or gene to account for such a dynamic cultural category. For the purpose of conducting research, psychiatry may find it useful to temporarily suspend belief in schizophrenia, and to focus biological investigations on groups of people categorized in other ways which are less steeped in our cultural history, for example people who experience hallucinations or who manifest thought disorder.

This modest suggestion runs counter to the dominant stream of neo-Kraepelinian psychiatry, just as does much of the writing in this provocative book. But it indicates quite practical implications of an archaeological analysis of this 'dynamic cultural category'. It suggests, for example, the importance of serious cross-cultural research, in which 'belief in schizophrenia' is at least held open for discussion. It argues for further research into the interplay of the idioms of science and moral agency in the shaping of the psychiatric subject and the trajectory of mental illness. And it suggests approaches to clinical and even biological investigations that are less constrained by the hidden contours of our linguistic and theoretical heritage. It thus sets forth a challenging agenda for psychiatry, the behavioral sciences, and anthropology.

Byron J. Good
Cambridge, Massachusetts
March, 1995

Preface

This study was carried out while I was employed as a psychiatrist at 'Ridgehaven Hospital'. I experienced a tension between my two roles—ethnographer and psychiatrist—similar in kind to that experienced by most anthropologists when they participate in the social group they are observing. Perhaps I felt it more keenly than most because the role of a psychiatrist was so conspicuous in Ridgehaven Hospital.

My education and professional training have oscillated between anthropology and psychiatry. After graduating in medicine and working as an intern in a general hospital, I completed undergraduate studies in anthropology. This period was followed by postgraduate training in psychiatry. After that I began working part-time at Ridgehaven as specialist psychiatrist and undertook this study as part of a doctoral programme in anthropology.

I thus brought to the study a fluency in the language of medicine and psychiatry. It was an undoubted asset but also an impediment; my familiarity with the world of the psychiatric hospital and its language often made it difficult for me to perceive the taken-for-granted assumptions on which that world was built. It was only with the assistance of my anthropologist colleagues, who continually insisted that I maintain a sense of curiosity about what I normally regarded as self-evident, that I was to make use of my cultural competence in an analytic way.

Being a member of the staff facilitated my entry into fieldwork. It gave me access to the clinical sphere of hospital life from which a nonclinician might have been excluded on

grounds of confidentiality. I was also drawn quickly into administrative domains of the hospital. Once it became known
that I was interested in studying how people wrote in case
records I was press-ganged into chairmanship of the hospital's
medical records committee, a position that thrust me into the
interface between the administrative and clinical divisions of
the hospital, an area of conflicting pressures. As the same
time, because I was already identified as a psychiatrist, I had
to work hard to establish myself as an anthropologist, which
involved bridging the social boundaries that separated the various professional and occupational groups. I found it fairly
easy to undertake field-work with psychiatrists, psychiatric
nurses, and social workers; but it was only by persevering that
I gradually gained the trust of domestic cleaners and pantry
maids. The most pronounced division within the hospital lay
between staff and patients. I was never adequately able to cross
this social chasm and be accepted as an anthropological researcher by the patients because at other times I might find
myself in a position of detaining these same patients to a
closed ward. I deliberately focused this study on the staff, although I tried, as much as possible, to incorporate into my
analysis the contribution patients made to our understanding
of hospital life and of schizophrenia.

My dual role as anthropologist and psychiatrist has given
me a personal experience, though a limited and benign one,
of the inner divisions within the person that become a focus
of this analysis. As the eminent social anthropologist Evans-
Pritchard (1973:1) observed:

> Perhaps it would be better to say that one lives in two different
> worlds of thought at the same time, in categories and concepts
> and values which often cannot easily be reconciled. One be-
> comes a sort of double marginal man, alienated from both
> worlds.

Toward a better understanding of inner division and marginality, I offer this book.

Acknowledgements

The same duality is embedded in my ancestry. My father combined dental research with cultural anthropology in a series of studies he carried out among the Wailbiri people at Yuendumu in central Australia. He sparked an interest in anthropology within me when, as a young teenager, I accompanied him on field trips to Yuendumu.

Of those who directly helped me with this work, my chief debt is to Roy Fitzhenry, who stimulated and developed my interest in the ethnographic study of modern institutions. Roy generously shared his ideas and his wide reading with me and provided rigorous and detailed criticism of this study as it developed. John Gray assisted me greatly in developing the skills of an ethnographer; and it was he, more than anyone, who forced me to question as an anthropologist what I as a psychiatrist took for granted. Issy Pilowsky fostered and supported this study from its beginning to its completion. Arthur Kleinman, Byron Good, and members of the Departments of Anthropology and Social Medicine at Harvard University offered careful criticism of this work during the period I was writing it up. My close friend, Don Pollock, who was at the time working on related problems in a study of a general hospital, continually extended the analytic scope of this work. Many others have given me encouragement and support, especially Nancy Munn and Renée Fox. More recently I have worked on this manuscript in association with my colleague Rod Lucas. At first Rod offered his skilled editorial assistance, but gradually his contribution developed into a critical analysis of the ethnographic data. Rod has a special ability to express anthropological and sociological concepts in clear English without sacrificing their complexity. As a result of his influence, successive versions of the manuscript became more readable and, at the same time, much more incisive and penetrating in their analyses of the psychiatric hospital and of schizophrenia.

The study was supported, in part, by a Neil Hamilton Fairley Fellowship from the National Health and Medical Research Council. I received the full support of my colleagues at Ridgehaven Hospital, which included financial assistance from the hospital research fund. In particular, the Chief Executive Officer encouraged this project from its inception to its completion, when he proof read the manuscript with his customary enthusiasm. I wish to thank the staff of the Schizophrenia Team, particularly the psychiatrists and trainee psychiatrists who showed great patience in being studied and tape-recorded, and in answering the many questions which I put to them, especially those where the answers seemed, at first, to be self-evident. The Team Leader not only subjected himself to my scrutiny but provided thoughtful comments on the research findings. The nursing staff, more than any other group, were enthusiastic about the research and willingly helped me at every turn. I am particularly grateful to the patients of Ridgehaven for the insights they gave me into schizophrenia and which I have tried to convey in this work. Anne McGrane gave many hours of time helping with the transcription of audio tape-recordings. Carla Fujimoto removed all the split infinitives from the drafts of this book and Judy Liney checked the proofs with precision.

My wife, Mitra Guha, with her physician's knowledge of hospital culture and her clarity of English expression, was the final judge.

1

Schizophrenia in context

Ridgehaven Hospital is a state psychiatric hospital in an Australian city. In 1980 one division, or 'Team', of the hospital was designated exclusively for the treatment of schizophrenia. This book is a study of the 'Schizophrenia Team', the clinical staff who worked on it, and the patients they treated. Its purpose is to develop a contextual understanding of schizophrenia by studying a clinical setting in which this disorder was experienced, diagnosed, and treated.

At the time of the study, Ridgehaven Hospital was widely regarded as a modern public psychiatric hospital that had very high standards of practice, the first such hospital to be accredited by the Australian Council of Hospital Standards. There was an *esprit* among the staff. This book is thus a study of hospital psychiatry at its best, not a critique of a custodial backwater. It is an opportunity to examine the place of modernity and progress in psychiatric treatment.

The book focuses first on the clinical staff of the hospital, who were members of different professions but worked together in teams when treating patients. It looks at three core professions—psychiatry, psychiatric nursing, and social work —comparing the different perspectives their members employed in their individual therapeutic work and when acting in concert as part of a treatment team. My purpose is to examine how the professions were organized in relation to each other within a psychiatric hospital, and how this organization influenced the way clinical staff approached patients and constructed them as cases of psychiatric illness.

Two of the basic tools of clinical work are writing and talking. The second part of this book looks at how the staff of Ridgehaven wrote and talked about their patients. It concentrates on assessment interviews and the ways in which these interviews were documented in case records, tracing the transformations that occurred from spoken dialogue to written record. I compare these written accounts of patients with the way staff members spoke to each other about their patients—that is, with what could be said but never written in the record. This section of the book poses a number of questions: What consequences do such basic clinical processes as diagnosis and treatment have for a person? What transformations are achieved in a person's experience and identity when he or she engages with an expert team of talking, writing professionals?

Ridgehaven was not only a place where patients were treated, it was also a site for the production of knowledge about psychiatric illness. The third part of this book looks at some of the prominent psychiatric theories of schizophrenia that have been produced by institutions such as Ridgehaven Hospital. To accomplish this task it is necessary to go back to the origins of the concept of schizophrenia itself, beginning with ideas that were current during the nineteenth century and that emerged mainly from European psychiatric asylums and universities. I trace how these ideas have changed during the twentieth century as psychiatric hospitals and their related institutions have themselves undergone change. These theories are not merely abstract ideas about schizophrenia found in textbooks or scientific journals; they have practical significance for patients. Thus I take a number of contemporary theoretical constructs and show how they are applied by clinical staff when they teach patients about their schizophrenia.

A standard method of studying schizophrenia is to proceed from illness to context, that is, to take the psychiatric category of schizophrenia as a given and show that it can have different clinical manifestations depending on the cultural and institutional context in which it occurs. This book turns that method on its head. It proceeds from context to illness. It begins with an analysis of a modern psychiatric hospital and shows how its organizational features have fundamental consequences for the way in which schizophrenia is constituted as a diagnostic category and a moral state.

There are important differences between this approach and that of labelling theory, which asserts that the hospital merely imposes a false and stigmatizing identity upon the patient. By contrast, I argue that the psychiatric hospital is a site where common-sense ideas about mental illness are concentrated and refined. Many of these ideas have currency within the broader community and are shared by patients and their families. Worked up into scientific concepts of schizophrenia they take on a distinctive objectivity and distance. When patients, during the course of their treatment, learn that they are suffering from schizophrenia, their experience of illness and of themselves is transformed. This book traces these transformations.

In the course of this analysis, schizophrenia is encountered in a variety of guises. For patients it is a multitude of experiences: confusing, unusual, often devastating, but also entrancing and sometimes quite mundane. Some patients may not even define these experiences as an illness at all. Family members speak of schizophrenia as a tragedy and, in the more recent context of deinstitutionalization, as a burden that strains their ability to cope. For clinicians it is a severe illness that is difficult to treat and that usually has a poor prognosis. Within the field of biomedical research it is a poorly understood syndrome at the basis of which is a brain disorder with genetic, cognitive, and neurophysiological aspects. To the antipsychiatrist it is a myth—an invention of psychiatry and the mental hospital as joint agents of social control. At a common-sense level it is madness. Many of these views are incompatible, and some of them are put forward and defended with great vehemence. These competing definitions point to fundamental ambiguities in the way reason, autonomy, and the person are defined in our culture. Advocates of each approach often assert their particular view as an exclusive truth, but it impoverishes schizophrenia to reduce it to one version or another. On empirical grounds it is more accurate to assert that schizophrenia is all these things; and that in order to understand it we must grasp it as a multiple reality. An objective of this study is to map out these multiple manifestations in order to develop an anthropological analysis of the cultural logic that generates them and that accounts for the various relationships between them.

In this book, no one view of schizophrenia is accorded priority. In particular, it is neither an apology for nor an attack on psychiatric definitions of schizophrenia. In much sociological literature the 'medical model' has been something to be dismissed out of court by marshalling contrary evidence. On the other hand, cross-cultural psychiatry has tended to treat the psychiatric definition of schizophrenia as an *a priori* entity and then proceed to show how it is variously experienced within different social groups or influenced by various cultural factors. Both in its dismissal by sociology and its unquestioning acceptance by cross-cultural psychiatry, there has been a failure to disarticulate and examine the psychiatric definition of schizophrenia itself in order to demonstrate how such a set of ideas and attendant practices can come to exist at all. This study seeks to burrow underneath medical, psychiatric, and sociological reasoning, to look at daily interactions between patients and clinicians, to examine the ideas that constitute schizophrenia, to locate these ideas within Western culture and institutions, and to understand the consequences for those who experience the disorder.

Ethnography and the interpretive approach to schizophrenia

To grasp schizophrenia in its various guises it is necessary to use an ethnographic research strategy. This provides the most sympathetic and exacting way of exploring relationships between ideas, the people who use them, and the settings in which they are used. Ethnography is a method of gathering data about people's everyday lives that requires the researcher to immerse himself or herself in their world. It is also a mode of analysis that accords a central place to interpretation. At one time it was associated solely with social anthropology and was of interest to medicine only as a curiosity. However, in the last three decades ethnography has increasingly penetrated medical research to the point where it is now acknowledged as an important and innovative research strategy, though it has not yet achieved the complacency that comes from being a conventional method.

Ethnography produces a different type of knowledge about schizophrenia than that produced by positivist clinical science. Within the positivist paradigm, a researcher gathers a group of patients, either an epidemiological sample or a case series. They are then 'measured' in terms of their clinical state, neurophysiology, psychological functioning, or sociodemographic profile. Techniques are standardized because the researcher's own interpretations are regarded as a bias that contaminates the findings. Clinical interviews are therefore structured into questionnaire and rating scale format, giving them a mechanical or instrumental quality. The chief technical concern is to conduct investigations that can be repeated reliably by numbers of researchers in varying contexts.

Positivist science produces a form of knowledge known as 'facts', which are attributed objectivity because they are quantifiable, replicable, and lie beyond the interpretive discretion of the individual researcher. Data are translated into variables and rendered into numbers in order to discover statistical correlation and test hypotheses. Cases are studied in sufficient numbers to allow the variety and range of patients' experiences to be eliminated by an averaging process. The purpose of such research is to study the illness by isolating it from its context. This is reflected in the style of research reports. The passive tense, abstract nouns, and technical language convey a sense of distance, moving the patient and clinician out of focus in order to bring a decontextualized disorder into focus. The method derives its mandate and validation from the spectacular success of twentieth century medicine in understanding the mechanisms of illness.

By contrast, ethnographic inquiry brings the context—the patient, family members, clinicians, and setting—into focus. As a field technique it depends on an intimate association with the group of people under study and is usually carried out by one or two individuals at most. Rather than seeking anonymity and distance, the ethnographer plays an active role in the group he or she studies. This strategy of engagement aims to elicit data that would be told only to an accepted member of the group, and it enables the researcher to observe at first hand the social processes of that group. Fluency with language is mandatory—in this instance, the language of psychopathology and psychiatric hospital argot. Observations are recorded in field notes, jotted at the time and written up in more detail within a day or so. I also found it useful to openly tape-record interviews in which clinicians assessed patients, as well as the case conferences in which the treatment of patients was discussed.

Ethnographic research pays special attention to ceremonial occasions such as, in this study, the weekly team meeting or the admission of a new patient into the hospital. Such ceremonies boldly display the values and social processes of the group. Texts are another valuable source of data, particularly the case records and the voluminous documentation produced within the hospital about the hospital itself, its organization, its public image, and its history. Open-ended questioning of patients and staff provides a source of data in which informants reflect on themselves and their practices. The focus of all observations is the culture and social organization of the hospital.

As an analytic technique, ethnography begins with the systematic description and analysis of recurring social interactions (for example, in this study the admission interview, the morning coffee break, or the team meeting), of organizational categories (for example, the trainee psychiatrist or the chronic patient), and of major social processes (such as the process of writing in case records). These data are employed to identify more general processes, cultural meanings, and problems that pervade the organization and give it its coherence and distinctiveness. These first-order generalizations are analysed in the light of higher-order theories, so the conclusions of the study are grounded in a dialectic of formal social theory and field observation (Glaser and Strauss 1967).

Ethnographic research recognises the importance of interpretation at every stage, from the collection of field data to the conclusions of the study. When a researcher writes down so called 'naked' observations, interpretive judgements are already at play in choosing what is relevant, omitting what is taken for granted, and couching the data in a prose style that ensures it is read as a witnessed fact. The analysis seeks to lay bare these interpretive processes, both those of the researcher and the group being studied. In the case of the researcher, it involves a reflexive process that takes the unstated assumptions that she or he brings to the field and seeks to make them explicit rather than mask them. Applied to the group, ethnography's chief concern is with the way people interpret and make sense of their world. In this study I was concerned with how people make sense of schizophrenia in the setting of a psychiatric hospital.

Ethnographic studies of the psychiatric hospital

Isolated ethnographic studies of mental hospitals were started during the 1930s, but the major, classical studies were carried out in the United States during the two decades following World War II. This was a time of reform and therapeutic vigour, of the kind that had periodically swept through asylums since their inception. Health policy determined that these inward-looking institutions, which had come to epitomize state oppression, should be opened to public scrutiny, democratized, and eventually dismantled. Ethnographers worked in collaboration with hospital administrators to articulate such state policy, and the perspectives they used to analyse hospital organization reflected this political context.

Thus Caudill (1958) expressed the reformer's view that the psychiatric hospital was in trouble because it was a small, static society, an enclosed system with interrelated subsystems, walled off from the larger world. Stanton and Schwartz (1954) had proposed a similar functionalist view of the mental hospital as an integrated social system that could achieve effective treatment of the mentally ill so long as its subsystems meshed in harmonious consensus. According to their analysis, which differed little from the thinking of hospital administrators of that era, failure was located in the covert disagreements and pseudo-consensus that were symptomatic of a malfunctioning system. Rushing (1964) also drew on the functionalist theories of Parsons and Radcliffe-Brown to study how members of different professions adapted to conflict in a university psychiatric hospital. Belknap (1956), when he documented the failure of a southern state mental hospital to achieve its own goal of humanitarian treatment of the mentally ill, pitted the abject

conditions of the hospital against an ideal of scientific psychiatry as a salvation. By embracing the contemporary enthusiasm for psychiatry, Belknap committed himself to the rational-
efficient model of hospital organization commonly espoused
by clinician–administrators. As a consequence, he was unable
to perceive that hospitals might have structured, though un-
intended, consequences that differed from their publicly
stated goals.[1] The most influential works were those of Goffman (1968), whose essays on the 'total institution' and the
underlife of the asylum were, respectively, an indictment of
state control and a celebration of the freedom-seeking self.

One study, *Psychiatric Ideologies and Institutions* (Strauss *et al.*
1964), deserves a more extended critical analysis because its
perspectives were not wedded to state health policy but derived instead from the theoretical school of symbolic interactionism. This school, which developed in Chicago over the
first half of the twentieth century to become a dominant paradigm of American sociology, is germane to the arguments
developed in this book. Symbolic interactionism stressed the
symbolic environment of shared ideology, meanings, and values that characterizes the human social world (Blumer 1971;
Rose 1971). Its principal theorist, George Herbert Mead
(1934), viewed social interaction as a mutually interpretive
process, based on the capacity of the individual to take the
role of the other person—to imagine how he or she might be
interpreted by the other. At a macrosocial level, symbolic interactionism posited a fluid model of society in which change
and conflict are integral to social structure, an explicit critique
of previous models of society as static and harmoniously functioning systems. At a microsocial level, it posited a 'self' that
was not only grounded in social roles but also a locus of re-
flexivity and creativity.

From this basis, Strauss (1978:31–8; Strauss *et al.* 1964:172–5)
argued that Goffman's view of the asylum was overly pessimistic. For Goffman the total institution was primarily coercive,

[1] See Etzioni (1960) for a critique of Caudill, Stanton and Schwartz, Belknap and
a number of others who have approached the study of mental hospital organization from a 'human-relations' perspective. They place too much emphasis, argues Etzioni, on communication and participation in decision making, and they
tend to see the mental hospital as an autonomous totality, at the expense of analyzing its structural location within the broader society.

and the patient's 'moral career' was fatefully determined by the hospital. He could define freedom only in terms of the distance individuals accomplished from institutional roles (Goffman 1972). Strauss accorded a more central place to the way members of an institution actively affected their own fate. For him, the institutional order was not an external force that controlled passive individuals. Individuals, including patients, participated in determining this order.

Psychiatric Ideologies and Institutions compared three settings: the 'chronic' section of a state mental hospital in Chicago, the 'treatment' section of the same hospital, and a private psychiatric hospital. In the chronic service, custodial care was provided for large numbers of patients by poorly trained staff. In contrast, the treatment service comprised wards that had been established in a spirit of reform. Each was well staffed by professionally trained clinicians who brought with them a zealous commitment to treatment. Three distinct psychiatric ideologies were evident in this hospital. One was a 'somatotherapeutic' ideology, which took a biological view of psychiatric illness and was associated with the use of physical modes of treatment such as electroconvulsive therapy. The second was 'psychotherapeutic'. It argued that psychopathology is caused by emotional trauma during the formative childhood years, and it advocated psychotherapy as a mode of treatment. Third, there was a 'sociotherapeutic' ideology whose proponents stressed the importance of environmental factors in mental illness. For them, the whole ward was a therapeutic milieu.

The state hospital was characterised by conflict and change. The treatment service was in conflict with the chronic service. Within the treatment service itself, each ward was in fierce competition with the others for successful cure rates and financial resources. Within each ward there were shifting alliances as different professional groups struggled to assert therapeutic dominance. The psychiatric hospital was an arena into which changing ideologies were introduced from universities and training institutions. Different ideologies generated conflict. As a consequence of this conflict, the ideologies themselves were sharpened and amplified. Thus the hospital was both a recipient of and a crucible for the production of the ideologies that influenced how patients were treated.

The private hospital was similar. Explicit and tacit negotiation between staff members was a pervasive aspect of hospital life. Rules emerged and then faded into the background. The institutional order was not simply a formal jurisdiction governed by fixed administrative rules; it had an informal area of negotiation as well. The whole order was negotiable, the rules being just one resource that people used in their negotiations. Patients too bargained with staff for discharge or privileges. Although there were recurring patterns in this web of negotiations, the negotiated order itself was in continual flux. According to Strauss *et al.* (1964:375):

> Such findings suggest that organizational theory, elaborated largely from studies of both bureaucracy and rather formalized industrial or governmental organizations, needs considerable modifications to be meaningful for hospitals. When professionals are brought together and enjoined to carry out their work in the same locale, concepts of structure (formal or informal) as relatively set systems of norms and expectations, are inadequate to explain resulting activity. The activity of interacting professionals is, we submit, largely governed by continual reconstitution of bases of work through negotiation.

Anselm Strauss's symbolic interactionist perspective is a point of departure for this study of Ridgehaven. Like Strauss, I view the psychiatric hospital as an arena of competing professional perspectives in which individuals actively negotiate institutional rules and meanings. However, my study has a number of objectives that cannot be addressed adequately within Strauss's framework because symbolic interactionism fails to deal with two important issues: one concerning taken-for-granted ideas of mental illness, and the other concerning the broader social and historical location of psychiatric knowledge. The social phenomenology of Alfred Schutz and Michel Foucault's analyses of power and knowledge, in turn, provide the theoretical means to address these two issues.

Taken-for-granted ideas and practices

Strauss pays insufficient attention to those ideas about psychiatry that are taken for granted by the people who work in the hospital. He uncritically embraces their terminology, tacit models, theories, and beliefs. Such ideas creep, scarcely noticed, into his analysis (Day 1977). For example, the staff of the state mental hospital stressed that although they did espouse conflicting ideologies there was an underlying bedrock of consensus. All agreed on the fundamental common goal, which was to cure or treat the mentally ill. Strauss takes this idea of consensus and incorporates it into his analytic model. With an optimism typical of the liberal political order of that era (Hall 1973), he views ideological conflict as a surface phenomenon that can always be resolved by negotiation, thereby reaffirming the underlying basis of consensus on which the social order rests.

Yet by scrutinizing the ethnographic data of his study more closely, it is possible to show how this abstract notion of consensus frequently masks tacit ambiguities, disagreements, and discrepant purposes, which are more often than not left unresolved. Even the concept of mental illness itself is used by Strauss in contradictory ways, yet this is never acknowledged. Ethnographic description within the book is replete with terms the staff used to typify patients. Such terminology is structured by two competing interpretive frameworks that are not differentiated in his analysis. One framework implies that the patient is a passive object who is a victim of psychiatric illness. The other framework implies that the patient can engage in consciously motivated action and is morally responsible for these actions. 'Acting out', a term commonly used in psychiatric hospitals, illustrates these competing frameworks because it can be employed in either sense. Used in the strict psychoanalytic sense, it refers to patterns of behaviour that stem from unconscious conflict, which means that the patient is not responsible for this behaviour. However, it is also used commonly within the hospital simply to describe behaviour the staff finds unacceptable, and in this usage the patient is held responsible for what he or she has done.

These are tacit expressions not of consensus but of an underlying tension within the discourse of psychiatry. On the one hand this discourse is rooted in the concept of psychiatry as a technical practice, which secures its licence and claims to efficacy from its scientific foundations and its relationship to medicine. On the other hand, it is anchored in the notion of psychiatry as a moral practice, as expressed in psychiatry's claim to be a humanistic enterprise that treats patients not as mere objects but as people with problems. As a technical practice, psychiatry objectifies the patient; as a moral practice it reconstitutes the patient as a subject. A more penetrating analysis of the data contained in *Psychiatric Ideologies and Institutions* would argue that conflict is located not only at the surface level of competing professional ideologies but also at the more fundamental level of a dynamic tension between 'scientific' and 'moral' domains, two antithetical background assumptions concerning the nature of mental illness. This tension is productive of ambiguity and equivocality in the definition and treatment of the patient.

In this study I focus on the taken-for-granted language of hospital practice and the background assumptions about psychiatric illness it implies. My interest in taken-for-granted knowledge is informed by social phenomenology, drawing particularly on the theoretical work of Alfred Schutz (1972) and a number of scholars who have applied his theory to ethnographic situations. As a philosophical school, phenomenology grew from Brentano's analysis of intentionality and his exploration of the apprehending, conscious subject. Of equal importance is Husserl's concept of the phenomenological reduction, or *epoché*, a method of putting the world in brackets or suspending belief in the everyday in order to grasp the essence of objects as they are presented to conscious thought. Twentieth century psychiatry has been influenced by phenomenology, especially through the writings of Heidegger, which have been taken up by Binswanger, Buber, and Laing to develop an existential approach that venerates the authentic, subjective experience of the individual patient (Benda 1966). The more significant impact on general psychiatry is through the clinical phenomenology of Jaspers and his pupils, with their concern for patients' subjectively meaningful experiences of psychopathology. More recently in England this approach has been appropriated by an empirical tradition, so much so that clinical phenomenology has now become synonymous with a method of classification and objectification of patients' experiences. Both the intense subjectivity of existential psychoanalysis and the remote objectivity of contemporary clinical phenomenology are side tracks leading away from phenomenology's central programme, which is to explore the foundations of man's subjective experience in a world of shared meanings (Husserl 1960:89–157; Ricoeur 1967:115–42).

Schutz's social phenomenology lays the groundwork for such a programme. It is a phenomenology of the mundane, everyday world in which we live (*lebensweldt*). In order to interact with others, argues Schutz, we adopt a 'natural attitude' in which we suspend doubt in the reality of this world. For Husserl, phenomenological investigation proceeded by putting our *belief* in the everyday world in brackets. For Schutz, the task of phenomenology is to discover how we put our *doubts* about the reality of this world in brackets. As social beings, we must work on assumptions, for example, that our perspectives are interchangeable with those of others, and that the world would be more or less the same if we saw it from the other's standpoint. Otherwise it would not be possible to accomplish practical projects in conjunction with others. The everyday world is, by and large, the world of work. It is dominated therefore by pragmatic motives. Hence Schutz's approach is relevant to understanding the organization of a psychiatric hospital because it directs us to look at clinical work as a practical activity. It directs us to examine the ordinary, daily round of duties, the common-sense reasoning of the clinical staff, and the tacit assumptions they make in order to process cases and get their work done. It leads us to inquire into matters that seem, to them, hardly worth asking about because they are so ordinary, natural, and self-evident—questions they never ask of themselves. In this way it elucidates the very groundwork of clinical psychiatry.

What is an unexamined resource for Strauss, the patient as a 'case' of psychiatric illness, becomes a main focus of this study. A case is more than simply an instance of an illness, it is a way of constructing a person. When a person is rendered into a case format, a particular temporal framework is invoked. The person is shaped into a 'case history'. He or she becomes an evolving narrative that begins with genetic endowment and proceeds through each stage of the person's life— gestation, neonatal period, childhood, adolescence, adulthood—culminating in the onset of the psychiatric illness. Mental health workers also think about cases using spatial metaphors. They regard them as having a deep core (the source of genuine emotions) and a surface zone (allowing for the possibility of a false façade).

On the basis of the ethnographic evidence from Ridgehaven Hospital, I demonstrate that there were tensions that lay beneath the case and that informed the way it was constituted. One of these was the tension between part and whole. Sometimes clinical staff treated a case as if it were divided into segments, each of which could be worked on separately; but when team work was required, the same staff reintegrated these segments back into a so-called 'whole person'. There was also a tension between object and subjectivity within the case, and this was related to the distinction I have drawn between psychiatry as a technical practice and psychiatry as a moral practice. On the one hand, a case was sometimes treated as an object, as if it were a mechanical thing without consciousness or motive—an 'it'. On the other hand, a case could be treated as a person, as someone who was endowed with subjectivity and volition.

These temporal and spatial dimensions and the underlying tensions between whole and part, object and subjectivity, are the principal taken-for-granted features of all cases treated in a psychiatric hospital by multi-disciplinary teams. This book examines their relevance to schizophrenia. Is schizophrenia located within the core of the case? Or can it be construed as a surface problem—a façade of symptoms the person can turn on or off at will? Does it affect just one part of the person, or can it pervade his or her entire identity? What are the implications for regarding schizophrenia as some sort of object or thing lying within the person? Is it possible to personify schizophrenia itself, as if it were another person lying within the patient?

Psychiatric discourse and practice

This study of taken-for-granted knowledge is balanced by an equal interest in explicit knowledge concerning schizophrenia: ideas about the illness that are formulated, taught, debated, and researched within the hospital and beyond. Whereas Strauss' Chicago scene of the 1950s and 1960s was torn by ideological debate between different schools of therapy, Australian hospitals in the 1980s and 1990s, like psychiatric hospitals the world over, have been dominated by diagnostic reasoning. Ridgehaven Hospital was an extreme example. It was subdivided administratively according to diagnostic categories, with one division to deal with affective disorders and another to deal with schizophrenia. This so called 'diagnostic streaming' linked illnesses to administrative arrangements so unambiguously that Ridgehaven could be taken as a case study in diagnostic reasoning and its relation to the institutional framework of psychiatry.

To explore this relationship, I move the analytic focus from ideology to discourse, drawing extensively from the works of Michel Foucault. In *The Archaeology of Knowledge* (1972), Foucault argued that a discursive formation, for example, psychopathology, is a heterogeneous collection of knowledge, the specificity, unity, and form of which should not be understood so much in terms of its internal logic or the conscious intention of its authors but in terms of the social and historical conditions from which such a field of statements emerges. This directs attention to the cultural domains within which knowledge is situated, the institutional sites from which it is dispersed, the socially validated status of authorities who define the categories of the discourse, and the status of its subjects. For Foucault, the importance of *nondiscursive* processes (such as institutional arrangements and economic forces) is that they form the very conditions of possibility for the *discursive* practices that produce and constitute knowledge. Thus the psychiatric discourse concerning schizophrenia emerges from within a broad complex of institutions: the psychiatric hospital, the university, professional bodies, state health services, legal codes and parliamentary acts, pharmaceutical companies, and associations for relatives of the mentally ill. Each specific version of schizophrenia in turn validates the particular projects of these institutions.

Symbolic interactionism has long been criticized on the grounds that its careful attention to the perspective of those

it studies leads to neglect of the structural framework in which
social interaction is embedded (Sharrock 1979:119). By viewing knowledge about schizophrenia as a discursive formation,
I am able to address these broader structural issues. At the
forefront of Foucault's approach to discourse is the problem
of power and its relation to knowledge, and this overcomes
my dissatisfaction with the way that an analysis of power is
neglected, in both symbolic interactionism and social
phenomenology.

Foucault begins to delineate the relationship between institutional processes and psychiatric discourse in *Madness and
Civilization* (1967). He argues that madness as a homogeneous
social category, a focus of state institutions, and an object of
theorizing emerged late in the course of Western civilization.
Its cultural origins took form when diverse mediaeval ideas
gave way to a unified theme of madness in Renaissance art
and literature. Its economic origins were in seventeenth century Europe, when the crises of nascent capitalism created
massive unemployment. In response to this situation, the idle,
the poor, and the vagabond were confined in houses of cor-
rection. Alongside them were the mad, who were exhibited as
exemplars of unreason. Psychiatric discourse took its form
from these cultural and economic spaces of unreason and confinement, where it discovered madness already prefigured and
presented to it. The isolation and confinement of the mad,
argues Foucault, preceded the rise of psychiatry, which only
entered the asylum during the early modern era as a reform
movement, making madness the object of twin discourses: a
moral discourse of salvation through individual responsibility
and a technical discourse of treatment through scientific
medicine.

Discipline and Punish (Foucault 1977) also addresses the relationship between institutions, power, and knowledge. It is
not solely concerned with mental illness, yet its relevance to
psychiatric hospital practice and knowledge is immediately
recognizable. It contains Foucault's major discussion of institutions of 'discipline' within the modern state and the forms
of discourse they produce. These include the asylum, the hospital, the workhouse, the prison, and the school—all built
around a regimen of discipline. They share a common deri-

vation from earlier monastic institutions, a common form of internal architecture enabling continuous and ubiquitous surveillance, and a common project, which is the shaping of marginal categories of people to become useful within the capitalist state.

Disciplinary power is not concentrated at one point, nor is it necessarily oppressive. Foucault writes of a more anonymous and diffuse network of power pervading an institution and permeating beyond its walls into society at large. It is exercised by means of minutely detailed observation and description, a so called 'micro-physics of power'. Disciplinary institutions are machines of meticulous observation, examination, measurement, and documentation. Within them, authorities observe and describe the distinctive qualities of their subjects (the mentally ill, the prisoner, the school child) and thereby constitute them as individuals. At the same time they exercise normative judgements, weighing one against the others and against institutional standards, toward the overall project of maximizing output and generating productive, useful people. Foucault's approach directs attention to the interview, the examination, the writing of a case file, and the personal biography of the subject as central to the exercise of power (Foucault 1977:184–94). He stresses that such power is not solely negative. It is a productive force that generates both useful individuals and forms of discourse. Thus disciplinary institutions are sites not only for the confinement and treatment of marginal categories of persons but also from where experts produce and disperse specialized knowledge about these categories.

At a micro-interactional level, I explore these themes by analysing the clinical processes of interviewing patients and documenting their case history. I compare the written language of the case record to the spoken language of psychiatry, which takes place in case conferences, ward rounds, and more informal settings such as the staff tea room. Written and spoken accounts of patients jointly form the clinical discourse. I map out these contrasting genres and demonstrate that clinical discourse as a whole characterizes the patient with schizophrenia as a marginal and anomalous category of person.

At a macrosocial level of analysis, I examine the scientific discourse on schizophrenia in order to highlight the relation between specialist knowledge and the various institutional bases of modern psychiatry. I show how changes in the knowledge that constitutes schizophrenia reflect a changing pattern of institutions that produce and disperse knowledge of mental illness. Ridgehaven is not only a site in which this changing knowledge is applied to cases, but also a site in which cases are accumulated and studied for the perpetuation of a discourse, as clinicians read the scientific literature on schizophrenia, convene seminars and teaching sessions, carry out research on patients, and write theoretical and popular dissertations on the subject. It is not only a hospital for the treatment of patients with schizophrenia but an organization for the reproduction of theories of normal and abnormal personhood.

Person, case, and schizophrenia

Foucault is concerned with the historical *constitution* of the conscious subject in modern Western thought and practice. However, his approach is inimical to the hermeneutic or interpretive tradition because it silences the participating subjects (Dreyfus and Rabinow 1982:164). In fact, Foucault (1980: 117) has argued that 'one has to dispense with the constituent subject, to get rid of the subject itself, that is to say, to arrive at an analysis which can account for the constitution of the subject within a historical framework'. Far from dispensing with it, this ethnographic study gives voice to the subject (here, the patient and the clinician). Its purpose in doing so is not merely to humanize the account of the hospital but to delineate how the subject is given form as a person with consciousness, intentionality, and identity. Thus there is a radical inconsistency between the two theoretical foundations of this book: Foucault's distancing 'archeology of knowledge' and a phenomenological approach that calls for an ethnographic treatment of interacting, meaning-giving subjects. I adopt a strategy of theoretical tension, maintaining these two perspectives in opposition to each other. I use Foucault to critique social phenomenology and use social phenomenology to critique Foucault.

This theoretical tension forms the basis for my analysis of schizophrenia as a pathological category of the person. Following Geertz (1983:59), I regard the concept of *'person'* as a universal category that 'exists in recognizable form among all social groups'. This usage enables me to employ the concept as an analytical tool and thereby focus attention on the distinctive representations of the person to be found in a psychiatric hospital. The *'case'* is one such representation of the person, itself having a number of forms, including the 'segmented case', the 'fully worked-up case', and the 'whole person'. When a diagnosis of schizophrenia is made, the person is imbued with yet additional cultural meanings that are rich in their diversity. He or she can become, for example, a 'person with schizophrenia', a 'schizophrenic', a 'chronic', or even a 'schizo'. The aim of this book is to examine these specific varieties of person, dissect the institutional practices by which they are constructed, demonstrate the psychiatric discourse within which they are constituted, and explore how they are variously endowed with subjectivity or divested of subjectivity.

Direction of the book

The sequence of chapters in this book is structured by the overall logic of its argument, which moves from social process to diagnostic category; from the organization of the hospital, to the construction of the case, to schizophrenia. The second chapter describes the hospital landscape and the history of the institution to show how space, time, and an ideology of progress are pervasive themes that give the hospital a sense of cohesion and a particular identity. The third chapter examines the unique features of each professional group and its distinctive approach to the patient; whereas the fourth chapter analyses the operation of clinicians in concert as a multidisciplinary team. The chapter on clinical writing includes a detailed analysis of a patient being admitted to the hospital with a diagnosis of schizophrenia. It examines the effects of documentation on the patient's experience of the disorder. Clinical talk is examined in the sixth chapter, with an emphasis on the language used to describe patients as they recover from acute psychosis and proceed to a course of chronic schizophrenia. The seventh and eighth chapters examine the historical emergence of the diagnostic category of schizophrenia during the nineteenth century and its subsequent development in this century, demonstrating how changing theories about its nature and cause reflect major social and institutional changes. The study returns, in the ninth chapter, to the interactions between clinical staff and patients in Ridgehaven Hospital. It focuses on an education programme in order to examine how these clinicians and patients together build up practical working definitions of schizophrenia. I show how they draw on a number of models of illness, moving deftly from one to another as they negotiate between themselves what schizophrenia means. The final chapter draws together the major themes of this book. It identifies two tensions—whole versus part and object versus subjectivity—that underlie and inform our cultural definitions of the person, the case, and schizophrenia.

The relevance of this book to clinicians is that it is an anthropological study of the day-to-day practice of psychiatrists, social workers, and psychiatric nurses. It demonstrates how important clinical decisions (concerning, for example, the prescription of drugs or the discharging of a patient from hospital) are based on unquestioned common-sense notions and taken-for-granted terminology.

For patients, the book is an attempt to clarify psychiatric thinking. It is difficult enough to have schizophrenia, and it is only fair that patients should not be burdened by psychiatric confusion about the meaning of this diagnostic concept.

For social science, this research is relevant to a growing body of literature concerning the relationship between illness, institution, person, and society. After the early ethnographies of mental hospitals during the 1950s and the subsequent scaling down of the older institutions, anthropological attention followed patients as they were discharged and struggled to find a place in the wider community (Scheper-Hughes 1979; Estroff 1981). More recently there has been a renewed interest in the psychiatric hospital (Rhodes 1991), now an increasingly medicalized institution with a more rapid turnover of patients. What is unique about the present study is that it explores the relationship between the modern psychiatric hospital and a specific diagnostic category. It employs the insights of Foucault, though not merely to illustrate his theory but to modify it by bringing it into confrontation with social phenomenology. It is a study of one of the important institutions in modern society for the definition of normal and abnormal categories of person.

Finally, the findings of this study are relevant to social policy. Ridgehaven Hospital, like many of its kind in the developed world, is currently transforming into a community service, in keeping with the aim to deliver a form of psychiatric care that is even more modern, humane, and relevant to patients' needs. It is anticipated that new community-based treatment units will be more refined and efficient versions of the teams at Ridgehaven Hospital. However, without attention to the basic problems and processes that are analysed in this book, these planned improvements may be only cosmetic.

2

Time and space in a progressive psychiatric hospital

Ridgehaven Hospital was located in a marginal zone on the edge of a major Australian city.[1] It had been built during the late 1920s on farming land at a distance of seven miles from the city centre. Surrounded by paddocks, it was intended that patients would engage in healthy outdoor work as part of their rehabilitation. At the same time it was accessible to visitors because it was located at the end of a metropolitan tram line.

When this study was carried out during the early 1980s, Ridgehaven Hospital had maintained its quasi-rural disposition. Although the suburbs with their network of bus routes had extended many miles past the hospital over the intervening fifty years, surrounding tracts of open farm land had been preserved as an agricultural research station, separating the hospital from the nearest housing estates. Two other institutions, a training centre for the intellectually retarded and a prison with its farm, were situated adjacent to the hospital. Slightly farther away were the city abattoirs. Four marginal categories—the mentally ill, the intellectually retarded, the criminal, and the slaughtered beast—thus shared a borderline space between city and country.

Progress

During the 1980s Ridgehaven Hospital was regarded as one of the most progressive psychiatric hospitals in Australia, and the idea of progress itself had become fundamental to the way

[1] I have altered the name of the hospital and the names of all wards and buildings within it.

22

the hospital defined itself. Its motto, *Ex Tenebris in Lucem,* captured the sense of movement from old to modern, from ignorance to knowledge, from evil to good.[2] Expressions of progress pervaded the brochures, biennial reports, and press releases through which the hospital projected its public image. These publications emphasized the advanced management practices of Ridgehaven and the modern treatments it made available to patients. Addressing the staff on the theme of organizational change, the Medical Director/Chief Executive Officer asserted: 'The only constant factor is change itself'. In this atmosphere of ongoing improvement, he sought to instil an ethos of 'striving for excellence'. Ridgehaven became the first public psychiatric hospital in Australia to be officially accredited by the Australian Council of Hospital Standards.

Of the public psychiatric hospitals within the state, it was Ridgehaven that set the pace for deinstitutionalization, the chief index of progress for such institutions. Accommodation for inpatients (measured in numbers of available beds) had declined from a peak of more than 1200 beds in 1952 to 414 in 1983. This reduction had been accomplished despite the fact that the hospital concentrated on the treatment of patients with severe psychiatric disorders such as schizophrenia and manic depressive psychosis, drug and alcohol dependence, personality disorder, and dementia. The number of patients admitted to the hospital, however, steadily increased and by 1986 was in excess of 2,000 patients each year. This admission rate, coupled with the decline in bed numbers, generated pressure on the clinical staff to discharge patients as quickly as possible to make way for new admissions. The most common length of inpatient stay was just 17 days. A progressive Mental Health Act passed by the State Parliament defined strict criteria for involuntary detention and facilitated mechanisms of appeal by patients; it thereby discouraged their long-term involuntary confinement.

Ridgehaven Hospital served a population of approximately 650,000 people. The annual budget in 1983 was $17.5 million

---

[2] Compare with the biblical rendition of this motto: 'that they may turn from darkness to light and from the power of Satan to God, that they may receive forgiveness of sins and a place among those who are sanctified by faith in me' (Acts 26:16).

(Australian dollars). There were 668 members of staff, more than two-thirds of whom were directly involved in clinical work. Increasingly, these staff and financial resources were being withdrawn from inpatient services to be deployed in outpatient and community work, mainly organized through Outreach Clinics located closer to where the patients lived. However, these changes did not represent a scaling down or redeployment of resources, as they occurred against the backdrop of steady expansion in the state's psychiatric services. During the preceding twenty years, five psychiatric wards, each of approximately twenty beds, had been established within general hospitals. Three large suburban community mental health clinics were set up. Two academic departments of psychiatry were founded. Although it was true that the number of patients residing in Ridgehaven had fallen dramatically, many of these patients had merely been relocated in the nearby training centre for the intellectually retarded, psychiatric hostels, and nursing homes. The 'deinstitutionalization' of Ridgehaven was thus a relocation of psychiatric services from the traditional space of the psychiatric hospital to a variety of new sites, and it occurred in the broader context of a major growth in the scope and complexity of institutional psychiatry (c.f. Castel, Castel and Lovell 1982:124–74).

This ethos of progress within the hospital and its goal of deinstitutionalization meant that ideas of change and movement were central to the way patients were evaluated and treated. The clinical staff conceived of their patients in terms of a trajectory, and the principal aim of their work was to have an impact on this trajectory—to keep the patient moving toward recovery and discharge. Under the constant pressure to discharge ('pressure on beds', as it was called) the staff would rapidly initiate pharmacological treatment to achieve the fastest possible improvement in a patient's mental state. They were encouraged to begin planning for a patient's discharge from the outset by including 'discharge planning' in the initial admission assessment. Patients who did not demonstrate improvement were soon characterized as 'treatment resistant' or a 'management problem'. Before long, the staff would arrange to transfer such a patient from an acute to a subacute or chronic ward of the hospital, although this avenue was often blocked because it was here that the pressure on beds was greatest. Rhodes (1991) has characterized the emergency psychiatric unit she studied in terms of its 'management of movement'. Its principal clinical aims were to change the patients' behaviour enough so they could go elsewhere: 'The process of disposition had a fascination and immediacy and held out a possibility of success compared with which speculation about larger causes of the patients' troubles seemed futile and discouraging' (Rhodes 1991:40).

For the clinical staff at Ridgehaven, the most rewarding patients were the 'acute' cases, who responded by improving, at least to the extent that they could move out of the hospital. The least rewarding were the 'revolving door' patients with 'multiple admissions', or 'chronic' patients, because they did not demonstrate any progress. They were devalued because their trajectories were circular or had come to a standstill. In an institution where change was expected, the moral evaluation of patients who showed little or no change became a significant problem for the staff, and in a subsequent chapter I examine the rich stock of terms and phrases that arose in response to this problem.

Ideas of movement and progress also pervaded the psychiatric professions. Career mobility conferred prestige on an individual, whether it be the upward mobility of climbing through the hospital ranks or the outward mobility from hospital employment to private practice. Professional bodies as a whole viewed progress in terms of advancing their own status, expanding their membership, and most of all securing their autonomy from other professional groups. Prior to World War II there were fewer than ten doctors with an interest in psychiatry in the state, and they were most often specialist physicians or neurologists. By 1983 there were 120 specialist psychiatrists, more than half of them working predominantly in private practice. Thus hand in hand with the expansion in government-funded psychiatric services came a remarkable growth in the private sector. The postwar period also saw the establishment of clinical psychology as a practising profession, psychiatric nursing as a recognized specialty, and psychiatric social work as a major component of social services within the state.

The ongoing momentum of change and innovation at so many levels within Ridgehaven Hospital reflected a broader ideology of progress within Australian society and more widely still within advanced capitalist states where economies are predicated on expansion (Berger and Luckman 1967:142). Gellner (1964) argues that such a belief in progress characterizes modern thought more generally. In contrast to 'episodic' notions of time associated with pre-modern thought, an 'evolutionary' doctrine of progress posits a view of time that is not morally neutral:

> Time could have been said to be 'morally neutral' in the historic perception of a society for whom excellence was just as likely to be found in the past as in the future. A society can be said to believe in progress when this symmetry does not obtain, when there is, at the very least, some predisposition to tie up *past* with *bad* (in one word: *backward*), and *future* with *good* (*progressive*). (Gellner 1964:3)

Histories of Ridgehaven

An official history of Ridgehaven was commissioned for publication for the year of the hospital's jubilee celebrations (Holt 1979). Working from archival and oral sources, the author organized this history into an evolutionary narrative wherein the negative aspects of the hospital were relegated to the past and its positive aspects located in the present or projected into the future. It was the story of a hospital that was evolving from the brutal custodialism of the past into the modern era of enlightened care and scientifically based classification and treatment. It was a local version of the more widely known progressivist histories of psychiatry, such as that of Zilboorg (1941).

The narrative began with a 1909 Parliamentary inquiry into the inveterate problems of overcrowding and undercapitalization at Albert Park Hospital, the state's only mental hospital at that time. The inquiry recommended the establishment of a second institution to be situated on farm land where able-bodied patients could be gainfully employed in outdoor work, thus facilitating their recovery while at the same time reducing state expenditure on the mentally ill by the sale of farm products. A suitable farm was purchased, but what with delays in the building programme, Ridgehaven Hospital was not opened to patients until 1929. With the advent of the Depression and the subsequent transformation from a rural to an industrial state economy, the ideal of a farm colony was never achieved. Like Albert Park Hospital before it, Ridgehaven soon became overcrowded. Large numbers of elderly, demented patients and severely intellectually retarded patients were 'dumped' there, to use an expression from a critical report (Stoller and Arson 1955). Buildings designed to accommodate 100 people were crammed with as many as 180. There was a combination of government neglect and public disinterest. The reduction of public expenditure on the mentally ill, a major rationale for locating Ridgehaven in an agricultural setting, exacted a toll on the patients. It led to them being poorly fed and clothed as well as subjected to recurrent epidemic infections. These early years were characterized by problems of violent behaviour on the part of attendants as well as patients and a pervasive atmosphere of therapeutic pessimism.

This was a depressing backdrop, against which a more favourable version of the contemporary hospital could be developed. Holt related how, amid these degrading, inhumane, brutal conditions, there emerged the figure of the modern psychiatric nurse—the embodiment of humane care. Moreover, into this oppressive institution of confinement, its buildings enclosed by wire mesh, came the reforming medical superintendent, who introduced the 'therapeutic community' movement, gradually unlocked the closed wards, and opened the hospital to the wider society. Community service clubs began to hold fêtes on the hospital playing field. Principles of rational classification were introduced. The patients were divided into separate medical categories—the demented, the intellectually retarded, the mentally ill—leading to specialization in the treatment of each group. Therapeutic pessimism and ignorance were dispelled by psychopharmacology and therapeutic optimism.

A former patient published an account of the hospital, incorporating the written reflections of various staff and ex-patients (Heaslip 1971). It was organized into the same trajectory of progress that was evident in the hospital's official history. Scenes of cruelty formed a counterpoint to the new age of humanitarian and scientific progress:

> [U]nknown to me, brilliant chemists had been at work. And the first boxes of Largactil were on their way to the mental hospitals of the world. And so I was privileged to witness . . . what I think of as the Largactil Revolution, right there on the job, amid my puddles of soupy water and slosh. The screams, the yells, the fights, the whistles blowing, my best friend being dragged kicking and struggling to be put in a strait jacket, all subsided to a marked degree. (Heaslip 1971:13)

For the purpose of this study, the relevance of such history is 'not whether the past occurred as depicted, but how it is called forth to make the present meaningful' (McHugh 1968: 24). During the period of my field-work, I noted that the staff sometimes characterized Ridgehaven as a 'dumping ground' or a 'bin'. They complained among themselves that it was used by other hospitals and by members of the community as a repository for their 'rubbish', rubbish referring to mentally ill people who were socially unacceptable and undesirable. Within the written histories of the hospital, this negative definition of Ridgehaven was essayed in vivid detail, but it was relegated to an earlier era rather than the present. In this way, the hospital histories encompassed divergent and often contradictory definitions of the hospital by arranging them onto a temporal framework of ongoing improvement.

Similarly, there was a tendency in hospital publications to minimize the extent to which it functioned as an institution of confinement and control. A Biennial Report stressed that only one-third of the annual admissions were by detention or custody order. The involuntary detention of patients was often rephrased as 'care' or 'therapy'. The main locked ward, for example, was called an intensive therapy unit. The official history addressed this need to play down the 'lock-up' functions of the hospital. Confinement was transposed to the past and depicted as having been rendered unnecessary by humane care on the one hand and modern medicine on the other. Yet it was still central to the functioning of the hospital. Seven of its seventeen wards remained locked. It could even be argued that the hospital's capacity for surveillance was more extensive than ever before, for the Mental Health Act now made provision for long-term monitoring of patients living in the community.

The problem of ineffective treatment too appeared in the official history to be a problem of the past, where it was deemed to stem from ignorance. Yet during the period of this study, treatment failure was an everyday problem faced by the staff. The many patients who could not be discharged and the even greater number who were repeatedly readmitted undermined staff confidence in the efficacy of the therapeutic and pharmacological 'revolutions'. In such circumstances, the staff often made sense of this problem by recourse to history. When confronted with a patient who remained in a psychotic state associated with violent behaviour, they would draw a comparison with what patients must have been like in the 'old days' before the introduction of modern treatment.

Hospital landscape

Progress was not only the central motif of Ridgehaven's histories, official and unofficial, it was also inscribed onto the landscape itself. A walk from the front to the back of the hospital was a passage back in time from the 1980s to the 1920s. The topography and architecture of Ridgehaven were spatial expressions of a temporal continuum.

At the time of the study, there were thirty buildings distributed over forty-eight hectares of grounds. Although some were devoted to administrative and service functions, most were inpatient wards, day-patient centres, or occupational therapy facilities. Drawing on a domestic metaphor, they were referred to as 'houses'. Houses were discrete geographical and administrative units of patient treatment. Each evoked an aspect of Ridgehaven's past, as they were named after former members of staff who had made significant contributions to the development of the hospital.

At the front of the hospital, the main entrance looked out onto a major suburban road and across several paddocks to the nearest suburbs. The modern facilities were located in this area, set on either side of a curved driveway so they faced the entrance at an angle. They contained admission wards for the assessment and treatment of acutely ill patients, and specialized facilities for the treatment of identified diagnostic groups. One focused on patients with major affective disorders, neuroses, and personality disorders. The other was Heathfield House, the main setting of this study; and it concentrated on patients with a diagnosis of schizophrenia. Both of them contained 'open' wards, and voluntary patients were treated there. The turnover of patients was brisk.

The back of the hospital communicated via an old orchard, now untended and overgrown, with a nearby centre for the intellectually retarded. Old buildings—literally the 'back wards'—were arranged in rows like barracks, connected to each other by a grid of covered walkways. This area had a rigid, stark appearance. 'Back wards' housed the chronic patients, for whom there were lower expectations of improvement and discharge. The turnover of patients here was sluggish. In contrast to the specialized treatment units at the front, the back wards usually contained a mixture of diagnostic groups, lumped together only by virtue of their common failure to improve. In this regard they were a reminder of how the whole hospital might have looked before the introduction of rational classification. 'Closed' wards, where involuntarily detained patients were confined, were also located in these buildings at the back of the hospital.

Heathfield House was Ridgehaven's most modern facility, having been commissioned in 1982. A single-storey building, it had a low, unobtrusive profile, surrounded and partly disguised by native Australian trees and shrubs. The architect aimed to achieve a 'domestic' atmosphere and thus strove to avoid any hint of 'institutional' design or resemblance to barracks. For this reason the length of corridors was kept to a minimum. The resulting floor plan was in the shape of a cross, the four arms containing an inpatient ward, a day patient centre, an occupational therapy facility, and an outpatient wing. The 'natural' aesthetic of the eucalyptus trees around Heathfield House was continued into the interior of the building. For example, there were wall hangings with gum leaf designs in khaki and green. At the centre of the cross was a light court constructed of large glass panels. It admitted natural sunlight to an indoor garden. The nursing and secretarial staff maintained the potted plants growing there. The architect had successfully achieved a feeling of spaciousness within Heathfield. In an effort to convey a sense of open communication with the exterior he had been careful to make sure that each room had a view to the outside. The front entrance and porch were obvious and faced the road, which led directly to the hospital entrance. Heathfield was an 'open' setting, being locked only at night.

At the intersection of the four wings, adjacent to the light court, was a reception desk and office area, the centre of operations for the Schizophrenia Team. A line of pigeon holes for incoming mail was located here, as was the photocopying machine and a control panel for piped music. The receptionist and stenographer typed clinical reports and collated patient statistics using word processors that were linked to the hospital's central record system. Psychiatrists, social workers, and occupational therapists had their consulting offices nearby; and when they went from any one wing of the building to another they walked through the central area. It thus formed a busy intersection constantly criss-crossed by people who would stop to catch up with one another as they opened their mail or handed the stenographer a cassette of dictation. For the Schizophrenia Team, this was a hub of information, including both official written reports and informal conversations about the patients and fellow staff members.

Heathfield House was designed to maximize efficiency. It contained a well equipped clinic room where patients were physically examined and blood samples obtained. The nursing stations within the ward and the day-patient centre were built for ease of observation. Large glass windows enabled nursing staff to look along the corridors or scan the dining and recreation areas. Although it incorporated these features, Heathfield House did not appear to be obviously set up for surveillance, which was more efficient for being invisible. In his discussion of disciplinary power, Foucault takes Jeremy Bentham's panopticon as the model for the modern institution, arguing that such institutions function as instruments of the disciplinary gaze: a modern, nonviolent, invisible mode of power that is mainly exercised by rendering its subjects visible and describable (Foucault 1978). A contemporary transformation of Bentham's panopticon, Heathfield House epitomized an open and gentle regimen of surveillance. Acutely ill patients—those undergoing their first admission to hospital or those who had relapsed and needed reassessment—were treated here for short periods. Most improved sufficiently to live outside the hospital, thereby attesting to the effectiveness of the Schizophrenia Team in Heathfield House and rewarding their optimism.

Elder House was a typical back ward. Some of its residents suffered chronic physical illnesses, some were periodically violent, and most exhibited some form of socially unacceptable behaviour. All were unable to care for themselves, and all were severely incapacitated by mental illness. For the staff, they were less interesting, less frequently seen, and less valued than the Heathfield patients because their condition was unlikely to change; most were considered incapable of living outside the hospital. Elder House was one of the first buildings to be erected. It was a large, foreboding two-storey structure, coated with peeling white paint and pigeon droppings. The staff described it as institutional in appearance. It was said to resemble a 'block house'. It was not immediately obvious where to find the entrance. What might have appeared to be a front door was in fact a service entrance for food and linen. The main entrance was through a small side doorway, courageously decorated by the nursing staff with potted plants. As a stylistic counterpoint to its dehumanizing architecture, the nurses of Elder House made an effort to inject a 'human touch' and a 'homely atmosphere'. On entering the ward, one felt cut off from the outside world. Narrow windows set high in the walls admitted little light. The office space, nursing station, and medical examination room were cramped, makeshift, and inefficient. The nursing staff experienced a sense of isolation. They felt that visits by psychiatrists and social workers to review and discuss patients occurred all too infrequently. Elder House, they said, was used as a 'dumping ground' for the 'treatment failures' or 'behavioural problems' of Heathfield House and the other acute wards. Once transferred to Elder, patients were quickly forgotten and neglected by the psychiatrists and social workers. Therefore a major task for the nurses was to guard against therapeutic pessimism and 'burn out', which they did by working steadily to achieve long-term rehabilitation goals for each of their patients. This had a heroic quality. The discharge of just one of their patients to a community hostel was cause to celebrate. It conferred a sense of achievement against insuperable odds. Ultimately, however, part of the floor in Elder House began to subside. The feeling among staff was that the building should be bulldozed. When it was closed, patients were moved to another building, which although of similar design and built during the same era was less dilapidated.

Located further toward the back, against the rear fence, was Oakley House, the main locked ward. Like Elder House, it was also a large, old building, clearly designed as an instrument of confinement with its locked doors, barred windows, and a high wire mesh fence around its courtyard. It was also obvious, once inside, that the building was purpose-built for surveillance. On either side of the main corridor was a row of seclusion rooms, each door containing a small window through which nursing staff could observe patients. The staff believed that the architecture itself frightened and intimidated patients. They regarded it as a vestige from Ridgehaven's past that would best be abandoned.

Integration of time and space

Bittner (1974) has criticized a number of sociological studies of modern organizations for the way they simply borrow common-sense ideas held by the people who work in them (such as the distinction between formal and informal spheres of organization) and use these ideas as analytical or theoretical constructs. Instead, Bittner suggests that the role of social science is to analyse such common-sense ideas in order to reveal the tacit, background assumptions that structure them but which are largely taken for granted by members of the organization. In this chapter I have looked at the way the people of Ridgehaven described their own hospital in order to reveal the framework of assumptions on which these descriptions were based. I have looked at oral and written accounts of the hospital—accounts provided by administrators, clinical staff, a former patient, and a professional historian. I have identified an underlying temporal framework on which each of these descriptions relied but which was rarely stated explicitly.

On the basis of this framework, negative aspects of the hospital were characteristically displaced back in time to the 'bad old days' and its positive aspects located in the future as goals toward which everyone worked. Thus the most familiar expression of this implicit time frame was the idea of progress. I have shown how 'progress' surfaced and resurfaced in diverse domains of hospital life. It could be found in the motto, the style of leadership provided by the Chief Executive Officer, the ethos of the hospital, and the history commissioned by its administrators. It provided a link to the wider community insofar as a modern progressive hospital is part of a modern progressive society. Medical science too was invoked in the form of 'science as progress', and as a result patients were represented as suffering from disorders soon to be solved by advances in psychiatric research. The way clinical staff categorized cases as acute or chronic was predicated on whether they demonstrated progress. The success or failure of professional careers and indeed of professional bodies as a whole was measured in the same terms.

Progress provided a stylistic unity that served to integrate an organization characterized by diversity, complexity, potential schism, and a sense of uncertainty resulting from continual change. Bittner (1974:78) argues that within large organizations such unifying themes order relationships between people who are too remote from each other to directly negotiate a *modus operandum*. People who are not within each other's sphere of influence can derive a general sense of working together to a common purpose. At Ridgehaven, progress provided a shared focus for the various divisions of the organization that were otherwise not connected. For example, the financial administrator, who was striving continually to improve the hospital, shared a common ground with clinicians striving to improve the lot of their patients, where otherwise they might have been at odds or perhaps never have met.

Not all aspects of the hospital could be integrated by this theme. There were more fundamental contradictions that could not be reconciled through the rhetoric of progress; in particular, contradictory ideas of the hospital as a bad place and a good place. Advocates for modern psychiatry promoted the view that the psychiatric hospital, at long last, had the expertise and resources to deliver effective treatment to those patients most in need, whereas advocates of deinstitutionalization argued that this same psychiatric hospital damaged the patients it treated. For the staff of Ridgehaven, this contradiction was condensed into a single question: 'If the hospital was evolving into an institution of unparalleled excellence, why were there plans to wind it down?' Nursing staff in particular, in an uncertain job market, questioned whether they should be striving for even higher standards or making alternative career arrangements. Thus there was a loosely organized but widespread body of sceptical opinion among the staff that expressed an articulate critique of the hospital and its goals. Deinstitutionalization was 'seen through' as a cynical cost-cutting exercise foisted on a hospital too weak to resist it by anonymous financial administrators from higher levels of government bureaucracy. The so-called advances of deinstitutionalization were redefined as a disgraceful failure to care for those who were incapacitated by chronic mental illness. By discharging patients indiscriminately, many were rendered vulnerable to financial and personal exploitation by unscrupulous people in the community. 'Some patients just need asylum', was the catch phrase of this critique.

Many staff also questioned the doctrine of escalating achievement. They expressed a view that things were getting worse not better. So-called improvements in the organization of the hospital were redefined pejoratively as 'increasing bureaucratic red tape'. More staff, it was said, created more meetings, more minutes, and more memoranda—but less time with patients. With increasing professionalization, there was an incessant movement of personnel through the hospital, which was seen to work against the building of therapeutic relationships with patients. How could trainee psychiatrists get to know their patients if they were always moving from one division of the hospital to the next as part of their training programme? How could nurses get involved if they were constantly shifted from one roster to the next or transferred from one ward to another? A counterhistory emerged in which the hospital was seen as regressing rather than progressing, gradually slipping backward in its ability to care for patients. In this version of history, the 'good old days' became a time when staff got to know their patients over many years like old friends. Senior nursing staff would sometimes point out the location of the vegetable fields formerly worked by the patients, now a car park. They would reminisce about how things were simpler in those days. Perhaps the staff were paternalistic, but at least the patients were secure.

However much it dismissed progress and deinstitutionalization, this alternative history of Ridgehaven still relied on the same implicit temporal framework to make sense of the hospital. It did not dispense with time but simply reversed the values commonly associated with its passage. Thus at an underlying level the temporal framework was a tacit resource used by everyone at Ridgehaven, advocates and sceptics alike, as a means of comprehending what to them were the good and bad aspects of the hospital. Statements about the past, present, and future were a means of conveying a moral evaluation of the work carried out within the hospital.

Time was expressed in terms of space and space in terms of time.[3] Together they formed a spatio-temporal unity that structured the landscape of the hospital, the distribution of its buildings, their architectural features, and their decor. Going to the back wards of the hospital meant going backward into the past. Returning to the front was a movement forward into modernity and outward into the community. Layered on top of this spatio-temporal continuum were several related gradients. The back buildings were decrepit, cramped, and unworkable; the front ones were smart, spacious, and efficient. The back was closed off from the world like an isolated backwater, looking across an agricultural setting that had not been used for decades. The front communicated openly with the busy world outside. The back wards were like living museums where people were still performing the same functions they

---

[3] See Munn's (1992) review of the cultural anthropology of time for a discussion of the integral relation between time and space.

would have carried out prior to the 'therapeutic revolution', whereas in the front wards people kept abreast of the latest developments in psychiatric practice throughout the world.

The spatio-temporal continuum was also a moral continuum. The distribution of patients across the hospital was a reflection of the moral worth they held for the staff. The more dangerous patients and those with behavioural problems tended to be concentrated at the back. Detained patients too were held at the back, whereas the proportion of voluntary patients was higher at the front. Diagnosis, the lynchpin of psychiatric treatment, was pertinent only to the patients in the front wards. The distinction between chronic and acute forms of illness, which was so central to the assessment of patients, was made tangible and visible because it coincided with the topographical distinction between back and front.

3

Professional domains and the dimensions of a case

Like the arrangement of buildings and the narrative history of the hospital's evolution, clinical work was structured in space and time. This chapter looks at the meanings that space and time had in the professional culture of Ridgehaven Hospital—how, for the clinical staff, they became a particular 'work space' and 'work time' (c.f. Zerubavel 1979). It examines three central professions: psychiatry, psychiatric nursing, and social work. Each differed in its structure, its characteristic mode of practice, and the way in which the work space and work time of its members was organized. These differences were reflected in the distinct perspective that each profession brought to bear on the people they treated. I examine these perspectives in turn and explore their implications for the way clinical staff rendered a person as a case of psychiatric illness.

The starting point of this discussion is a sociological argument about the nature of the professions. Sociological research in this field initially focused on the characteristic traits of the professions. They included special skills, a complex and abstract body of knowledge, prolonged training, and an ethical or altruistic orientation. More recent scholarship, especially the work of Freidson (1986:20–40), argues that such research tended to reiterate the ideology employed by professionals to justify their prestige and defend their institutional power. It failed to analyse the economic and political power of the professions in relation to the state. Freidson (1970:71–84) argues that it is autonomy of practice, by which he means 'legitimate control over work', that is the paramount feature of professional organizations. Whereas Freidson was concerned with autonomy and power at the macroscopic level of professional organizations and their relation to the state, I redirect and extend this analysis by examining the manifestations of professional autonomy and power in the day-to-day work of a psychiatric hospital. In this clinical context, the main expression of power was the capacity to define cases of psychiatric illness. From this power flowed the means to distribute cases across the hospital.

Since World War II Ridgehaven had seen a striking growth in the absolute number of professional workers, the number of professional groups represented, and the internal differentiation within each group. This growth was part of a more generalized expansion in the professions devoted to 'processing people' (McKinlay 1975), which occurred in developed economies as they became more oriented to the production of services rather than goods. In this climate of expansion, each profession at Ridgehaven mustered its unique body of knowledge, promoted its 'characteristic professional act' (Strauss and Bucher 1975:13), and marshalled its distinctive definition of the case in order to establish autonomy vis-a-vis the other professions. As a confederation of developing professional groups (Freidson 1971:19–38), the hospital organization was characterized by division and competition. Thus I am describing a modern organization that was essentially schismatic, and I argue that this schism was reflected in the way it constructed its principal product, the case, as a segmented object. My general thesis is that the institutional structure was isomorphic with the structure of the case.

The 'construction' metaphor is deliberate. It does not refer to fabrication or falsehood, because what is constructed is incontrovertibly real (Berger and Luckman 1967). It conveys the idea that the hospital takes a person and builds layers of clinical assessments and professional definitions in and around that person until he or she is made into a case. It also invokes the antonym 'deconstruction', and it will be argued that in the process of making a case clinicians carved the person into various component parts or segments and disarticulated these segments one from another in order to examine them more closely. The metaphor of the case as a structure is also apt because it draws attention to the way in which clinicians attributed basic spatial and temporal dimensions to a case, although they were largely unaware that they were doing so. To differentiate these case dimensions clearly from 'work space' and 'work time', I refer to them as 'case space' and 'case time'. A case, for example, was treated as having a surface and a core, was divided into epochs, and was given a trajectory.

During the course of this discussion, I use the term 'patient' to refer to any person who was treated in the hospital because this term was most commonly used by the staff of Ridgehaven. At the same time, I distinguish ethnographically between the 'case', the 'patient', and the 'client', three different constructions of a person that remain unexamined in most scientific discussions of psychiatric illness. By analysing what is normally taken for granted, I aim to elucidate some of the conceptual structures that make psychiatric work possible and that enable particular cultural meanings to be bestowed on a person when he or she is treated in hospital for psychiatric illness.

Professional domains

Psychiatry

Psychiatry was the most autonomous of the clinical professions in the hospital, and this derived from its connections outside the hospital; most importantly, from its status as a specialty within the profession of medicine. As Willis (1989) has shown, it is the medical profession that has dominated the organization of health care delivery in Australia, chiefly by virtue of state patronage. Psychiatrists at Ridgehaven were employed by the state and had achieved high remuneration, for they were represented by an effective industrial body. Furthermore, their collegiate body, the Royal Australian and New Zealand College of Psychiatrists, acted in a powerful advisory capacity to state and federal legislatures and administrations. As a corollary, only psychiatrists and their juniors, the trainee psychiatrists and medical practitioners, had certain types of statutory power, for example, the power to prescribe medication and the power to detain patients in hospital against their will under the provisions of the state mental health act. Within Ridgehaven Hospital, the profession had further maintained a position of authority by fulfilling official administrative roles.

Psychiatrists had occupied key executive positions since the inception of the hospital. In thirty years, their ranks had increased from just two—medical superintendent and medical officer—to a steep pyramid that went from the chief executive officer downward to his deputy, and then on to team leaders, senior psychiatrists, psychiatrists, trainee psychiatrists, and nonspecialist medical officers.

Despite the hierarchy, the individual practice of qualified psychiatrists was not subject to strict supervisory control. Reflecting this autonomy, psychiatrists could be held individually responsible at law for their actions, although there was only one such civil action by a patient against a psychiatrist during the period of this study. Nevertheless, psychiatrists frequently employed a rhetoric of legal culpability to defend their clinical decisions, claiming that they were the ones who would have to appear in court if anything went wrong. So compelling was this rhetoric that other professions began to seek the right to be sued.

Psychiatric knowledge took precedence over that of the other professions. Ridgehaven was a teaching hospital affiliated with a university medical faculty, and its psychiatrists held simultaneous appointments as clinical lecturers. The education of trainee psychiatrists and medical students was centred around cases. Because this instruction took place in case conferences, the other professionals who were present formed an audience for the pedagogic task of psychiatry. Student nurses, social workers, occupational therapists, and psychologists did receive clinical training in the hospital, but this teaching did not take place in case conferences. Hence at the level of case formulation, it was psychiatric knowledge, rather than nursing or social work knowledge, that was displayed to the gathered professions as the dominant body of knowledge.

There was a steady flow of qualified psychiatrists out of the hospital into private practice, and those who remained behind had ample room for promotion. These opportunities for career mobility were coupled with a high degree of geographical mobility during the course of day-to-day work. In large measure, psychiatrists were responsible for setting their own work agenda, especially their starting and finishing times. They moved about within the hospital from ward to ward and then perhaps drove away in the afternoon to work in another hospital or in private practice, all the while connected to the hospital switchboard by an electronic paging device. In the case of the general hospital, Freidson (1970:115) has argued that the extension of work outside hospital space determines specialist dominance within it: 'The physician is not so much part of the hospital as the hospital is part (and only part) of the physician's practice'. Likewise for an emergency psychiatric unit, Rhodes found that part time work in private offices conferred greater prestige as well as control over space and time within the unit because 'status was correlated with mobility, privacy, and distance from the patients' (Rhodes 1991:30).

Mobility was a basic structure of specialist practice that was built into the earliest stages of training. Trainee psychiatrists had a distinctive freshness and élan because they were advancing rapidly in their careers. They were birds of passage, working in any one place for no longer than nine months as they 'rotated' from section to section within the hospital, and from hospital to hospital, gaining experience in different branches of psychiatry. The movement of trainees was known colloquially as the 'clinical rotation'. Medical students rotated faster. They had a six-week attachment to the hospital before moving on to learn about another medical specialty.

Nonspecialist medical officers embodied the converse of mobility. They usually worked in one section for many years and had no structure of career advancement. They were often doctors who had abandoned the specialist training programme, or sometimes immigrant doctors awaiting full registration.

These temporal and spatial aspects of work influenced the way the medical staff viewed the people they treated as cases. Trainee psychiatrists approached cases as ongoing trajectories to which they would become attached for a few months. Accomplishing involvement, making a difference, and then withdrawing smoothly was fundamental to their work. Fully qualified psychiatrists were attached to cases for much longer, although on the Schizophrenia Team, where some patients were treated for decades, even a ten-year involvement might represent only one phase of a patient's career. Nonetheless, knowledge of a patient that had been accrued over years was a resource which, in combination with specialist expertise, was used to stamp an authoritative definition on the case. In a typical division of clinical labour, psychiatrists provided long-term knowledge of a case yet remained in the background, supervising a succession of trainee psychiatrists who were responsible for the day-to-day treatment. The medical officers possessed the same longitudinal knowledge but lacked the specialist expertise of the psychiatrist, and there was no one of more junior rank to stand between them and the patient. Long-term knowledge was thus a source of authority, provided it was combined with accredited expertise and the capacity to work through more junior staff.

The consulting room was the primary work space of psychiatrists and trainees. While they did talk to patients briefly in the ward or see them in the corridor 'on the run', the characteristic encounter, the psychiatric assessment, was conducted behind closed doors in the privacy of the consulting room. Psychiatrists and trainees saw their patients intermittently, at intervals of days or weeks for inpatients, and weeks or months for outpatients. In Heathfield House the suite of consulting rooms in the western wing was physically separate from the ward on the eastern side, and nurses discouraged patients from loitering in the west wing corridor. Because rooms were in short supply they were coveted and, once occupied, defended vigorously. Decor included psychiatric texts and journals, which defined this room as a space of professional knowledge. A reproduction of a favourite painting on the wall or a small family photograph on the desk defined it as a personal space. Medical students, who had no access to offices, had to interview patients in various nooks and corners of the building, which in a junior and makeshift way approximated both the privacy of the consultant psychiatrist's office and its distance from the ward. On arrival, each new batch of medical students was given a guided tour of the nooks of Heathfield House by the charge nurse.

Psychiatrists (and, in decreasing measure, the trainee psychiatrists and medical students) were able to achieve *distance* from patients. Their offices were separate from the wards, and their contact with the patients was intermittent rather than continuous. Between psychiatrist and patient stood the other

ranks, particularly the trainee and the nurse. The abstract
forms of knowledge used by psychiatrists also had a distancing
effect, especially the classificatory system, which enabled them
to approach a person as a diagnostic category.[1] In the longer
term, psychiatrists usually left their patients behind as they
pursued careers that led them up through the hospital ranks
or away from the hospital altogether.

Although distance conferred 'objectivity', it also rendered
psychiatrists vulnerable to charges of remoteness and lack of
involvement. Their response was to claim an 'in-depth' knowledge of their cases. It was as if a case itself had an inner space,
and psychiatry had privileged knowledge of its deeper regions.

An orientation to the deep interior of the case was evident
in the demeanour of psychiatrists at their work. Interview
etiquette—making the patient feel comfortable, the sober attitude of concern, the open-ended question, the establishment
of a 'trusting alliance'—was primarily aimed at eliciting inner
mental symptoms. In clinical parlance, a thorough assessment
was described as a 'depth interview'. It was said to 'tap' the
inner or deeper emotions. The adept clinician was said to 'un-
cover', 'bring out', or allow the patient to 'open up', as in the
expression, 'He opened up and out it all came'. What
emerged were the 'underlying' thoughts, feelings, or delusions the patient had been 'covering up' or that had been
lying 'deeply buried'. The metaphor of industrial mining
structured many of these expressions, and the patient's
thoughts and feelings were referred to as 'material', as if they
were a substance. When it was difficult to elicit this 'underlying
material', the process was sometimes called 'prising it out',
and when this became a long-term project it was called 'chipping away'. These common-sense ideas held by psychiatrists
about their work had their counterpart in the popular view
that psychiatrists possessed an uncanny ability to 'see right
into' a person or to 'read a person's mind'. The psychiatrists'
depth perspective was thus reinforced by patients' ideas of
what was happening during an interview.

These everyday metaphors were given academic legitimacy
by theories of 'depth psychology', referred to as 'psychody-

[1] See Armstrong (1984) for a historical perspective on abstraction and distance in
medical diagnosis.

namics' or, more colloquially, 'dynamics'. The Freudian psychodynamic construct of the person as comprising successively deeper layers, from conscious to preconscious to unconscious, was sometimes called the onion skin model of the person.[2] Gaining a deep psychotherapeutic understanding was likened to peeling off successive layers. Psychiatrists claimed an exclusive mandate to practise psychodynamic psychotherapy and defended it by telling cautionary tales about nonpsychiatrist colleagues who attempted this form of treatment and consequently got out of their depth. The tales related treatment 'disasters' that occurred because these colleagues lacked awareness of how the patient's unconscious mind and early relationships with parental figures could affect a therapist (a phenomenon called transference) and how that therapist could unconsciously react (counter-transference). In essence, these problems were attributed to untrained therapists not having sufficient skill in understanding the deeper aspects of either the patients or themselves.

Through a detailed enquiry known as the Maudsley history (after the London hospital where it was encoded and enshrined), a case was constructed as having depth in time as well as in space. The centrepiece of the 'Maudsley' was the developmental history, a biographical narrative that extended deep into the patient's past, commencing prior to the patient's conception and birth and culminating in the present. In onion skin terms, each successive experience was layered onto earlier experiences. Thus the metaphors of 'case time' and 'case space' were mutually defining. What lay deep within the patient (case space) was buried deep in the past (case time).

As part of their penetration of the case, psychiatrists had a special interest in previously undisclosed information. The privacy of the office encouraged disclosure. This generated a case history that was, in part, a collation of personal secrets, whose twin guardians were the ethics of confidentiality and non self-disclosure on the part of the psychiatrist. Secrets were primar-

---

[2] Compare with Littlewood's (1986:42) discussion of the Russian doll model of the person as a 'basic psychological or physiological core surrounded by a series of envelopes awaiting unpacking'.

ily sexual: pubertal feelings, masturbatory fantasies, homosexual experiences, and, most importantly, incest.

The interior regions of the case were the main site of psychiatry's indeterminate knowledge—knowledge that could not be taught 'by the book', but which could only be learned by direct experience over long periods of time.[3] There were many words to describe such knowledge, including clinical judgement, acumen, intuition, psychological mindedness, or a sixth sense for a patient's underlying dynamics. Jamous and Peloille (1970:112–20) have identified indeterminate knowledge as a personal attribute of the professional, his or her biography or personality characteristics. These authors contrast indeterminate knowledge with technical knowledge, which is public and transmissable because it can be set down as a precisely formulated, rational code that may be openly communicated to those in training and even to people outside the profession. Jamous and Peloille's particular study examines the ratio of 'indetermination' to 'technicality' in the development of the medical profession in France, but their broader concern is to identify a contradiction in the production of professional knowledge, a contradiction that pits rationality against autonomy. They argue that as a consequence of specialist knowledge being rendered into prescriptive rules the expertise of a profession becomes accessible to outsiders, thereby opening the profession to the possibility of external control. The alternative strategy of locating expertise in the personal qualities of individual professionals allows a profession to assert a monopoly over its field and exert control over external appraisal.[4] Atkinson, Reid and Sheldrake (1977) view indeterminacy not as an absolute or objective trait of a profession but as a claim made by members of that profession in

[3] Compare with Polanyi's (1958:69–248) notion of 'tacit knowledge', that is to say, 'knowledge that is acquired through practice and that cannot be articulated explicitly' (Kuhn 1962:44).

[4] See also Johnson (1977:100–4) who argues that the contradictory forces of 'technicality' and 'indetermination' stem from a contradiction in the way the professions are structured within modern capitalism. Professionals derive income from their labour and, like all collective labourers, are subject to the routinization of work (technicality). On the other hand, they are 'associated with the global functions of capital', especially the surveillance and control of the work force. Accordingly, they are protected by means of 'indeterminacy' from external control of their own work.

order to secure autonomy of practice: 'To the extent that knowledge is defined as "indeterminate", the practices of an occupation's members will be treated as nonaccountable ... as beyond the scrutiny of fellow professionals and laymen alike' (Atkinson et al. 1977:257–8). For psychiatrists at Ridgehaven, indeterminate knowledge always involved the deeper aspects of the case. A psychiatrist possessed of clinical acumen was capable, by working on a hunch, of identifying an underlying psychosis that might be missed by others. Similarly, an 'intuitive grasp' of the 'underlying dynamics' of a case was the hallmark of a good psychiatrist. Those with a 'capacity for empathy' could, through awareness of their own feelings, reach into the patient's inner feelings and understand them. Each of these examples involved a core psychiatric expertise that, because it was indefinable, secured psychiatry's monopoly over the interior of the case.

Psychiatry exercised jurisdiction over the major internal divisions of the case, the most basic division being that between body and mind. With its focus on the body, a biological organism, psychiatry invoked its medical authority in a tangible way. As doctors, psychiatrists were licensed to examine the body and 'open up' its interior spaces to view. While there was passing interest in the skin, the physical examination was mainly orientated to the internal organs, the heart and lungs by means of the stethoscope and the brain and nervous system by means of the ophthalmoscope, tendon hammer, and neurological examination. Only doctors could authorize technical investigations such as electroencephalography, computerized axial tomography, or magnetic resonance imaging, which displayed two dimensional images of the brain. Psychiatrists claimed an advantage over other mental health professionals by asserting that only they had the training and expertise for accurate diagnosis in cases where the symptoms and signs appeared to be caused by psychiatric disorder (such as schizophrenia) but were actually caused by an underlying physical disorder (such as epilepsy or a brain tumour).

By contrast, psychiatry's prerogative to define the mind was neither exclusive nor legally authorised. It was subject to challenge by other professions such as psychology, or could easily be watered down to the common-sense notion of 'what everyone knows about other people's thoughts'. As a result, psychiatrists had to reassert their prerogative constantly by declaring that by dint of special training and experience in the 'mental state examination' they possessed a superior method of observing, recording, and interpreting the thoughts, perceptions, and feelings that lay deep within the patient's mind. Members of other professions were capable of appreciating only the patient's more accessible thoughts and feelings. Nevertheless, because psychiatry's claim to the mind as an exclusive work site was always tenuous, there was a tendency to fall back on its medical stronghold, the body. Thus statements about a patient's mental state often had a biological reference, as when a psychiatrist pointed to the mental experiences that resulted from a biological depressive illness. It was largely a matter of psychiatric discretion to determine the relative mix of body and mind for each case and to adjudicate, for example, on whether a stressful emotional state triggered a biological illness or that illness caused the emotional state in the first instance.

Another division within the case lay between illness and 'personality'. The definition of illness was also a psychiatric prerogative. Although other professions had an informal warrant to advance diagnostic opinions when talking with their colleagues, only psychiatry was licensed to make formal diagnostic statements of illness that could be entered into the official case record. These statements had legal implications, for example, authorizing the enforced detention of the patient within the hospital. They also had administrative implications. Because functional treatment units at Ridgehaven were organized on the basis of diagnostic classification, psychiatry determined the distribution of patients throughout the hospital. Moreover, the 'illness' was not just a segment of the case, it encompassed the case itself. The name of the illness was the name of the case, for example, a case of schizophrenia. Psychiatry's power to define a person as a case of illness was central to its dominance over other professions.

'Personality' was the obverse facet of this dichotomy. It referred to long-standing traits that characterized persons, their distinctive behaviour, and their habitual way of relating to others. Whereas illness was episodic, personality was enduring.

Psychiatric patients were classified according to standard personality types—paranoid, histrionic, obsessional, borderline—each with their symptomatic behaviour patterns. This way of typifying persons relied on metonymy, the use of a partial feature to refer to the person as a whole. For example, a history of childhood truancy, drug taking, and promiscuity during adolescence and crime during adulthood were evidence of a sociopathic personality, which was regarded as the total identity of the person, both as an enduring trait discernible throughout the person's life and as a pervasive trait, affecting all aspects of the person's behaviour.

Illness and personality were defined by mutual exclusion. What was not illness was personality. Psychiatrists moved the boundary back and forth in their role as definers of the illness/personality ratio of the case: more illness implied less personality. Each item of a patient's behaviour—a particular style of relating to staff, an angry mood, a suspicious attitude—could be ascribed to either illness or personality. A typical psychiatric discovery was to diagnose an underlying psychiatric illness that was responsible for behaviour formerly attributed to personality. Alternatively, what had been seen as an illness could be recast as a manifestation of personality factors, as in the following case discussion of a woman I have called Judith.[5] Judith had, until then, been treated for a schizophrenic illness over many years. The treating psychiatrist reported to the team:

> Well Judith wants to sign herself out. It's hardly surprising. I
> saw her this morning and, um, said that I didn't think she had
> schizophrenia or any chronic psychotic illness of that nature
> and I suggested to her that her problems really were problems
> of personality and of relationships, and that if she wanted her
> relationships to turn out differently then she was going to have
> to change within herself, and *that* was a long-term process. She
> really has a histrionic personality disorder. She was telling me at
> great length about the number of men that are making sexual
> advances to her, and that they are all after her. And just the
> amount of time she's taking up with us—you know she's being
> really very seductive, and she talks about rape and incest and
> anything she thinks will interest us, just to get more time. So I'll

[5] Names and personal information that might identify individual members of staff or patients have been altered throughout this book.

see her after this, but, um, I doubt if staying in hospital any longer is going to serve any purpose. If there is a psychosis I think it is a psychogenic psychosis ... you know, a brief reactive psychosis, because it settles so quickly on so little medication, and it was so clearly related to all the environmental stresses.

In sum, psychiatry was the most autonomous and powerful of the mental health professions at Ridgehaven Hospital. Psychiatric practice was relatively independent of supervisory control and largely immune to interference from fellow professional groups. Psychiatrists were relatively independent of patients too. They were able to work at a spatial, temporal, and organizational distance from the daily lives of their patients and eventually move away from them altogether. The counterpart to this distant vantage was a unique psychiatric perspective which viewed a case as having a spatial dimension (with a deep interior core) and a temporal dimension (its extended background history). The depths of case space and case time were the domain of psychiatry, a domain of secret knowledge generated within the privacy of the psychiatric encounter. At these depths, psychiatry presided over the division between body and mind and stood guard over the interface between illness and personality.

Psychiatric nursing

Psychiatric nursing was less autonomous than psychiatry. It was an emergent profession (Strauss and Bucher 1975) that was moving toward independence from the traditional Nightingale stance of being the handmaiden to medicine. This change was evident in the transfer of nursing education from hospital campuses to tertiary institutions in order to produce university-qualified nurses. It was embodied in the development of a distinctive core of nursing theory and research. Postgraduate education in nursing showed a growing interest in management, with the aim of propelling nurses into health administration. In clinical practice, there were two important developments that signalled a drive toward autonomy. First, nurses had achieved the designation 'consultant', and could be called to give an opinion on a case (Stickey, Moir, and

Gardner 1981). Second, there was a change from 'task-oriented' to 'case-oriented' practice. Although they had long been treating patients, nurses had hitherto been unable to play a role in the definition of sick people as cases. Now, instead of being responsible for performing a few tasks (say, measuring blood pressure and temperature) on all patients in a ward, a nurse would carry out all tasks on a few patients. As a result, nurses could now treat their charges not merely as patients but as cases. To perceive a person as a *patient*, one who suffers and passively receives care or treatment, was different to perceiving that person as a *case*, an instance of illness that is a suitable object for professional consultation. Finding a niche in the case was a crucial step in the establishment of autonomy for the nursing profession, and it would subsequently develop into an impetus for recognition as 'case managers' (Kanter 1989).

The political organization of psychiatric nursing outside the hospital lacked unity. Membership of the Australian Congress of Mental Health Nurses was not obligatory, nor did this body exercise any regulatory authority. In industrial terms, nurses were divided between no less than three labor organizations. Within the hospital the pyramid of ranks, like that of psychiatry, consisted of eight steps, from director of nursing to deputy, to supervisors, charge nurses, deputy charge nurses, to registered psychiatric nurses, student nurses, and finally enrolled nurses, a lower echelon with shorter training and little clinical responsibility. Instead of appearing as a pyramid, this ranking might be depicted as a flower vase with a broad base (there were 380 nurses at the hospital) and a bottleneck that restricted upward mobility at midcareer. Whereas for psychiatry the gradation of ranks represented the possibility of upward movement and autonomy, for nurses it represented career stasis and loss of autonomy through the strict surveillance of line management. At Ridgehaven there were many registered psychiatric nurses who were waiting, year after year, for promotion to deputy charge nurse, and a number of them developed a sense of disillusionment and detachment known as 'burn out'. Nurses did not have the option to move out into private practice: self-employment was restricted to those few who had sufficient capital to buy a private nursing home. With the reduction in hospital bed numbers that accompanied de-institutionalization, there could be no expansion of nursing jobs within the hospital. The one significant outlet was community nursing. Compared to their hospital-based counterparts, grounded in the wards, the community nurses had an enthusiasm and prestige that came from their location at the leading edge of the 'community movement' (c.f. Gray 1986). Their daily round of work took place in the suburbs, which were positively valued as 'the community', in contradistinction to the hospital as an 'institution'. With the possible exception of these community nurses, it was not possible for psychiatric nurses to achieve distance from the patient or from the hospital.

By means of schedules, rosters, and close supervision of clocking on and clocking off, nursing administrators exerted strict control over the work time of each nurse. Nurses were rostered on duty for two days followed by two days off duty, with a resultant cycle of engagement and disengagement. A pair of nurses would work jointly but alternately on a case: when one was off for two days, the other was on for two days. Although they left notes for each other, they did not actually meet. A good working relationship ('I like working opposite him') required a joint approach based on a common understanding of the patient.

Whereas psychiatrists worked individually and saw patients intermittently, nurses related in pairs and groups to their cases. The individual nurse–patient mode of treatment involving privacy and confidentiality was used so infrequently on the Schizophrenia Team that when it was, it was specifically prescribed as giving the patient some 'one-to-one' or, with tongue in cheek, some 'deep one-to-one'. The phrase 'deep and meaningful one-to-one' was sometimes used by nurses to ridicule colleagues who indulged in this individual form of counselling.

Wards were staffed around the clock with day and night shifts. Thus nurses worked not only in tandem with their opposite numbers but also in conjunction with fellow nurses on contiguous shifts. Each shift overlapped with the next by means of a 'hand-over' meeting in which nurses gave a brief update of the patients in their case load. Pertinent, practical information was handed on, and at the same time nurses not directly involved with a case would add their own observations. In this way, nurses jointly worked out a common approach and a common definition of each patient. An experienced charge nurse would unobtrusively comment from time to time in a hand-over meeting, and thereby make fine adjustments to the tone of the entire nursing team toward problematic cases. Unlike the intermittent and individual psychiatric involvement in a case, nursing involvement was collectively continuous. 'The psychiatrist sees them for an hour, we have them for the other twenty three'.

Hospital-based nurses worked an entire shift in one ward, the principal therapeutic space for patients and the principal working space of nurses. Through the 'ward programme' with its sequence of activities in different rooms—the morning meeting, activity time, afternoon tea, free time—nurses managed the space and time of the ward and husbanded the patients within it. They did not have private offices. Furthermore, the ward decor did not identify individual nurses but emphasized the group. Photocopied cartoons about overworked nurses or humorous posters about a team of efficient staff (depicting a troupe of monkeys) adorned the nursing station.

The status of psychiatric nursing, the distinctiveness of its practice, and the uniqueness of its perspective on the case, were defined in terms of *proximity* to the patient. This concept was exemplified by the intimate nature of nursing tasks in relation to the body, such as the giving of medication by mouth or injection. In keeping with the etymological derivation of 'nurse', the relationship between nurse and patient was often likened to a nurturing bond between parent and infant. When admitting a patient to the ward, nurses itemized clothes, money, and possessions, recorded the distinguishing features of the patient's appearance and any identifying marks on the body, and then made sure the patient was cleaned and fed. For dishevelled patients, this process might mean putting them in a bath, giving them a good scrubbing, and putting their clothes through an industrial washing machine. In contrast to the doctors' physical examination, which looked into the interior compartments, nurses largely worked on the surface of the body.

Working at close quarters to patients' bodies, nurses were responsible for controlling violent behaviour that took the form of self-mutilation, suicide attempts, or physical attacks on others. They had an extensive, though uncodified, body of practical knowledge concerned with the constraint of violence in ways that ensured no damage would come to the patient, staff, or other patients. Strategies ranged from 'talking some-one down', to 'sitting on a patient' without getting hurt, to the extremely dangerous instances when a small group of nurses would have to enter an isolation room behind a mat-tress held as a shield, pressing the violent patient up against the wall. In a situation of extreme violence, psychiatrists stayed outside the room, writing up orders for major tranquillizers to be given by injection. From time to time, inexperienced trainee psychiatrists would attempt to help by entering the melee, but the nurses soon expelled them because, not being part of a well trained formation, they got in the way, placing themselves and the nurses at risk. From their practical knowl-edge, nurses derived the power to define the level of danger in each case, and this definition prevailed over psychiatric as-sessments. A nursing decision that a patient was too dangerous to be in an open (unlocked) ward would always override a psychiatrist's wish to keep the patient there.[6] Whereas psychi-atrists distributed cases among the Teams on the basis of di-agnosis, nurses, on the basis of their determination of danger, moved cases from one ward to another along the gradient of closed to open.

Closeness to the patient, on the other hand, was a threat to status. Controlling violent patients rendered nurses suscepti-ble to being labelled as guards. Among the nurses working in the closed ward, this was the subject of humorous banter. Tack-ling a patient and bringing them to the ground was called 'one-to-one therapy' in jocular reference to individual nurse counselling. Furthermore, cleaning, clothing, and feeding pa-tients could sometimes be dirty and contaminating, and there-fore degrading. There was also an idea of social contagion expressed in the semihumorous lay person's idea that if you spent too long in close contact with 'mad' people you ended

---

[6] Compare with the account by Strauss *et al.* (1964:110) of 'ward shape', whereby nursing staff decided which type of patient should be treated in each ward.

up going 'a bit funny' yourself. Nurses dealt with this problem through humour, such as the oft-heard dining room quip that if you ate the patient's food it would poison you. There are many ways of interpreting this pithy joke, but it always drew laughter because it broached the normally unspoken fear of contagion. Within the joke the identity of the nurse merges with that of the patient by virtue of sharing food to the extent that the nurse develops a typical paranoid delusion of the food being poisoned. The distinction between nurse and patient is blurred by means of a role reversal, but at the same time recreated and reinforced because it is only a joke.

Proximity also rendered nurses vulnerable to being compromised ethically. Their work was so physically close to patients that the relationship could be misconstrued as sexual. The practical danger of this misconstrual to a professional's career was the risk of being deregistered and losing one's livelihood. I was not aware of any nurse having had sexual relations with a patient during the time of this study, yet cautionary tales abounded. One concerned a legendary nurse with a ravenous sexual appetite. It was reputed that she had sexual intercourse with psychotic patients in the deserted upstairs wing of a back ward. As in the dining room quip, identities are blurred within this tale in that the nurse exhibited an unbridled sexuality often attributed to psychotic patients. Whereas the quip tickled the nurses' sense of humour, the story also shocked them and thereby served a warning function. Although it was said to have happened in a bygone era, the story maintained a steady currency over the years because it reinforced the fragile and ambiguous boundary between nursing proximity and sexual intimacy.

Nurses were thus vulnerable to the danger of pollution by dirty patients, the danger of social contagion by mixing closely with 'madness', and the physical danger of being assaulted. Proximity threatened nurses with a blurring of boundaries and was therefore dangerous and polluting in the more fundamental sense of these concepts, as developed by Mary Douglas (1966:113). Proximity rendered their professional identity ambiguous and brought them to the point where they could cross basic cultural boundaries within the hospital—boundaries that divided staff from patients.

Yet proximity was also the strength of nursing. Psychiatric nurses described their intimate work with patients as basic, practical, and caring. This meant that it was logically and temporally prior to the work of any other profession, as in the maxim: 'You can't give psychotherapy to someone who hasn't eaten'. Such sayings emphasized the esoteric nature of psychiatrists' work and showed how dependent it was on the nurses' 'basics first' approach. An orientation to what was simultaneously fundamental and intimate was expressed in the term 'basic nursing care', which distilled the essence of the nurses' work. Although formulated during the 1920s by Bailey (see Mark 1980:34), the term still had currency among Ridgehaven Hospital nurses.

Whereas psychiatrists worked at a distance from the patient but countered the charge of remoteness by claiming an indepth perspective on the case, nurses worked up close to patients and countered the contaminating aspects of this proximity by extolling their pragmatic approach. From this practical stance, nurses claimed a unique knowledge of patients, captured in the assertion, 'We know what they are *really* like'. They could detect whether or not a symptom was 'genuine'. According to nurses, patients could present a façade to a psychiatrist and could easily maintain it for an hour, the length of a standard psychiatric interview. Having returned to the ward, it was not long before they revealed what they were 'really' like to the twenty-four hour scrutiny of the nursing team. Nurses used a light-hearted classification that was based on the length of time patients could maintain a false front before they revealed their true colours—this patient having a two-hour façade, that patient having a ten-minute façade. 'Presentation' was another term used to describe how patients put on a 'face' for the staff. It might be said of a patient that 'she presents well superficially, but underneath is quite psychotic' or, conversely, he 'presents with all the right psychotic symptoms but is actually quite resourceful in getting what he wants'. Nurses took particular note of patients as they engaged in activities that were not expressly clinical or therapeutic. Credence was placed on these observations as reflecting patients' true behaviour. For example, when a psychiatrist gave the opinion during a case conference that a patient was actively psychotic, it was effectively refuted by a nursing observation that the patient had organized a game of netball for fellow patients on the hospital playing field, behaviour that was hardly compatible with active psychosis.

The nurses' capacity to observe patients over time and in different contexts thus conferred an authority to define what was 'real', 'true', 'genuine', or 'actual' about a case.[7] The nurses' particular version of 'reality' was a practical, common-sense one. It was grounded on observations of the everyday world of the patient. In his essay 'On Multiple Realities', Schutz (1962:207–59) argued that 'the reality of the world of daily life' is *the* paramount reality, more fundamental than other realities that lie within the world of theatre, play, dreams, or scientific theory. When there was a conflict between nursing and psychiatric definitions of a case, the practical perspective prevailed over more theoretical formulations.

Like psychiatrists, psychiatric nurses talked about cases in spatial metaphors, as if they had a surface zone and a deeper core. Unlike psychiatrists, who largely focused on this inner core and its various divisions, nurses were primarily concerned to discriminate between the superficial veneer and the underlying reality, between what was false and what was genuine. Whereas psychiatrists presided over the deeper regions of the case, nurses exercised discretion at the surface of the case. By knowledge of the surface, I do not mean superficial knowledge but a capacity to see through a façade. This view was in keeping with their work on the body surface, which focused on a patient's appearance, personal possessions, and clothing, rather than internal organs. The same orientation applied to case time. Unlike psychiatrists, for whom knowledge of the patient's early developmental history was crucial because it gave a time depth to the case, nurses' strength lay in their ability to comment on what the patient was like in the 'here-and-now'. This idea has been elaborated within nursing theory. Rogers has developed a concept of the 'relative present' based on a nonlinear view of time, according to which, 'the key to

---

[7] Rosenthal and McGuinness (1986) write of 'contactfulness' as a central aspect of nursing. It combines proximity to the client, nurturing, and observation; and it asserts the privileged position of nurses to provide 'objective facts' and to define 'reality'.

resolving emotional problems, whether they originated in the past or in the person's anticipation of the future, resides in the client's perspective on the present' (Reed 1987:26). Thus in both time and space nurses valued a surface rather than a deep knowledge of the case.

Their indeterminate knowledge also focused on the case surface, and they talked about this knowledge using tangible or sensate metaphors. Following an admission to hospital, it was commonplace for a clinical team to wait for several days until the nursing staff could 'get a feel for the patient' and only then proceed with major treatment decisions. The older psychiatric nurses were said to have been able to 'smell schizophrenia' because they worked so close to the patients, although no such claim was made by the nurses working at Ridgehaven during this study. The capacity for olfactory diagnosis was nevertheless compatible with the focus on the surface, which characterized all nursing claims to an exclusive zone of expertise.

Nursing knowledge was not highly theorized. Individual nurses quoted authors such as Maslow (1970) and his idea of a hierarchy of needs (starting from the physical and extending to the psychological, the social, and ultimately the spiritual) but did so mainly to defend their 'basics first' orientation. In the main, nurses did not sprinkle their clinical conversations with the names of theorists, as did the trainee psychiatrists. Such knowledge was dismissed as esoteric, and nurses who employed it were lampooned by nursing colleagues as 'playing psychiatrist.' One form of insult was to damn a fellow nurse with faint praise as 'really dynamic', in sarcastic reference to his or her excessive preoccupation with depth psychologies. Instead of giving deep psychotherapy, nurses saw their chief contribution as providing common-sense counselling and helping patients with activities of daily living. Within academic nursing, efforts were being made to advance the profession and to secure its independence from medicine by developing a distinctive nursing theory that would overcome the problems created by overdependence on the medical model (Hall 1988). However, such abstract knowledge created a distance from the patient, potentially undermining the chief sources of nursing power, proximity, and pragmatism. In response to this dilemma, conceptual frameworks were developed that linked theory with practice (Magan and Mrozek 1990) and placed special emphasis on 'reality' (O'Toole 1981:12):

> In reality, theory must be pragmatic to be useful and practice must be theoretical to be tested. . . . The invention of practice theory involves two simultaneous and complementary processes. The first is practice itself, that is, a clear explication of nursing by those who practice it. The second is research or scientific inquiry about practice.

Another response to the dilemma was to develop an interest in ethnographic research, no surprise for a profession with a long-standing interest in the patients' everyday world, common-sense reasoning, practical problems of living, and participant observation.

In the first section of this chapter I showed that psychiatrists, with their autonomy from other professions and from the patient, could work individually, privately, and from a distance, and accordingly defined patients in terms of deep case space. Here I have shown that psychiatric nurses, whose profession was less autonomous, could not establish this distance and privacy. Their power to define cases was derived from their collective proximity to patients. On this basis they could claim privileged knowledge of what I have called the surface of the case. For psychiatry, a patient's actions were seen as *symptoms* of underlying forces, be they biological or psychodynamic. Nurses would characterize the same actions as *behavioural*, indicating that the patient was trying to elicit a response, especially from the nurses themselves. They said of patients who were good at this that they 'knew how to push all the right buttons' in the staff. In the psychiatric version, actions stemmed from inside; in the nursing version, actions were oriented to the outside.

Another important difference was that psychiatrists tended to view patients as passive and controlled by their psychiatric illness, whereas nurses tended to see them as more active and capable of exerting control over their mind, their illness, and its symptoms. Thus case surface was to case depth as being in control was to being controlled. What psychiatrists said was 'thought disorder' nurses could call 'evasiveness'. What psychiatrists diagnosed as 'catatonic mutism' could be redefined by nurses as 'refusing to talk'. The psychiatric category of 'acute dystonic reaction' (a side effect to major tranquillizers in which the patient's eyes turn upward) was often referred to by nurses as 'putting on the look-ups'. A critical turning point in a case trajectory was when nurses started to redefine a patient's symptoms as 'largely behavioural'.

The distinction between passive and active constructions of cases had implications for what they were called. Some nurses had stopped referring to cases as patients and begun to call them 'clients'.[8] To use the term 'patient' was to place emphasis on the illness and the suffering, as indicated by its etymology. It also connoted passivity and invoked the idea of submission to medical domination and knowledge. The term 'client' construed the person as more active and implied an idea of therapy as a contract voluntarily entered into by two free agents.[9] The commonly used phrase 'empowering the client', conveyed the idea that a person could take control of his or her illness, life, and relationships with mental health workers. At the same time, for nurses it preserved a power and knowledge differential that is implicit in any professional–client relationship. When working in conjunction with psychiatry and drawing on the traditional doctor–nurse alliance, cases were 'patients', but when establishing professional independence in opposition to psychiatry, nurses redefined cases as 'clients'.

Social work

In terms of autonomy of professional organization and autonomy of individual practice, social work at Ridgehaven Hospital occupied a position halfway between psychiatry and nursing. Unlike psychiatrists, fully qualified social workers were subject to some supervision from their seniors, but it was not the intense scrutiny experienced by the registered psychiatric nurse.

[8] See Mark (1980) for a developmental history of nursing appellations for mentally ill people (from 'lunatic' to 'patient' to 'client'). Forchuk (1989) discusses the different phases of the nurse–client relationship within a conceptual framework developed by the nursing theorist Hildegard Peplau.

[9] Taussig (1980) argues that the practice of contracting serves to mystify relations of inequality within the clinical encounter, preserving professional dominance while at the same time producing a fiction of patient autonomy.

In terms of their ability to determine the schedule of their daily work, they also occupied an intermediate position between the *laissez-faire* approach of psychiatry and the rigid rostering of psychiatric nursing.

Far from being homogeneous, social work was a 'profession in process' (Bucher and Strauss 1961:325), as it was undergoing rapid change and comprised segments with different backgrounds and interests. There were two distinct echelons at Ridgehaven Hospital, each with a separate provenance. The senior social workers were recent arrivals to the hospital. They were young, university qualified, and would all soon move on to other hospitals or academic positions because, like the psychiatrists, they had career mobility, limited only by the lack of opportunity for private practice. The junior social workers were older and had worked in the hospital for decades. Their promotion was constrained by a career structure of only four ranks, which could be depicted as a flattened pyramid. Many had started their careers as psychiatric nurses, become 'mental health visitors' (a kind of community nurse) with the first wave of deinstitutionalization during the 1960s and 1970s, and ultimately entered the base grades of the social work profession across a series of bridging courses, through which they had upgraded their qualifications. What they lacked in higher qualifications was compensated for by their long-term knowledge of the older patients, accumulated in some instances over a twenty-year span. Their enduring relationships with these patients often looked more like friendships, especially to the young seniors who saw it as their supervisory role to introduce notions of case work—assessment, planning, setting aims, interventions, and evaluation—in order to redefine such relationships as therapeutic.

In Heathfield House the social work offices were located near the central 'light court', midway between the psychiatrists' offices and the ward. They were semiprivate spaces. Two people frequently shared a single office. The characteristic decor—a desk piled high with government application forms—indicated that the social worker remained the chief intermediary between the welfare state and the disabled. Social workers did not contest office space like the psychiatrists. Instead, they competed for hospital cars because the suburban home or hostel, not the private office, was their primary work space. The number of hospital cars was limited, and the cars were distributed each day from a pool. Social workers vied for their use with community nurses, as each group strove to define itself as the profession with prior claim to 'the community'. Among social workers there was a grumbling conflict over cars between the young seniors and the old juniors, which came to a head when one of the latter managed to reserve the use of a particular car every day and, to make matters worse, personalized it with carpets and other forms of automobile decor.

Whereas there were straightforward assumptions within the hospital about what doctors and nurses did, the role of the social worker was less clearly delineated. Davidson (1990) argues that social work, as a comparative newcomer to hospital practice, has not fully established its niche vis-a-vis the other professions; and as a consequence social workers commonly encounter ambiguity and role blurring. At Ridgehaven, members of the social work department worked for many years on the development of new protocols for patient assessment, the purposes of which were to both standardize professional practice and demonstrate the distinctiveness of their contribution and knowledge.

Social work knowledge was hybrid: partly pragmatic and partly abstract. As pragmatists, they were allied with nurses in their disrespect for abstruse ideas, and they made this clear by the way they valued those psychiatrists who displayed a more pragmatic approach. Social workers prided themselves on their personal knowledge of hostels, boarding houses, and nursing homes where patients without family support could live after being discharged. They built up goodwill with the managers of these establishments by a form of delayed reciprocity known as 'juggling' or 'swapping' in which they would arrange to transfer one difficult patient from a hostel into the ward and then later ask the hostel manager to accept another difficult patient from the hospital. In this way some social workers developed a reputation for being able to 'place' even the most difficult and objectionable patients (the so-called 'placement problems'). These practical skills were highly valued by the other professions because they facilitated the movement of patients out of the hospital.[10] Movement was valued therapeutically because it indicated progress and recovery and made way for new admissions. It was valued administratively as patient turnover, which was an indicator of the quantity of work done and served as statistical justification for the hospital budget. The power of social workers to distribute patients outside the hospital rendered them indispensable to the other professions. When social workers planned the partial withdrawal of their labour in the context of a potential industrial dispute, refusing to place patients was their first strategy because it allowed them to continue caring for and supporting patients while quickly bringing the central work of moving patients out of the hospital to a standstill.

At the same time, practical social work activities, such as driving patients to government departments or helping them secure financial assistance, could be status degrading. These tasks could be construed as a demeaning form of service: 'running errands' or 'providing a free taxi service' (c.f. Ruzek 1971:217; Ben-Sira and Szyf 1992:371).

In addition to these practical forms of knowledge, which were a source of both kudos and debasement, the senior social workers had tertiary qualifications in liberal arts with a major component of theoretical sociology. During the 1970s it was this group who, with copies of Goffman in hand, carried radical sociology to the psychiatric hospital. In the 1980s, when this study was carried out, eclecticism, 'systems theory', and an 'ecological approach' were the core theoretical ideas (Siporin 1979). A patient was viewed as just one element within the family and just one node within the wider social network; and was sometimes called the 'identified patient' to convey that he or she was merely representative of an entire system that was malfunctioning. Social work's unique contribution to the case was the family assessment, the purpose of which was to develop an understanding of the 'family dynamics'. It was important that this assessment be carried out in the patient's own environment—hence the central importance of the car and the 'home visit' to social work practice. Social workers'

---

[10] Roach Anleu (1992:30) shows that the performance of practical tasks is an important resource for social work when asserting independence from medicine within a hospital setting.

indeterminate knowledge was concerned with the 'flavour' or atmosphere of the home. Just as nurses claimed a special knowledge of patients from round-the-clock observation in the ward, so social workers claimed a distinctive knowledge by observing patients in the context of their families during the outpatient phase. As social workers emphasized, the greater part of their illness was managed outside the hospital: 'You only see them while they are in hospital; we see the rest of their lives'. On the Schizophrenia Team, this point was illustrated by the special contribution that social workers could make to the understanding of a patient's psychotic symptoms. They were often able to demonstrate that what was regarded by psychiatrists and nurses as a delusion was, in part, consistent with the patient's reality. It was a matter of uncovering what was called the 'element' or 'kernel' of truth contained within a delusion. For example, a social worker might discover that a patient's seemingly delusional belief in a spouse's infidelity was indeed justified.

Social workers were concerned to demonstrate the interactions between a patient's personality, their schizophrenic illness, and their family. To do so they employed a form of causal reasoning, reminiscent of Newtonian physics, as if illness, personality, and family were mechanical forces that influenced each other. Thus they showed how certain family dynamics could exacerbate a patient's psychotic symptoms or, alternatively, how a severe schizophrenic illness could place immense strain on an entire family, pushing them beyond their coping capacity.

In addition to this causal reasoning, social workers employed a form of moral reasoning when evaluating a patient's family and its relation to his or her illness. A family could either be described in positive terms as 'supportive', 'concerned', 'understanding', 'coping', or 'sensible'; or it could be described negatively as 'pathological', 'enmeshed', 'over involved', 'noxious', or 'over stimulating'. A schizophrenic illness, too, could be ascribed moral value, as when it was described as 'malignant', 'nasty', or 'destructive'. When a family was described in positive terms the corresponding description of the patient's personality or illness was usually negative. Joyce, a woman in her late fifties, was admitted to Heathfield House with a relapse of a long term paranoid schizophrenic illness. She had developed delusions that she was a Gypsy. In the case discussion she was described as a 'weird character' who 'kept lots of rabbits' and 'had not been outside her house for 16 years'. Her family, by contrast, were described by the social worker as 'sensible and supportive'.

In another typical permutation, the family situation would be described as pathological, the patient's personality as vulnerable, and the illness a result of these forces. Sudachanh Littlejohn, a young woman from Thailand, was treated at Ridgehaven for a florid psychotic illness that manifested in behaviour such as prostrating herself on the lawn outside the ward and standing for long periods of time facing East, her palms held together with thumbs touching her forehead, as if assuming a posture of prayer. This was understood partly in the light of her psychosis and partly in the light of her cultural and religious background. She was described as a 'mail order bride' because she had met her husband through an introduction agency, married in Bangkok, and emigrated to Australia shortly thereafter. Her personality was said to have an 'hysterical flavour'. Her husband had 'obsessional traits' and was described pejoratively as a 'dreadful man' who 'blames doctors for his wife's illness'. Sudachanh experienced sexual difficulties and was said to be 'trapped in a marriage which has no future'. In the case formulation she was thus construed as a vulnerable person who was at the mercy of her husband. Her schizophrenia was thought to be driven by this dynamic and, as the social worker said, 'Sudachanh could not possibly get better with all this going on'.

I have identified *distance* with psychiatry and *proximity* with nursing. *Context* was the hallmark of social work. Whereas psychiatry focused on a deep view of the case, and nursing discriminated between the surface presentation and the underlying reality, social work exercised its power to broaden the definition of the case such that it included the family and the wider social network. The examples of Joyce and Sudachanh Littlejohn suggest that for social workers there was an implicit moral economy within this broader definition of the case, as if there were a finite quantity of goodness and badness that was apportioned between the family, the personality, and the illness.

Cutting across professional domains

I have shown how work time and work space were managed by the professions to achieve autonomy and distinctiveness. However, these categories of psychiatric hospital life were so fundamental they often undercut professional domains and formed the basis for interprofessional alliances and conflicts. All those who had worked at the hospital for many years, the old-timers, had a long-term perspective on cases that united them, irrespective of profession, and distinguished them from those who had recently joined the hospital and who would soon move on. On the Schizophrenia Team a psychiatrist, a medical officer, an older social worker, and the nurse in charge formed such an interprofessional alliance. All had worked together 'since the year dot' and had a common basis of reminiscence about what the hospital used to be like in the good or bad old days. Another psychiatrist (myself) had worked there for only six years and in this regard had more in common with a young senior social worker and the deputy charge nurse. All would shortly move to positions outside the hospital. When he was working out who would work with whom, the leader of the Schizophrenia Team put several old-timers together in one group and the more recently ap-pointed staff members in another. Although he did not make explicit that he had taken into account the time frame of the staff members' careers, this dimension was taken for granted in his calculations. He merely said that the two formed 'nat-ural' groupings and that he believed members of each treat-ment team would be able to work well together.

Work space also cut across professional boundaries. Social workers and community nurses were allied because they shared the same work space outside the hospital. This pro-vided grounds for a common way of understanding patients. Such spatial structuring of work was so pervasive that it threat-ened to override professional distinctions altogether; and as a result these two groups needed to reiterate their differences constantly. Community nurses pointed to the patient's body as their separate space ('We give injections, social workers do not'), whereas social workers identified the assessment of the family system as their own domain, lying beyond the capability of the community nurse.

Case time and space

This chapter has examined how the daily routines of mental health professionals were organized in time and space to perform work on a person so that he or she could be treated as a case of psychiatric illness. As a consequence of these routines and perspectives, the case itself was attributed spatial and temporal dimensions. A patient who had an interest in semiotics and art criticism expressed this eloquently when he said that the Team at Heathfield House had access to the 'internal geometry' of patients.

Team members paid close attention to the definition and redefinition of case time. The most common example was the way retrospective case time (the background history) was reorganized to transform an acute case into a chronic case. This was a matter of showing that the initial signs of illness began much earlier than had been hitherto recognized. What appeared as a sudden onset some months prior to hospital admission would become recast as a more insidious onset with its roots in the patient's adolescence, childhood, or even in the earliest origins of his or her personality. Such reframing of past time lowered clinicians' expectations concerning the patient's prospects for future recovery. This point is illustrated in the case of Peter, a twenty-four year old man who had a six month history of becoming introverted, withdrawn, and preoccupied with religion. He suddenly developed ideas that he had been reincarnated, and that one of his sisters was a Hindu goddess and the other a water spirit. When admitted to the hospital, a week later he was observed to be thought-disordered and floridly delusional. In a case conference three weeks later, a trainee psychiatrist reported that he was just as delusional as on the day of admission, and that he had not developed any insight. The psychiatrist reformulated Peter's case, beginning with a question directed to the trainee that he then answered himself:

When would you say the illness started from his history? You
know I wondered, from the sound of it, whether it goes back
longer than we realize. Even right back to the time when he
changed his name. Perhaps that was the response to some sort
of idea. . . . It sounds, from the history, that it is a chronic
schizophrenic illness—process schizophrenia—in which case
the condition we are going to get him back to isn't as good as
it would be if it were a first break, you know, with a good premorbid personality.

Prospective case time (the future trajectory) was also the focus
of intense work. This topic is subjected to detailed analysis in
Chapter 6.

The professions also aligned themselves in relation to case
space. Clinical psychology, the fourth profession, was engaged
in a feud with psychiatry of the type that has long characterized the relationship between these two groups internationally
(Brody 1956) and that reached a special intensity at Ridgehaven Hospital. Psychology formed an alliance with nursing
against psychiatry at the case surface. Psychologists spoke and
wrote against the validity of all forms of psychiatric deep
knowledge, including Freudian psychodynamics. They argued
that diagnostic streaming was irrelevant and that the hospital
should be reorganized into functional units that addressed patients' problem behaviours. This orientation, with its roots in
academic psychology, particularly the behaviourism of Skin-
ner, was close to the nurses' view that patients' actions were
often behavioural rather than caused by illness. To the psychologist, treatment was seen in stimulus–response terms as
reinforcing desired behaviours and extinguishing maladaptive
ones, rather than treating the underlying psychopathology or
addressing the underlying psychodynamics. One ward for the
treatment of adolescent patients with behaviour problems became the stronghold of this psychology–nursing alliance. Most
other nurses maintained the age-old alliance with psychiatrists,
who for their part argued that the stimulus–response idea was
a superficial 'black box' model of the person, as if to say there
were nothing inside. It failed to take into account the 'meaning-giving' processes that lie within humans and mediate the
perception of such stimuli and modulate the responses. Thus
these internecine squabbles within the hospital turned on the

definition of the principal spatial parameters of the case—
here, depth versus surface.

Depth, surface, and breadth, defined by psychiatry, nursing,
and social work, respectively, were the three fundamental dimensions of case space. Within this space, the case was divided
into segments. Body and mind formed two such segments.
Another primary division was into illness and personality,
which, with the addition of social work, became a tripartite
division into illness, personality, and family. The temporal divisions of the case into epochs—developmental history, present complaint, future prognosis—were no less striking. The
case was also ascribed a client/patient ratio that rested on a
more fundamental active/passive ratio. Nurses and social
workers vacillated between these two constructions (client and
patient), but psychiatrists insisted on the latter. Irrespective of
these contested appellations, all shared the concept of 'the
case', and all took for granted its fundamental spatial and temporal parameters. Finally, I have shown that the most potent
metaphors that structured clinicians' thinking about cases,
such as the onion skin model, occurred when case time and
case space were brought together into a mutually defining spatio-temporal unity.

A struggle for professional autonomy influenced the way the
clinical staff at Ridgehaven Hospital defined people as cases
of psychiatric illness. Each profession emphasized its unique
perspective. Each profession exercised power by defining cases
in its own distinctive way, thereby controlling the movement
of these cases. From its depth perspective, psychiatry defined
the core features of cases and determined their distribution
within the hospital on the basis of diagnosis; from its surface
perspective, nursing developed a behavioural definition of
cases and moved them along a gradient from closed to open
wards; from its ecological perspective, social work defined
cases in terms of environmental context and controlled their
placement in the community.

The social structure and culture of the psychiatric hospital
thus endowed a person with particular meanings that rendered him or her into a case. The most striking aspect of a
case was that it was dissected, triangulated, and quartered into
a matrix of cross-cutting divisions. The schismatic hospital or-

ganization with its autonomous professional domains, its intraprofessional conflicts and interprofessional alliances, its social divisions of work space and work time, was reflected in this multifaceted cubist object—the segmented case.

4

Clinical teams and the 'whole person'

I have examined the division of psychiatric labour and the assertion of distinctiveness among the mental health professions as they jostled for autonomy and power, resulting in a hospital characterized by organizational schism and, at the level of case formulation, a fragmented construction of the person. Running counter to this schism was the integration of mental health professionals into multidisciplinary teams. The psychiatric hospital was thus characterized by theme and countertheme—the rhetoric of professional autonomy versus the rhetoric of team work. Each demanded the other in the same way that parts demand a whole but a whole also demands its parts. The division of labour was in keeping with ideas of psychiatric treatment as a technical practice, where efficiency was enhanced by specialization and differentiation. Teams, on the other hand, were an expression of psychiatry's claim to be a humanistic enterprise, to treat people as individuals. Only a team, it was said, could treat the 'whole person'.[1]

At Ridgehaven Hospital the staff were enthusiastic about teams as a means of engaging their personal involvement. Teams were a channel for individual commitment in a large organization where alienation and disenchantment might have otherwise prevailed. The staff often characterized the hospital as a bureaucracy in the pejorative sense of red tape, referring to the rules that blocked personal initiative and to the imperative to document everything they did. Alienation from the hospital was countered by commitment to a team. Whereas the hospital was large, the team was small. If the

---

[1] See Matthews (1960:51) for a typical example of the thinking that links 'the team concept and the concept of the human being as a total person in his total world'.

hospital was impersonal and rank-ridden, with titles as the pre-
ferred mode of address ('Dr So and So'), fellow team members called each other by their first names. Whereas the hospital had rules that governed and restricted, the team had a
'spirit' which encouraged involvement and initiative.

With few exceptions (see Moffic *et al.* 1984:63), the psychiatric literature in this area merely endorses the perceived
benefits that flow from teams, these being organizational integration for the hospital and a feeling of personal involvement for individual staff members. These benefits are extolled
with a degree of enthusiasm and reverence that betrays a commitment to team values rather than a capacity for critical analysis (see, for example, Bowen, Maler, and Androes 1965). The
sociological literature, too, largely affirms these values:

> When members of a team have different formal statuses and
> rank in a social establishment, as is often the case, then we can
> see that the mutual dependence created by membership in the
> team is likely to cut across structural or social cleavages in the
> establishment and thus provide a source of cohesion for the es-
> tablishment. Where staff and line statuses tend to divide an or-
> ganization, performance teams may tend to integrate the divi-
> sions. (Goffman 1959:82)

To a large extent, the literature on teams relies on a theoretical perspective that emphasizes attitudinal conformity, stability of the system, and corrective balance.[2] Conflict is understood in terms of malfunction, an impediment that must be
overcome to restore the smooth operation of the team.[3] A
medical metaphor is commonly employed, as if a team were
a person and conflict was a symptom of illness or psychopathology (see Nason 1981, 1984:32–5).

In this chapter, I develop an analysis of teams that acknowl-
edges their integrating function but at the same time accords
a more fundamental place to conflict and power in their organization. I begin by asking how the profession of psychiatry

---

[2] The literature is directly aligned with or indirectly informed by 'functionalism',
a theoretical school most closely associated in medical sociology with Talcott
Parsons.
[3] See Sands, Stafford, and McClelland on interprofessional conflict (1990:70), Malone (1991:220) on demarcation disputes, Davidson (1990:231) on role blurring,
and Holzberg (1960:88) on ambiguity in command structure.

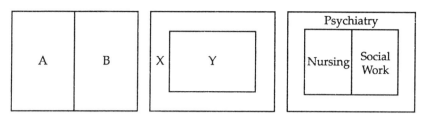

Fig. 4.1. Emcompassment. (Adapted from Dumont 1980:242.)

dominated other professions at Ridgehaven. Psychiatrists occupied key positions in the hospital bureaucracy, yet they
could not exercise imperative forms of authority, as first described by Weber. They could not override the autonomy that
had been achieved by the other professions in respect to industrial representation, hiring and firing, training, and disciplinary action against members. Given these constraints, psychiatric power took the form of hegemony rather than
bureaucratic authority.[4] The team was the principal arena in
which psychiatric hegemony was exercised. This is because psychiatric knowledge, especially diagnostic reasoning, defined
the team, its name, its intellectual tenor, and the *raison d'être*
of its work. Other professions did not overtly submit to control
by psychiatrists. Rather, they consented to participate in a team
defined by psychiatric knowledge.

Although it was only one part of the team, psychiatry identified itself with the team as a whole and defined its limits.
Psychiatry thus established hegemony by encompassing the
team. Dumont (1980:239–45) shows how the relation between
a whole and its parts may be complementary or hierarchical.
He illustrates complementarity by means of a rectangle divided into two equal elements, A and B (Fig. 4.1). Hierarchy

---

[4] My understanding of psychiatric hegemony is informed by the work of Gramsci,
who shows how particular groups within civil society create a web of institutions
and ideas that dominate 'subaltern' groups and secure their active consent to be
dominated (Gramsci 1971:80fn). Although Gramsci's work is a macroscopic
analysis of the modern state as a totality and the role of intellectuals, prestige,
and knowledge in sustaining capitalist society (1971:56fn), the core elements of
his thesis–domination, consent, and the central role of ideas—can be applied
to the analysis of power, as it is exercised at a microscopic level within a psychiatric hospital. Frankenberg (1988:328) shows how Gramsci's exploration of hegemony anticipated Foucault's studies of the 'capillary, diffuse, uncentralized'
nature of power in the institutions of the modern state.

is illustrated by a rectangle divided into two areas, Y and X, where Y is an inner rectangle totally enclosed by X, a surrounding border area. The elements X and Y are distinguished from each other, but together they form a unified whole. X is identical with this whole. As a consequence, X is different from Y but also encompasses Y. Hierarchy, for Dumont, is this combination of unity and distinction. X represents the whole at the same time that it is only one element of this whole.

In each of the major team forums—the team meeting, case record, and case conference—psychiatry encompassed the other professions (as represented in Figure 4.1 by the way it surrounds them). By this I mean that it circumscribed, summarized, and synthesized the clinical contributions of the nurses and social workers. Power, in this context, was the capacity to shape and summate a joint definition of the case. From this flowed the means to deploy fellow professionals around the case. Furthermore, by defining the total compass of the team and its outer limits, psychiatry was able to exclude other powerful groups within the hospital from exerting control over cases, particularly the 'administration' and the profession of psychology. Sources of potential conflict were thereby excluded from the central clinical arena within which cases were defined and patients treated.

The aim of this study of team organization and psychiatric hegemony is to ask what implications they might have for the way cases were defined. The body of this chapter examines how the processes of integration, encompassment, and exclusion pertained to the way members of a multidisciplinary team thought about and worked on cases of psychiatric illness.

Psychiatric hegemony

Diagnostic streaming and the psychiatric identity of teams

Multidisciplinary teams arose within Australian mental health services during the 1960s as part of a widespread expansion and reform of psychiatric hospitals throughout the developed world. Strauss *et al.* (1964:125) describes how, during the same era and with the same éclat, teams were introduced to reform a state mental hospital in Chicago. Comparable changes had already taken place in general medicine (Engel and Hall 1971: 81), having first occurred in hospitals caring for the chronically ill (Arney and Bergen 1984:83). In general hospitals, the team was known as the 'unit' or in Great Britain, drawing on imagery from corporate capitalism, the 'firm'. Outside hospitals, solo practices were replaced by group practices and polyclinics. These changes were indicative of a shift during the postwar era from the doctor–patient relationship to the team–patient relationship. They reflect more broadly the extent to which the team model has permeated modern society: in sport, military organization, science, and medicine.

At Ridgehaven Hospital, functional divisions arose during the 1960s and subsequently evolved into teams. The first specialist units were formed to treat groups of patients classified according to age (intellectually retarded children, adult patients, and the elderly). For the adult group, there was a further division between acute and chronic. An 'Acute Team' treated those who were likely to return to a productive life in the community, and a 'Rehabilitation Team' cared for those who were unlikely to achieve this. In 1980 a newly appointed Medical Director/Chief Executive Officer introduced 'diagnostic streaming'. The former Acute Team would now treat patients with a diagnosis of affective disorders,[5] neurotic disorders, and personality disorders; and it became known as the 'Affective Disorders Team'. The Rehabilitation Team would predominantly treat patients with a diagnosis of schizophrenia and thus became the 'Schizophrenia Team'. Nevertheless, it was not feasible to stream all patients purely by diagnosis. Vestiges of the older acute/chronic classification therefore carried forward into this new era of diagnostic streaming. Although the Schizophrenia Team was equipped with a modern admission ward, it also inherited many of the decrepit buildings at the back of the hospital housing the longest staying patients (including some with a diagnosis of affective disorder). Although diagnostic streaming was regarded as a bold, progressive initiative, its realization could not escape the un-

[5] This grouping included diagnostic categories such as major depression and manic depressive disorder.

derlying temporal and spatial structures of the hospital. These structures imbued the Schizophrenia Team with a 'chronic' identity. Schizophrenia was already defined as a chronic illness with a poor prognosis, and this new organization accentuated the association with chronicity.

Psychiatric diagnosis, as a basis for classifying patients, was not imposed as a new order. It was inlaid into the pre-existing categories that were taken for granted by the staff. It merged with the inherent spatial and temporal dimensions of the hospital, with its old back wards and new admission wards. By association with these intrinsic dimensions, the very idea of a Schizophrenia Team was largely accepted as a 'natural' and logical arrangement. Psychiatric hegemony was thereby ensured by the acceptance of diagnosis—a psychiatric preserve —as the rationale of team formation. Hegemony was given tangible form in the way the major buildings were earmarked for specific diagnostic groups. Through the new teams, diagnosis was writ large on the hospital landscape.

Encompassment and egalitarianism

The various wards, day centres, and clinics allocated to the Schizophrenia Team and the functions they served have been set out in Table 4.1. The three core professions—psychiatry, psychiatric nursing, and social work—were organized into four 'Mini Teams', a designation that conveyed the idea they were miniature replicas of the larger Schizophrenia Team. Each Mini Team was led by a psychiatrist and included a trainee psychiatrist, a social worker, and a nurse. Psychiatry was thus represented by two echelons. The psychiatrist and the social worker were permanent members, whereas trainee psychiatrists were attached to Mini Teams on a rotating basis. In Heathfield House the nursing rosters were coordinated with the Mini Team organization, allowing individual nurses to be assigned to a particular Mini Team for several months at a time.

Dr Halliday was Team Leader of the Schizophrenia Team, a position that could be filled only by a psychiatrist. However, the official authority vested in this position was not sufficient

Table 4.1. *Treatment facilities of the schizophrenia team*

Facility	Description
Wards	
Heathfield House	Acute ward for the assessment and treatment of newly admitted patients (24 beds)
Forest House	Subacute ward for rehabilitation of patients requiring longer periods of hospitalization (20 beds)
Elder House	Chronic ward housing patients who were unlikely to be discharged (20 beds)
Outpatient clinics	
Outpatient Clinic	For psychiatric follow-up treatment (300–400 attendances per month)
Modecate Clinic	For delivery of a long-acting injectable major tranquillizer (300–400 attendances per month)
Day centres	
Heathfield House Day Centre	Mainly for young adult patients (30–50 places)
Rehabilitation Day Activity Centre	For older, more debilitated patients (20 places)
Residences	
The Lodge	Hostel accommodation with nursing supervision several miles from the hospital (24 places)
Community houses	Three houses, each accommodating three residents; two on the hospital grounds and one in a nearby suburb (9 places)
Occupational therapy centres	
Heathfield House Occupational Therapy Centre	Low-key activities for newly admitted patients (20 places)
Occupational Therapy Activity Centre	Simple work-oriented activities for young, impaired patients (20 places)
Industrial Therapy Workshop	Work for those capable of a higher level of activity (110 places)

to explain his dominance within the Team because psychiatrists, including Dr Halliday, had no direct jurisdiction over nurses and social workers. Yet as a hard working clinician, he commanded widespread loyalty. On a sporting team he would

have been a playing captain and in warfare a combatant officer. He was rarely challenged or resisted because he had his
'sleeves rolled up' and was 'in the same boat' as everyone else.
Most staff called him by his Christian name, James. There was
widespread acceptance of his leadership because it was
couched in egalitarian terms, to which all subscribed without
question. Egalitarianism was a powerful means of coordinating
others, not only because it drew on the rhetoric employed by
nurses and social workers in their own case for equality but
also because it harnessed a pervasive theme within Australian
culture. 'In Australia, hierarchy receives its import in a logic
of egalitarianism' (Kapferer 1988:14).

James was also the leader of one of the four Mini Teams.
He was directly involved in the treatment of patients, just like
the trainee psychiatrist, the social worker, and the nurses who
were members of his Mini Team. This Mini Team, in turn, was
on the same footing as the other three Mini Teams, each treating approximately the same number of patients. En masse the
patients were described as a 'clinical load', and it was axio-
matic that each Mini Team should carry its fair share.[6] The
load was not lightened because James was the leader of the
larger Schizophrenia Team. Rather than conceiving of the administrative aspect of the Team Leader's role as the exercise
of line authority, he presented it as a specialized service, attending Team Leader meetings, preparing annual reports,
and making submissions for new initiatives, which he carried
out on behalf of the other members. Stated this way, such
duties were not envied. They were seen as the necessary evil
of dealing with the bureaucracy on behalf of clinicians in order to free the latter to get on with their work.

James was not only one of the workers; he embodied and
encompassed the Team by identifying himself with the Team
as a whole. He was the appointed Leader when the Schizophrenia Team was created. He was regarded as its founder and
architect, and it was usually referred to as 'James' Team',
rather than the Schizophrenia Team. At a lower organizational
level, he was similarly identified with his Mini Team. It was
called 'James' Mini Team', not 'Janice's Mini Team', Janice

---

[6] See Zerubavel (1979:117–23) on 'fairness' as an egalitarian value of distributive
justice in the hospital workplace.

being the social worker who worked with him. The Schizophrenia Team was thus a whole that comprised parts. Each
part, in turn, was a whole comprising even smaller parts, the
clinicians. The principles of wholeness and encompassment
thus pervaded the Team: at each organizational level there
was a whole encompassing a smaller whole. Through James,
these principles of wholeness and encompassment were identified with psychiatry at each level. The Team was not based
on the model of an organizational tree, where the trunk,
branches, twigs, and leaves ramify out and where each level is
different in nature from the next. It would be represented
more accurately by a Russian doll, the largest doll containing
several similar (but smaller) dolls, each of which encompassed
other dolls, and so on.

Encompassment became a value to which the team aspired
in its work. In James's vision, the team should embrace all
aspects of patient management. Arney and Bergen (1984:87)
have pointed out that the very notion of management is all-
encompassing. It is much broader than the notion of treatment. It embraces all aspects of patients' lives, taking into consideration their total situation: income, occupation, where
they live and with whom, and their emotional relationships
with their families. Whereas individual clinicians treated patients, teams managed them. James's policy was to develop a
'comprehensive service' that provided 'total patient care', and
to this end he developed new services to be delivered by additional small-scale teams. The Schizophrenia Team thus grew
internally by spawning more teams, for example, a Family
Therapy Team and an Education Team. As a consequence, the
Team had a growing, enveloping, totalizing quality. Had anyone, year by year, opened the Russian doll for inspection,
more mini dolls would have been found inside.

Encompassment and egalitarianism were reproduced each
week at the 'Team Meeting'. This was a regular Friday morning staff meeting of 20 to 30 people, seated in a large circle
in the Heathfield House Occupational Therapy Centre, the
only room large enough to accommodate them. A nurse at-
tended from each treatment facility, ward, centre, and clinic;
representatives of each profession were present; a member of
every Mini Team was there. The entire Schizophrenia Team

was represented. James chaired the meeting, and on one occasion he explained its purpose thus:

> This is a team meeting in which we deal with clinical matters to
> do with patients. It is a communication meeting, and I hope it
> would also give us a sense that we are all working together as a
> team managing patients together.

The meeting was informal, without written agenda. It always
began and ended with convivial chatter. Once it had started,
staff members often set up side conversations with those sitting
adjacent to them. It was common for several conversations to
be held while the main business continued. James did not
attempt to stifle this talk, which in a more formal setting would
have been frowned upon as a distraction. He exercised a tolerant chairmanship that consisted mainly of framing the meeting by opening and closing it. One after the other, the nursing
representatives reported on 'patient movements' (that is, the
patients who were admitted into or transferred out of their
area), and 'problem patients' (patients who disrupted the routine of clinical work). Sometimes the reporting went according to a set order that was based on the organizational structure of the Schizophrenia Team (from acute ward to subacute
ward to chronic ward, then the centres, clinics, professions,
and Mini Teams). Sometimes the reports were just given
around the circle. Nurses were not reporting to their superiors
or to the psychiatrists or Team Leader but to the meeting
itself—that is, to the Team. Any case could be opened up by
any participant for a more general discussion, and from time
to time the Team Leader entered these discussions as a clinician rather than as chairman.

The egalitarian ethos of the team was displayed in the
round circle discussion, the informality, and the right of any
member to report or pursue any issue. Psychiatric hegemony
was displayed in the way James defined and framed the meeting and thereby gently shaped how the Team defined itself
and its cases. The sheer size of the meeting, the large circle
of chairs, and the continual reports of patient movements,
conveyed an impression of the Team as a large, enveloping,
cellular whole with patients flowing in, out, and around its
components.

Involvement and exclusion

Processes of involvement and exclusion are apparent in the 'topography' of the Schizophrenia Team, with its central core, its peripheral reaches, and areas outside its ambit. Heathfield House was the heartland of the Team. Official visitors were shown through this complex because it contained the Team's most modern facilities: the acute ward, outpatient clinic, Modecate clinic with on-line computer facilities, and suite of consultation rooms. It was the pride of the Team. So strong was the ethos of involvement at Heathfield that even nonclinical workers were included as Team members, thereby bridging a gap between professional and occupational groups. Rebecca, the stenographer and receptionist, was entrusted with clinical information because she routinely handled case records and typed psychiatric reports. She was the first point of contact for patients, either by telephone or face-to-face across the reception desk, when they wanted to see their psychiatrist or social worker. The latter regarded her as capable of exercising sound judgement as to whether patients had a genuine need to see them or they were merely making a nuisance of themselves. She became the gatekeeper between patients and staff, letting the deserving patients through and keeping the frivolous ones out. The clinical staff had confidence in her because she erred on the side of caution and when in doubt would quickly arrange for a patient to see their psychiatrist or social worker. Although she had no clinical training, she was increasingly attributed the indeterminate qualities that were normally reserved for clinicians: discretion, compassion, judgement, and experience. She was involved as a central member of the Schizophrenia Team.

Domestic workers who cleaned the ward and prepared patients' meals were officially nonclinical staff, which meant that they were not permitted to talk to patients about their problems or to talk to nurses about patients. Most importantly, they were not permitted to read case records. As such they were not members of the Schizophrenia Team, yet they were unofficially included in what nurses sometimes called the 'Ward Team'. The smooth running of the ward necessitated cooperation between domestic staff and nurses. The work of the domestic staff brought them into close contact with patients. To do their work safely they needed information that was, strictly speaking, clinical. Who were the patients who might unexpectedly attack them while they were polishing the floor? Which patients might be incontinent over this newly polished floor? Nurses, for their part, depended on domestic staff for information about patients. It was often the domestic worker who, during the course of her cleaning, first discovered that a patient had tried to flush tablets down the toilet. As she glided the polisher across the floor in the patients' recreation room, she might overhear conversations of a type that would immediately die down when a nurse entered the room. Cleaners were often the first to know that a patient was planning to leave the ward secretly or to kill himself, and they readily passed this information on to the nurses.

To cooperate in this way, nurses and domestic workers shared a language of common-sense terms that they used to typify patients. One set of terms had to do with patients' potential for violence: 'stroppy', 'quiet', 'off', 'fragile', 'about to go off'. Another set of terms concerned the likelihood of them making a mess: 'well behaved', or 'grotty'. Because domestic staff had no training in nursing or psychiatric terminology, this nontechnical language was the only one possible. Moreover, it was a specific form of language used within the hospital when staff members were defining their relationships in terms of equality, solidarity, friendship and 'mateship' in the workplace. Following Malinowski, this mode of talk is usually referred to as 'phatic' communication (Goody 1980:127). It united domestic workers and nurses in the common purpose of safely and cleanly completing the practical round of daily work, and it incorporated the domestic workers into the Schizophrenia Team.

In contrast to the central position occupied by Heathfield House, the Schizophrenia Team also had its peripheral reaches, in both a geographical and an organizational sense. At the periphery, team principles were diluted and replaced by traditional forms of organization, such as the ward or the department (for example, the Occupational Therapy Department). Forest House was the subacute ward, an old building at the rear of the hospital lying at the considerable distance of a five minute walk from Heathfield House. The nursing staff in Forest considered that they and their patients were neglected by the psychiatric and social work staff. It was difficult, they said, to convince anyone to walk or drive across the hospital to examine a patient and confer with the nurses. They criticized psychiatrists and social workers for losing interest in patients once they were transferred to this ward. Isolated in this way, Forest House became a bastion of nursing dominance. The work of nurses was ward oriented rather than team centred, with the case load of a single nurse spanning the patients of several Mini Teams. There was a robust programme of nurse-initiated education and group therapy. Nurses ruled that the other professions must see their patients outside group therapy hours, and that a patient could not be withdrawn merely for a social work or psychiatric interview. Thus in Forest House team principles and psychiatric hegemony gave way to ward principles and nursing dominance.

This was even more evident in Elder House. Here the very principle of diagnostic streaming was suspended, for Elder contained the most chronic of patients, irrespective of whether they had an affective disorder or schizophrenia. In Elder House there was no rhetoric of team work or progress. Thus as one moved across the Schizophrenia Team, from centre to periphery, from front wards to back wards, from acute patients to chronic patients, the team principles faded and psychiatric hegemony dissipated.

Some groups within Ridgehaven Hospital stood outside the team boundary altogether. I have previously described the antagonism between psychology and psychiatry, bridged sporadically by cross-professional friendships. Psychology resisted the power of psychiatry to deploy the other professions around a case. The head of the Psychology Department did not allocate clinical psychologists to the major hospital Teams lest they become subject to psychiatric control. They were deployed independently of the Teams in community treatment settings, behaviour modification programmes, and research. When the work of psychologists brought them into contact with psychiatry, as for the neuropsychological testing of patients, a strict consultation model was applied. It enabled psychologists to provide opinions while preserving their professional independence. Psychologists explicitly criticized the Teams at Ridge-haven, viewing the so-called equality between team members as a mask for psychiatric authoritarianism. Research carried out in the Department of Psychology demonstrated how the staff could function more effectively if diagnostic streaming (a psychiatric jurisdiction) ceased and the hospital were rearranged into divisions that dealt with patients who had similar functional impairments (a psychological jurisdiction). Psychiatrists, for their part, were happy to keep psychologists at a distance by excluding them from membership of the Schizophrenia Team.

Administrative staff were also excluded from teams. Whereas junior clerical staff such as Rebecca were included, senior administrators who could potentially exert an influence over clinical work were deliberately kept out. Control over cases was thereby contained within the team. For example, a conflict developed between the Schizophrenia Team and the Medical Records Department over the issue of discharging patients. Patients who were legally confined to the hospital for long periods were usually placed on 'trial leave' in preparation for complete discharge. While on trial leave and living outside the hospital they were still classified as inpatients for statistical and legal purposes. This practice created problems for the Medical Records Department because the number of apparent inpatient cases was always higher than the number of patients actually residing in the hospital. To contain this problem of cases outstripping patients, the head of the Medical Records Department issued a directive that cases on trial leave for longer than a month would be formally discharged from the hospital. Although this problem might appear to have been a minor clerical matter, it was an issue of some significance because it had to do with control over the movement of patients and the question of who had the power to admit or discharge them from hospital. James responded that it was a policy issue that should be decided by the Schizophrenia Team. He asserted that until such a decision had been reached the discharge arrangements would remain a matter of clinical discretion. One strategy to deal with conflict was thus to exclude its source by defining it as external to the Team—the legitimate arena in which clinical decisions were made about cases and their movement into and out of the hospital.

Team members made jokes at the expense of those they excluded, underscoring the process of exclusion. Such joking frequently took place at the Team Meeting because it was in this setting where people worked on the Team's identity. The issue of who had the power to discharge patients was used as an opportunity to lampoon the 'bureaucrats'. At one Team Meeting, a nurse reported that a patient on trial leave had been readmitted to hospital but as a result of a clerical error was assigned a new record number. The clerk who processed her admission had been unaware that she was still officially an inpatient. Here was an instance of a patient becoming two cases. Using a characteristic deadpan technique, the nurse said that the Medical Records Department wanted to know what to do about it. Amidst gales of laughter the answer came back, 'Discharge one of them!' She then drove the joke home: 'Yes, but Medical Records want to know which one'. By ridiculing administrators, this humour reasserted the right of the Team to control the definition and distribution of cases. At this same time, it reflected the capacity of the hospital to turn patients into cases, to objectify them, and even to multiply them.

Conflict between the three core professions could not be dealt with by excluding any of them because they were all indispensable components of the team. It had to be contained within the team and consequently had a long-term but low-grade quality. Social workers, for example, complained that psychiatrists and nurses spent too much time talking about patients within the hospital and that the Team Meetings were taken up with repetitive, circular discussions about the movement of these patients from one ward to the next. Eventually, social workers simply stopped turning up at the weekly Team Meeting. Though excluding themselves from this main Schizophrenia Team forum, they remained actively involved in the work of the Mini Teams.

Nursing conflict with psychiatry, which revolved around status, was chiefly expressed through an enduring pattern of jokes within the Team Meeting, the same type of joke surfacing month after month.[7] The three or four nurses who were

---

[7] Compare with Rhodes' (1991:7) discussion of the way staff employed humour to distance themselves from the power that suffused their relationships with each other and with patients.

informally licensed to joke were men who were senior in years but not in status, not yet having been appointed deputy charge nurse. These nurses were caught in the promotions bottle-neck. Their status *vis-a-vis* psychiatrists was ambiguous, and their humour lampooned psychiatrists by misconstruing them as pa-tients. While waiting for James to arrive to start the meeting, one of them quipped: 'Dr Halliday sends his apologies from St An-thony's [a rehabilitation centre for alcohol addiction]. Can someone please minute that and sign it "Dr McCusker" '. The comedy routine allowed public expression of conflict but min-imized its effect on working relationships between the two pro-fessions by containing it within a joking frame.[8]

I have argued that for psychiatry hegemony was achieved by encompassing the multidisciplinary team and stamping it with its own particular identity. The team was also used to involve less powerful groups in clinical work, such as the domestic workers and the junior clerical staff, and to exclude more pow-erful groups from this arena, such as the senior administrative staff and psychologists. Similar processes of encompassment and exclusion of conflict pertained to the day-to-day clinical work of Mini Teams. They were evident in the two main fo-rums of the Mini Team: the case record and the case conference.

Two forums: case record and case conference

Encompassing the record and excluding conflict

After working individually with their patients, members of the Mini Team wrote reports that were assembled together into the case record. The record was the joint literary product of the multidisciplinary team. Each case record entry was the discrete contribution of an individual clinician and was clearly identified with the name and profession of the writer, for ex-ample, 'Social Work Assessment—M. Sincock'. Entries were dated and always referred directly or implicitly to the previous

---

[8] Coser (1979:106) shows how humour among hospital professionals brings ambi-guity and conflict to the surface at the same time these problems are collectively laughed off.

entries of fellow clinicians as well as anticipating subsequent entries. In this way they were strung together into a multi-authored narrative that was a true chronicle, as it represented the patient as a temporal sequence: the background 'case history' and the ongoing 'progress'. I have previously referred to these temporal structures as *case time*.

In the record, case time provided an underlying framework that integrated clinicians of different professional backgrounds. They fitted together because each had an allotted place in the narrative sequence, the trainee psychiatrist's admission history coming first, the nursing entry coming second, and so on. Psychiatry encompassed this narrative by framing and summarizing it. Each time a patient was admitted to hospital, the first entry (admission assessment) and the last entry (discharge summary) was written by a trainee psychiatrist. Anyone skimming through an old set of case notes to see what had happened to a patient during a previous admission would tend to read the discharge summary rather than the case note entries themselves, not the least reason being that the discharge summary was typed and therefore legible. Psychiatry, nursing, and social work all made an equal contribution to the written definition of a case; but in addition psychiatry reserved the power to write an overarching definition of all the definitions, including its own.

To achieve an integrated, synthesized definition of the patient, it was important that the differences of opinion that frequently arose between staff members *not* be recorded. Conflicting opinions were excluded from the case record because it was a legal document that could be used as evidence in litigation. A breakdown of this rule occurred when a psychiatrist attempted to transfer a physically ill patient from Ridgehaven to a general hospital and became alarmed and angry when a senior psychiatrist from that hospital declined to accept the patient. The Ridgehaven psychiatrist wrote critically of the general hospital psychiatrist in the patient's case record. The implications of this indiscretion were driven home to her when the patient died. Had there been an inquiry into the cause of death, her written criticism might have placed her in a position of testifying in court about the possible role played by that senior psychiatrist in causing the patient's death. Although this situation did not occur, and indeed such a consequence never occurred during the period of my study, the potential for it happening produced a highly circumspect style of writing about colleagues.

The case record was thus a testament to consensus. In most instances it accurately reflected agreement among team members. However, even when they disagreed about a patient, the record maintained a semblance of consensus.

Disagreement was encoded in understatement, so it was evident to the staff within the hospital but not to outsiders. Nurses kept alternative records intended for nursing eyes only, one being a Nursing Care Plan, which was written in pencil on a separate sheet of paper. Only when a patient was discharged from the ward was a final version written in ink for inclusion in the case record. The earlier pencilled versions provided nurses an opportunity to record what they called their 'real feelings' about patients and colleagues. As an example, a nurse wrote in pencil to another nurse (John) about a patient (Jill) who was deteriorating and whose husband was dissatisfied with the treatment:

> Much deteriorated. Requires <u>URGENT</u> review. Please push this, John, as these guys aren't very happy with the way things are going.

With its underlining and use of capital letters, this note was an expression of exasperation that a patient was seriously relapsing because a trainee psychiatrist needed to be 'pushed' several times before he would do anything. In the case record itself, the same nurse wrote discreetly:

> Husband and Jill feel her condition is worse than when she was admitted. Jill appears to require some treatment review.

In the rare event of a judicial inquiry, this note could not be used as evidence that the trainee psychiatrist was negligent, yet for insiders who knew how to interpret understatement, 'appears to require some treatment review' was read as an implicit criticism of the trainee psychiatrist.

Encompassing the case conference and containing conflict

In Heathfield House, each of the four Mini Teams held a weekly case conference lasting one to two hours, during which current inpatients (between six and ten) were discussed. The purpose of the case conference was to review each patient's history and progress and to jointly decide on a plan of management. It was chaired by the psychiatrist who, as in the written record, framed the discussion of each case. The psychiatrist routinely asked the opening question ('Who have we got today?' or 'The other one we've got is Mrs South; can you tell us about her?') and brought each discussion to a close ('OK, that's that patient; who do we have next?'). As each Mini Team member reported a case assessment to the conference, the others would inquire and probe to elicit more details. Rights of inquiry were mainly vested in the psychiatrist, but anyone could ask for more information.

Just as there were distinctive prose styles that characterized a psychiatric case record, there were recognizable forms of clinical oratory at the case conference. The first was the 'case presentation'. Usually delivered by a trainee psychiatrist, its purpose was to introduce the patient's case history to the Mini Team. Its format adhered closely to that of the written case history, and trainees mostly read directly from the case record. The 'case discussion' was another recognizable form of oratory. It sounded more informal because it was structured by the fluid conventions of conversational repartee, rather than by the preordained format of a case presentation. Its objective was to forge a consensus 'team definition' of the patient which presaged the third form of case oratory, 'planning management'. This discussion comprised a more terse form of talk that was concerned with practical decisions (for example, which antipsychotic drug to use, what further information was required, when to discharge the patient) and with the disposition of Mini Team members in relation to further tasks (for example, the trainee to follow up investigation results, the nursing staff to work on illness education, the social worker to meet with the patient's daughter). It was usually the psychiatrist who 'pulled together' a case discussion in order to settle on a management plan, with the final decisions being

entered into the record in abbreviated note form by one of
the other team members. The case conference was thus an
excursus that took off from the case record and eventually
returned to it.

Amid the case presentations, discussions, and formulation
of management plans, the case conference also served as a
pedagogic forum for psychiatry. The psychiatrist would take
specific details of a case as a point of departure to illustrate
more general psychiatric issues for the trainee psychiatrist.
The case conference did not serve this function for nurses or
social workers; and as a consequence they formed an audience
for the education of trainee psychiatrists. The following is an
example in which the psychiatrist, Murray, taught Tim, a new
trainee psychiatrist, about the classification of schizophrenia.
The others listened in.

> *Murray*: So that's it then. The diagnosis is clear. There doesn't
> seem to be any doubt he's got schizophrenia.
> *Tim*: Do you go to great pains to classify the schizophrenia that
> they present with?
> *Murray*: I distinguish between schizophreniform psychosis and
> the sort of *DSM-III* schizophrenia, because it has got prognostic
> implications.
> *Tim*: Schizophreniform psychosis?
> *Murray*: Schizophreniform psychosis is an acute psychosis.
> *Tim*: It's an affective . . . ?
> *Murray*: Well no. But the chances are they'll get back to their
> previous functioning. They may or may not have another break.
> And it's important to distinguish the schizo-affectives because of
> the different treatment. Lithium might be helpful, and the
> management's different. You could just distinguish those three
> things. But within the schizophrenia, I guess you should know
> whether they're paranoid or chronic or whatever. We don't
> have simple schizophrenia any more.
> *Tim*: I must get a copy of *DSM-III*.

By these means psychiatry set the framework, the inquisitorial
mode, and the intellectual tenor of the case conference. These
were the specific media of psychiatric hegemony.

Although conflict between team members could be excluded from the record, it was more difficult to eliminate it
from the case conference. Even subtle differences of opinion
became obvious in this forum. It was readily apparent, for ex-

ample, if a team member's assessment of a patient ran counter to the way the others viewed the patient. A person's tone of voice would quickly betray when his or her attitude toward a patient was inconsistent with that of other team members, perhaps being too cynical and dismissive, or naive and gullible, in comparison with the others. Nevertheless, apart from the repeated use of pointed questions to reveal a colleague's problematic attitude or inadequate work performance, only limited remedial action was possible. I studied one instance of protracted conflict in a Mini Team, although it is not possible in this book to discuss its details lest the antagonists be identified. (Some forms of conflict cannot be documented in a written ethnographic record for the same reasons they cannot be documented in the case record.) Nevertheless, I can report in general terms that one individual was identified as the source of the problems, and arrangements were made to have this person reprimanded by senior members of the appropriate professional department in the form of counselling. Shifting the responsibility in this way was an attempt to preserve the Mini Team as a conflict-free zone. Counselling had no impact, however, and the Mini Team members eventually came to the alternative solution of walling off, and working around, the person concerned (c.f. Freidson and Rhea 1972:198).

Team definition of the case

Case presentation

I observed a range of case conferences on the Schizophrenia Team and followed one Mini Team week after week in order to study the sequential processes whereby a common team definition of a case was achieved. The following discussions about Miss Treloar took place over four weekly case conferences. During the first week, Murray, the psychiatrist, began:

> *Murray:* Right, who else is there? Mrs Treloar, or Miss Treloar should I say?

The case presentation by Tim, the trainee psychiatrist, was brief because it was only one day after Miss Treloar was admitted to the ward, and he had not yet obtained a full case history. Reading from the case record, he began:

> *Tim:* Miss Treloar is a 64-year-old woman who came in with para-
> noid schizophrenia. This is her first admission here. She has
> had a run-in with her neighbours after she was rather pointedly
> doing her karate exercises outside the block of flats in quite a
> threatening way. [The others smiled in amusement at this.] She
> has a number of delusions concerning her neighbours, saying
> that they want to hypnotize her for their sexual benefit, or to
> have sex with her while she is asleep. She is inappropriately
> concerned with the goings-on of the people who live in close
> proximity to her. She has a past history of a similar episode, ad-
> mitted either here or to Albert Park Hospital, so this is the sec-
> ond episode. She has a well encapsulated psychosis. It's just
> when she reacts against her neighbours that things get out of
> hand.

Murray interrupted at this early stage of the case presentation. He had arranged Miss Treloar's admission to hospital and knew the details.

> *Murray:* This episode was precipitated by her stopping her med-
> ication. She gradually went off over a period of time with ideas
> of reference and other psychotic ideas. She has no insight at
> all. I put copies of the letters she has been sending to the
> neighbours in the case notes. She writes that she is being tor-
> tured with hypnotism and psychology daily, and being made a
> public scandal of on radio and TV. She was telling me yesterday
> she was perfectly well and going home now, but we have to get
> her a bit more settled and give the neighbours a bit more time
> out.

Margaret, the social worker, reported:

> *Margaret:* I have spoken to two neighbours who were very fright-
> ened of her. Her GP [general practitioner] said that she was
> very good at her martial arts. [Everyone laughed.] She does her
> karate routine with all those special shouts they do outside the
> neighbours' unit [apartment]. She comes up to the windows
> and doors and leaves notes on the doors threatening them. All
> the neighbours are elderly. There is no way they have any boy-
> friends. One of them is meant to cohabit with a Frederick
> Swanson, but he doesn't even exist, according to them.

The eccentric and the bizarre were normally unremarkable for the staff of Heathfield House, yet with these images of a

64-year-old woman practising martial arts, sexuality among a group of elderly people, and a nonexistent man, the serious tenor of the case conference quickly erupted into one of hilarity and amazement. Within moments the psychiatrist restored a tone of sober concern.

> *Murray:* It is a sad story. She was the one who looked after her parents and stayed with them until they died. She functioned well before. She has an impressive list of things she does, like going to bowls and church and so on. She needs to be treated. She would be better on Modecate and she might be more accepting of Modecate from her GP. She would accept anything at the moment to get out of here. Once she is out it might be different though.

By the first case conference the Mini Team had accomplished an opening case presentation, and the psychiatrist had countered the potential for comic absurdity by setting a tone of clinical concern and therapeutic engagement.

'Full work-up'

Within a week, Miss Treloar's case had been fully worked up. The trainee psychiatrist, the nurse, and the social worker had conducted comprehensive assessments, observations, and investigations in their respective areas of expertise. The objective of a full work-up was to cover every facet of a case. Between them, the members of the Mini Team were able to explore the deeper aspects of the case, its surface appearance, and its broad context—all the various dimensions of case space that were mapped out in Chapter 3. In terms of case time, team members encompassed the totality of the case from its developmental origins to the present.

A full work-up was the basis for the claim that a multidisciplinary team looked after the whole person. In the psychiatric literature this holistic enterprise was called the bio-psycho-social approach (Engel 1980). Its ideal product was represented diagrammatically as a series of concentric circles with biology in the centre, surrounded by an intermediate zone of psychology, and then an outer ring of social and cultural influences, the background fading out into the universe (Fig. 4.2). The multidisciplinary team thus surrounded the case by de-

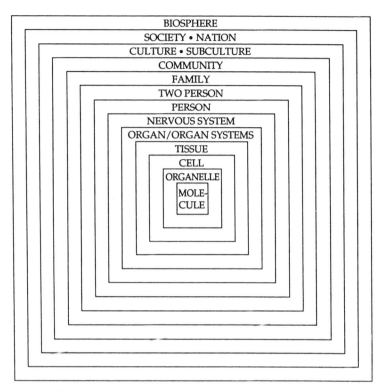

Fig. 4.2.   Bio-psycho-social model. (After Engel 1980.)

fining each of its facets and by occupying each conceptual level of the system in which it was located.

In practice, it was not possible for every team member to give a full report of the assessments they had undertaken. Time permitted only a brief summary of the salient points. Tim reported in the second case conference that he had checked Miss Treloar's thyroid function. He now had a full background and developmental history. Leslie, the psychiatric nurse, reported that Miss Treloar had teamed up with another woman of her own age. He said she basically wanted to leave and was willing to say anything that would get her out. Margaret had seen Miss Treloar's sister and brother-in-law and reported that they did not want her to come out of hospital yet. The neighbours, said Margaret, were exasperated, yet there was nothing they could do about the situation because she owned her home and they could not evict her. She had even clashed with the people at church. Murray quipped, 'She probably threatens the minister with a karate chop'. His statement signalled a shift in the tone of the discussion, acknowledging the absurdity of her martial arts and legitimating the humorous resignation that had been immanent in this case from the beginning.

Miss Treloar was then invited into the case conference to meet the Mini Team. She showed a doughty resilience and announced in a forthright, breezy style that she wanted to leave because she was 'big enough, old enough, and ugly enough' to look after herself. Murray, in reply, commented wryly on her expertise in karate. She responded with a knowing smile, saying that the only time the men in her neighbourhood paid attention to their wives was when she threatened them with a kick or two. She added that she had a range of musical instruments but had been stopped from playing them after 10 p.m. When Murray asked if the neighbours were upsetting her, she referred to them as 'dirty stop outs' who woke her up at night when they came home late. They were trying to get her married off, especially 'old Fred', who was pushing her into marriage. After Miss Treloar left the room, the discussion focused on the fact that she was still preoccupied with sexual themes and that 'old Fred' did not exist.

Epigrammatic appraisals

With the full work-up now available and the patient having met the Mini Team, the subsequent case discussion comprised an exchange of 'epigrammatic appraisals'. These were brief elements within a swiftly flowing conversational exchange. Their hallmark was an abridged rather than discursive style of talking. The speaker assumed a detailed knowledge of the case but summarized this knowledge in a compressed utterance, sometimes a word or a phrase, sometimes a short vignette. I have coined the term 'epigrammatic appraisal' because the staff had no term for this type of clinical talk, although it was sometimes called 'putting the patient in a nutshell'. The lack of formal designation suggests that these important elements

of clinical decision making were taken for granted and lay in
the domain of common-sense reasoning. Whereas the case
presentation format was thought about, written about, and explicitly taught to trainee psychiatrists, the format of the case
discussion and the salience of epigrammatic appraisals was sel-
dom reflected on at all.

Three typical epigrammatic appraisals are listed below. They
pertain to Miss Treloar and were offered by Mini Team members during the second case conference. In order to present
them in a list, I have had to remove them from the conversational context in which they occurred.

1. *Tim:* She functions reasonably well, it's just that she terror-
   izes the next-door neighbours.
2. *Margaret:* She can cope with her illness, she can get on top
   of it, but she gets on top of everyone else as well.
3. *Leslie:* She gets enjoyment out of annoying people.

Epigrammatic appraisals were often illustrated by relating
brief but telling interactions with the patient. To make the
point that the patient was in control of the situation, Margaret
related how she herself had been tricked by Miss Treloar. Margaret had driven her home to collect her clothes; and although there was ample time to get everything, when they
arrived back at the hospital Miss Treloar announced she had
'forgotten' her shoes, necessitating that Margaret drive her
back the following day.

The striking feature of epigrammatic appraisals was that
they employed lay language, even though they might contain
technical psychiatric terminology. I have shown how lay terminology formed a language bridge between nurses and domestic cleaners, who had had no clinical training. The epigrammatic appraisals of the case conference were also a form
of phatic communication that served the same purpose of solidarity among staff. However, unlike the language of domestic
cleaners, they had a pseudo lay quality. They were a clinician's
version of how an untrained lay person might talk about the
mentally ill. Here was a group of sophisticates deftly using
simple language. It bridged differences between professions
because it was an egalitarian style of talking that touched on
an area common to all members of the Mini Team—the es-

sentially 'human' aspect of the case.[9] A social worker explained it in the following way: 'Sometimes I don't have the right language. I'm all at sea. I have to fall back on my common sense'. Common-sense language also drew attention to professional expertise in a paradoxical way. Its 'layness' hinted at the speaker's specialized skill, and its brevity belied the detailed command of the case that the speaker was holding in reserve. It exhibited the power of professionals to summarize and encompass all that was known about a case.

The team definition of the case was usually constructed in runs of epigrammatic appraisals coming one after the other in the rapid interchange of speakers in a case conference. At other times, one member of the team, often the psychiatrist, would 'put it all together' into a 'thumbnail sketch'. The case of Eleanor, who was admitted to hospital one week after Miss Treloar, illustrates such a condensed team definition. At the case conference three weeks after her admission, the psychiatrist began with the following thumbnail sketch, synthesizing the previous assessments and appraisals of Mini Team members:

> *Murray:* Eleanor is a nineteen-year-old girl with a paranoid psychosis in the context of family problems, a difficult adolescence, and the brother having an osteosarcoma [bone cancer]. She took lots of drugs and that didn't help.

When a patient was already well known to the Mini Team from previous admissions to hospital, the case discussion began, not ended, with such a definition:

> *Murray:* The last patient is Bruce. He's as mad as ever.
> *Margaret:* But he's taking his medication and that's the main thing.

Just as the team encompassed its members, so the team definition encompassed a case. It produced a totalizing definition of a case by means of a full work-up; and at the same time it encapsulated, summarized, and reduced a case to a few phrases, putting it 'in a nutshell'.

---

[9] Compare with Strong (1979:82–3), who shows how the unexplicated language among colleagues in a clinical setting uses a 'we' orientation to create a shared consensus.

Intonation and key

The intonation employed by individual speakers was an important aspect of the case discussion. Forging a team definition of Miss Treloar was effortless because, with the exception of Murray's seriousness at the first case conference, everyone spoke about her in the same amused, exasperated tone. They rapidly concurred that she was eccentric and incorrigible, and that her illness was a problem only insofar as it was a nuisance to those around her. When each member of the Mini Team was speaking in the same tone of voice, the details of what they were saying fell into agreement so smoothly that this agreement was unremarkable and taken for granted.

I have used the term 'tone' to refer to the quality of individual voices in a discussion. When the tone of these separate voices was in accord, the conversation struck a common key. By 'key' I refer to the overall manner, mood, or spirit of a conversation. Speech that is otherwise the same in regard to setting, participants, message, or form may differ significantly in key, as between mock or serious, perfunctory or painstaking (Hymes 1972:62). I have already identified common-sense language as the medium of team agreement because it was taken for granted and it bridged professional differences. In the same way, the conversational key had a unifying effect. It went largely unnoticed and was a dimension of language and its interpretation to which everyone had access. Appreciation of the key did not rely on professional training. The key of a conversation provided team members with the capacity to communicate a metacommentary on how individual statements within it should be interpreted. The statement that a patient 'has been admitted three times this year' could be interpreted as evidence of the severity of the illness if the conversational key was one of concern; if it were cynical, it might be evidence of the way the patient took advantage of the free accommodation provided by the hospital. Key was thus a background feature of the clinical discussion that guided its interpretation, uniting disparate elements into what was sometimes referred to as 'the feeling of the team' or 'the mood of the meeting'. Whoever set the key of the discussion shaped the formation of a consensus team definition of the patient.

For the reader of this book, I cannot provide any direct indication of conversational key because it relies on vocal rather than verbal cues; yet it was a striking feature of the audio tape recordings that I made of the Mini Team case conferences. By listening to these recordings I was able to identify, for example, a mood of dismissiveness and irritation when the staff were discussing a patient who was considered to be staying too long in hospital and 'using the system'; a feeling of gravity and urgency when discussing an acutely psychotic patient who required immediate treatment with electroconvulsive therapy; or a tone of disgust and sadness when talking of the sexual abuse suffered by a patient when she was a child. I identified these qualities by the same processes of interpretation used by team members themselves. However, conversational key was such an unnoticed background feature of the discussion that, for the purpose of this study, it was necessary for me to consciously attend to it and make notes on it as I listened to the recordings. The tape recorder also conferred the advantage of being able to compare one case with another or to compare two discussions of the same case separated by several weeks. I was also able to identify sudden key shifts within a single conversation, as in the example of Miss Treloar where there was a rapid change from comic to serious. Without these techniques I, like the team members, would have taken these shifts for granted. Unlike the case presentation or the written case formulation, the key of case discussions was not the subject of analytical or didactic discourse in the hospital. It was in this untheorized, common-sense domain that consensus became possible.

Deploying team members around the case

The formulation of management plans was predicated on establishing general guidelines as to how the team as a whole would be deployed around the case. These guidelines were referred to as the 'team approach'. They were couched in terms of pragmatic strategies to deal with particular situations: 'what we do when Bruce goes off his Modecate' or 'how we usually admit Daisy Peng':

> *Murray:* When Daisy Peng becomes psychotic she can become very very sick very quickly, and we tend to bring her in and detain her immediately before she goes right off. Last time she went and hid herself inside the roof of a church and had to be brought in by the police.

The team approach set the level of involvement for all team members.[10] For example, the team as a whole worked at a distance from Bruce, not trying too zealously to cure his schizophrenia but keeping it more or less contained by making sure he took his medication. For Eleanor the approach was one of active involvement. All team members worked closely with her to treat the symptoms of her schizophrenia and to help her cope with the impending death of her brother.

In the case of Miss Treloar, the Mini Team had disengaged by the third week because they had jointly decided that intensive involvement would be pointless. When the team approach was to disengage from a patient who was still overtly psychotic it was not written in the case record because to do so would run counter to the injunction to care for patients. It would have been unthinkable to write in the case notes: 'Our approach to Miss Treloar will be to let her slip through our fingers and hope that nothing goes wrong, but we can always readmit her if it does'. This approach was nonetheless explicit in the management plan that arose from the case conference:

> *Murray:* We will just have to wait and hope the Modecate does some good and try to think of something. Perhaps we can increase the Modecate. We have a week to go before her detention order runs out.

A week later, members of the team talked in a tone of amused resignation when her case came up for discussion.

> *Murray:* She's no better. Perhaps we should just tell her not to do any more of those karate kicks and stop all that shouting. But she *won't* be changed. . . . It's a hopeless endeavour.
> *Leslie:* She says all the right things, she's got them off pat.

[10] See Kadushin (1962:517–31) on involvement, although his analysis is based on a static model. Goffman's (1968:79–80) notion of 'involvement cycles' is more dynamic, but the diversity among staff members is reduced, in his account, to a one-dimensional 'staff world'. Neither approach recognizes the importance of the team in modulating staff involvement with patients.

Murray made another suggestion that someone should talk to the secretary of the residents' association.

> *Margaret:* That's all been done. There is nothing we can do to change the situation unless we put it to her in a more firm manner, tell her to stop the karate. . . . She has a purpose to do the opposite of what people ask her to do. . . . If you stopped one thing she would start another. . . . The old ladies in the flats are constantly ringing me, and now they're getting paranoid. The blind one accused me of taking one of the letters.

By the following week Miss Treloar had been discharged, and her case was brought up by Tim who reported with a groan, indicating that what he had predicted had been confirmed; he had received a telephone call from Miss Treloar saying she was not coming for her appointment. No active follow-up was arranged. This management plan was not written, but it was nevertheless definitive. It had been developed as the result of a concurrence of epigrammatic appraisals that were united in a common key, assembled into a team definition, and put into effect as a joint team approach of disengagement.

The extent to which teams encompassed a case varied. In the instance of Miss Treloar, the Mini Team employed a 'hands off' approach and the degree of encompassment was minimal. For problematic cases that did not flow smoothly to recovery or discharge, the Mini Team responded by intensifying its encompassing activities, performing detailed reassessments and exploring additional dimensions. When this was not sufficient to contain the problem, other elements within the Schizophrenia Team were recruited. The patient might be referred to the Patient Education Group to fill out the educational dimension. The family might be referred to the Family Therapy Team. Additional psychiatrists, nurses, and social workers became involved, forming a second therapeutic line around the case. That is, when the Mini Team by itself was not able to encompass the case, successively higher levels of team organization were invoked. For the most difficult patients, every significant member of the Schizophrenia Team was involved in one way or another, the case ultimately being surrounded by what James called the Team's 'comprehensive service'. Thus for mild cases the level of encompassment was accordingly mild, but for the so-called management problems, encompassing processes were recruited with greater intensity and at higher organizational levels until the case was contained.

Since Goffman (1968:13–115) delineated the features of 'total institutions', psychiatric hospitals such as Ridgehaven have undergone deinstitutionalization. In place of the traditional structures described by Goffman, the team has emerged as an organizational form that, par excellence, enables the same totalizing approach to patients through its capacity to forge an encompassing definition of the case. Compared to Goffman's institution, teams are more modern and less oppressive, yet they are also more efficient in their capacity to produce total knowledge of the patient.

Because the power to deploy its members around the case was vested in the team, it was primarily the team that intervened when its individual members took a course that deviated from the agreed approach. The most common problem was overinvolvement with patients. It occurred most frequently among inexperienced staff or among psychiatric nurses whose intimate work with patients lent itself to a high degree of personal attachment. In such cases their reports to the case conference were out of key. Overinvolved Mini Team members would be pulled back into alignment by use of banter or ridicule. The novice would be teased for his or her gullibility and the nurse for 'playing therapist' or 'going off and doing his own thing'. At the same time, the specific patient who was the subject of overinvolvement was usually denigrated as being 'seductive', thus reinforcing the naivety and vulnerability of the clinician.

As with the definition of the case, the psychiatrist did not explicitly dictate the deployment of other professionals. Throughout the transcripts of thirteen case conferences there was no instance of a psychiatrist giving orders. Psychiatric control over the deployment of team members was limited to questioning each one about the course of action they wished to take ('What is the treatment plan? Is she getting involved in the ward programme?') and making suggestions as to how it could be done ('It might be nice to involve her in some of the occupational therapy things such as cooking.'). At a subsequent case conference follow-up questions might be asked about the progress of that intervention. The psychiatrist thus directed the various tasks of management by means of tentative suggestions. It also fell to the psychiatrist to raise questions concerning the approach that the team as a whole should be taking in regard to a case, thereby setting the overall agenda for action: 'I wonder if we aren't missing the boat here? We need a complete review of her case. I think we need to start again'.

At the time of this study, psychologists and nurse educators were beginning to raise objections to the power of psychiatry to control the deployment of other professionals through teams. Within nursing, these objections have led to the development of the 'case manager' concept (Kanter 1989), according to which a designated person has the explicit role of co-ordinating the work of other professionals. There was no reason, it was argued, why the case manager should not be a nurse (Nehls *et al.* 1992), though this argument has been strenuously rejected in the psychiatric literature (Leigh 1987: 86; Westermeyer 1991). In this way, the nursing profession challenged the hegemonic processes I have outlined. It sought to identify sources of power that were normally taken for granted and render them explicit. By raising them as a subject for debate within the sociopolitical arena of state mental health services, the profession aimed to make them a focus of political and industrial action.

Power of teams to define cases

Power that is taken for granted

This chapter and the previous one have been concerned with professional power and knowledge, and their role in the definition of cases of psychiatric illness. This concern developed from the ideas of Foucault regarding power as a productive rather than a repressive force that creates domains of knowledge within the institutions of the modern state. In Chapter 3, I showed how the power of individual professions was expressed by the assertion of autonomy, and how this led to a segmented version of the case, which comprised a number of partial definitions. On the basis of these definitions, the different professions controlled the distribution of cases within the hospital, its teams and wards, and beyond the hospital in the community. In this chapter I have demonstrated how power in a team context was expressed in terms of hegemony and encompassment, and the capacity to exclude other powerful groups from the clinical domain. By these means, the conflict that was integral to team organization could be excluded or at least contained. The profession of psychiatry controlled how the team as a whole defined a case and thereby controlled the deployment of fellow team members, especially the degree to which they were to become involved in a case or disengaged from it.

In accordance with Foucault, this ethnography demonstrates that within the modern hospital power is diffuse and decentralized, and best understood by examining its techniques in minute detail at the local level (c.f Rhodes 1992). However, the danger of a slavish adherence to Foucault's intellectual programme is twofold. First, because of the historical and ethnographic specificity of Foucault's analyses to France, with its centralized and authoritarian state organization and religious traditions (Gaines 1992:10), his ideas can provide only limited directions for the study of other cultural settings. Hence the concept of hegemony has been required to analyze the particularities of egalitarianism in Australian psychiatric teams. Second is Foucault's reliance on texts and a 'history of ideas' approach, which may lack explanatory specificity when applied to the study of everyday social interaction. An uncritical application of Foucault's method can lead to 'a systematic reduction of all social processes to largely unspecified patterns of domination' (Merquior 1985:115). Foucault's frequently quoted notion that power is infinitesimal, everywhere and nowhere, can be used to say everything and nothing.

This analysis avoids that danger by identifying the everyday life of the hospital, with its taken-for-granted assumptions, as the specific domain in which patterns of domination emerged. It has shown how psychiatrists can dominate the team and enlist a consent to leadership through the mundane activities of opening and closing case discussions, unself-consciously directing the conversational key of meetings, asking pertinent questions, routinely writing the first and last entry in a case record, and summarizing and condensing a case. This chapter has demonstrated that psychiatric classificatory knowledge, taught to all in the case conference, was the dominant set of ideas that defined team work and identified the team itself. Irrespective of professions, team members subscribed to the idea of a Schizophrenia Team because it seemed 'natural', and was even made tangible by the arrangement of buildings within the landscape of the hospital. These modes of power can be specified because the analysis is based on ethnographic methods that give privileged access to the assumptions of everyday life. They identify the unnoticed aspects of daily work—the common-sense language, tone of voice, conversational key—by which social workers, nurses, and psychiatrists enacted power. This focus on common-sense reasoning also reveals the practical consequences of power for patients in the way they were distributed and for clinicians in the way they were deployed.

Reconstructing the whole person

A major argument developed in this chapter is that the processes through which interprofessional relationships were mediated by multidisciplinary teams had a significant bearing on the way cases were defined. It was in the team setting that the different perspectives of each profession were integrated. The various segments of the case were put back together. The team could also encompass a case in its entirety, mapping out its every dimension. Team work, it was claimed, was all-embracing. The team could provide a 'comprehensive service', a 'complete work-up', and 'total patient care'. The final product of team work was a particular version of the case known as the 'whole person'. Wholeness itself was predicated on processes of exclusion. Patients were invited to make a contribution to the case conference. However, as in the example of Miss Treloar, the crucial discussions took place before and after she joined the meeting. When patients' views of their problems were in accord with those of the team they were incorporated into the case, but where they conflicted with the team definition they were excluded. For example, when patients adopted a spiritual interpretation of their illness or denied that there was any illness at all, these views were not given any credence by the team.

Cases of psychiatric illness were thus defined in a way that reflected the organization of the multidisciplinary team. The case and the team served as models for each other. Each was based on the idea of parts in relation to a whole. A team had its component professions, and a case had its corresponding segments. A team also formed a larger whole and accordingly claimed to treat the whole person: 'As the team contains its factions, it contains the whole patient' (Nason 1981:34). Just as teams were likened to people, healthy or sick, so people were seen to function like teams. A healthy, integrated, conflict-free team was a model for a healthy, integrated person.

This correspondence between the idea of a team and the idea of a person had implications for the way treatment was conceptualized. These were especially relevant to schizophrenia and its treatment. When talking about schizophrenia, both clinicians and patients employed a metaphor of disintegration, expressed in such phrases as 'cracking up', 'going to pieces,' 'falling apart,' 'psychotic disintegration', or becoming 'loose at the edges'. An acute psychotic episode could be called a 'break'. The person with schizophrenia was a fragmented object. When carrying out their individual assessments, members of the various clinical professions, each with their unique perspective, produced a segmented case that mirrored this fragmentation. By means of integration and encompassment, the multidisciplinary team united these component professions and, at the same time, reconstructed the case as a unified, whole object. Hence recovery was called 'reintegrating', 'coming together', 'containing the psychosis', or 'sealing over'. If coming apart was a metaphor for psychiatric illness, being further taken to pieces and then being put back together again by a team of professionals was a fundamental process of psychiatric treatment. Psychiatric case work involved deconstructing and reconstructing a person; alternating between parts and whole; disassembling them into bits and pieces and then putting them back together into a 'whole person' again. For patients, this was the most powerful effect of being treated by a team.

5

Documenting a case: the written construction of schizophrenia

Writing is central to psychiatric work. A common sight on the wards of the Schizophrenia Team was that of the staff hard at work, writing in the case records. So fundamental was writing to the interaction between clinicians and patients that if the case records were misplaced work ground to a halt until they were recovered or a temporary file established.[1] This chapter examines the clinical staff as they interviewed their patients and made entries in the case records. It analyses the processes through which these clinicians constructed written definitions of cases, processes that were so fundamental to clinical practice that they applied to all patients, irrespective of diagnosis. Because the material is drawn from observations of work on the Schizophrenia Team it focuses on the written definition of schizophrenia. The chapter aims to show that as much as psychiatry was a 'talking cure' it was also a 'writing cure'. Clinical writing did not merely describe the treatment of patients, it also constituted the treatment (c.f. Silverman 1975:287).

Cycle of interpretation

At the heart of clinical work was a cycle of talking and writing, of face-to-face interaction and documentation or, to use hospital argot, 'seeing patients' and 'writing them up'. The

---

[1] The idea of a 'literacy event' is relevant to understanding clinical interaction in a psychiatric hospital. Heath (1982:93) defines a literacy event as 'any action sequence, involving one or more persons, in which the production and/or comprehension of print . . . is integral to the nature of participants' interactions and their interpretive processes'.

common-sense view held that 'seeing' was primary and 'writing up' was a derivative record of that interaction.[2] Raffel (1979:19) describes this assumption as follows: 'Events are not seen as produced by the records but the record is seen as produced by the events. . . . The events can occur and remain unrecorded, but the record cannot occur without the events'. This view fails to take account of underlying interpretive processes that occur at each phase of the cycle of talking and writing. The work of Ricouer (1976:1–44; 1979:73–80; 1981: 145–9), especially his distinction between the interpretation of speech and the interpretation of writing, provides a useful framework for understanding how this cycle operates in a clinical context.[3] An interview was a dialogue in which meanings were negotiated between a clinician and a patient. The clinician then interpreted these meanings in order to make notes on the interview. Because the notes now formed part of a permanent record, they were distanced from that immediate context in which they were produced, and their subsequent interpretation was influenced by other factors.

The conventions of clinical writing were a major influence. A psychiatric admission history comprised several parts, each with its own characteristic style of writing. This chapter examines a number of these styles—for example, an abbreviated idiom that resembled a short-hand form of notation, and a characteristic intermediate form of typification that was used to form a bridge between lay and professional ideas of mental illness. Such structural features shaped the way in which clinicians wrote about their patients and how this writing was interpreted.

Ricoeur (1979:86) emphasizes that the meaning of a text also resides 'in the sense of its forthcoming interpretations'. When writing in case records, clinicians anticipated who might

---

[2] Within the social science literature on psychiatric records, analysis has often been limited to questions of whether clinical records provide an accurate description of patients and therefore whether they are innocent or harmful to these patients (Rosenhan 1973, 1981).

[3] Whereas the meaning conveyed in speech is fleeting, writing fixes meaning in a more permanent way. During spoken interaction, meaning is largely identified with the subjective intention of the speakers; but once inscribed in text, it may become independent of the author's intention. For Ricoeur it is a relative semantic autonomy that distinguishes writing from speech because, with speech, meaning is tethered to the situational context of interaction.

read them in future. In part, they were writing for themselves because the records served as an *aide memoire*. They also wrote for fellow team members who read the case notes before they interviewed a patient. Case records could also be read outside the immediate clinical context. As administrative documents there was a requirement for the diagnosis to be entered and coded in a format consistent with the International Classification of Diseases (World Health Organization 1978), thereby fulfilling the hospital's statutory obligations to provide quantitative information to a national bureau of statistics. Case records were also the principal means whereby professional bodies exercised supervisory control over members (Freidson 1970:101; Daniels 1975). At peer review meetings, clinicians scrutinized each others' records to find evidence of emotional or judgemental writing—for example the exasperated entry, 'Patient presents to hospital yet again' or 'This patient is ? depressed ? bloody minded'. In the context of peer review, disorganized notes were jokingly characterized as 'schizophrenic' or 'thought disordered'. The ideal record portrayed the clinician as a rational decision maker whose emotions were restricted to empathy and care. Case records thus described patients in a language that was, in part, a reflection of the need for professionals to define themselves in polar opposition to psychiatric illness. Hospital staff were also aware that anything they wrote in the record was legally binding (Garfinkel 1974:120), which tended to produce a formal, or 'frozen', style of writing (Scott and Lyman 1968:57). Assessments and decisions were couched in terms of 'standard practice', the routine defence should a clinician's treatment be subjected to scrutiny and the records subpoenaed by a court.

These requirements to document a case in a way that conformed to the conventions of clinical writing and that anticipated a variety of future readers influenced the interview conversation, determining the questions the clinician put to the patient: 'It is not that records record things but that the very idea of recording determines in advance how things will have to appear' (Raffel 1979:48). The interpretation of written knowledge shaped what was spoken; the interpretation of spoken knowledge, in turn, shaped what was written, and so on.

Thus the cycle of writing and talking was complete. It could be entered at any point, but it was most common for clinicians to begin by reading what was already contained in the record and then ask questions of the patient on the basis of this written information.

Patients, too, were involved in this cycle and thereby enlisted to the task of producing their case records. However, control of the written definition of cases was confined to the professional. The team of clinicians remained the authors of the record, and its ownership was vested in the hospital. Although they were involved in the process of documentation, patients could not directly read or write in the notes and were thereby separated from the written account. This had important consequences for the way they spoke.

For patients, an interview was an encounter with a clinician who referred to the case records, put questions to them in light of what was already documented, and then made further notes in the record. By repeated exposure to this cycle of reading, talking, and writing, patients learned what was germane to the record and amenable to documentation. Thus the written definition of the case influenced how patients articulated an account of themselves and their illness.

The core of this chapter analyses a series of assessment interviews by which a patient was admitted to Heathfield House with a diagnosis of drug abuse and schizophrenia. I compare transcriptions of audio-tape recordings of the interviews with the entries in the case record that were being written as these interviews proceeded, a method previously used by Cicourel (1974). It allows direct comparison between the written account and the conversation on which it was based. The example of Paul Lawrence was chosen for detailed analysis because he was regarded as a 'typical case'. He already had a well documented record of previous admissions to the Schizophrenia Team, and he illustrated the interaction between what had previously been written and what was talked about on this admission. However, my analysis elucidates processes that were not exclusive to Paul and draws on observations of interviews with many patients treated by the Schizophrenia Team. The cycle analysed here was fundamental to all interviews.

From document to interview

Dr George, a trainee psychiatrist, was the Duty Medical Officer (DMO) for Ridgehaven Hospital when Paul Lawrence arrived with his mother at the admission desk. Before meeting them, Dr George gathered background information on the case. The nurse in the admission area told him that Paul had been brought to hospital from a country town by his mother, who earlier that day had discussed the situation by telephone with Dr McCusker, Paul's regular psychiatrist. Dr George then read the nursing log book:

> Referred to see DMO by Dr McCusker. Patient brought to GP [general practitioner] by mother for assessment and probable admission. Admissions before to Heathfield House for schizophrenia, currently an OP [outpatient] of Dr McCusker.

Next, Dr George quickly perused the case records, concentrating on the typewritten discharge summaries. They documented a two-year history of schizophrenia with 'auditory hallucinations', 'thought disorder', 'flat affect' and 'social withdrawal'. There had been three admissions to Ridgehaven since the illness began. Just prior to seeing Paul, Dr George rang Dr McCusker, who confirmed that he had spoken with Paul's mother and arranged for him to come to hospital. His mother thought that Paul had been abusing prescription drugs and was worried about him becoming uncontrollable. On the basis of this background information, Dr George made the first entry in the case record under the heading '*Ref*:', which is an abbreviation of 'Referral'. (Dr George's case note entry, which he wrote as the interview proceeded, is shown in Figure 5.1.)

Like all patients, Paul was thus first approached through his case record. In their daily work, the clinical staff routinely came to know a case by reading the case record before they ever met the patient face-to-face. Only in contrived situations, for example, when being tested as part of a professional examination, did they interview patients without having access to the case records. This was known as 'seeing a patient blind', an acknowledgement of the importance of the case record as

RIDGEHAVEN HOSPITAL

RECORD OF CONSULTATION

PATIENT'S NAME Paul LAWRENCE
UNIT NUMBER 011095

STICK LABEL HERE

DATE: 25·7·84   TIME: 5:30 pm
SEEN BY: Dr· George
PRINCIPAL THERAPIST Dr· McCusker

Re: Mother phoned Dr McCusker this AM. as pt. has been using LSD (? no. of times) + ? other drugs. He took 10 serepax tabs. last night + slept till 10AM today. He had been crying + + uncontrollable, ? psychotic again ? compliance of Modecate. LMO on leave.

History from Mother (Mrs. James)

Son living on own 3-4/12 due to conflict c̄ step-father → makes Mother upset as she'd like to care for him. Mo. a nurse — she can't discard him. Poor peer group — involved c̄ drugs Girlfriend of 1/52 told mother, Paul says he wants to get off drugs, but finds it hard. 125 mgm Modecate due 3/7 ago Paul living on own as caretaker of friend's house.

In last 3/52, appeared drunk (Mo. never suspected drugs. supplied by shopkeeper), abusive, hitch hiked to Yarami to get drugs. Has become involved c̄ seasonal workers on drugs, looking for free bed. Looked "high", which upset step-father. Sits i a daze → ? hallucinating. Mo. found a cup of coffee in a saucepan in the oven, often wanders. Last night. Irresponsible re work, feeding dog etc. "forget" to turn up + meet solicitor last Friday re driving offence. Mo noticed this irresponsibility in last 2 years but at age 12, Mother remarried + I-P problems occurred in the house c̄ 2nd hb. Mo. divorced Paul's father who was a violent schizophrenic about 14-15 years ago. Paul has one sister in Albert Park c̄ same condition. 2 other children — no ψ history. The 2 youngest have become ill c̄ schiz.

History of Presenting Complaint — 4/52 drug taking — Avil, Serepax + Mogadon, L.S.D. (marijuana). Used marijuana ≈ 2 oz/week regularly since age 16. Stopped alcohol use 2/12 ago, except occasional beers. Presenting Complaint — Feels angry, hyperactive + "high". Feels unable to control how many drugs he uses unless he's in a controlled environment. Drugs keep him mellow, more relaxed i̅ I-P relationships. Sees life as a series of "habits" in the drugs. c/o hearing a voice occasionally c̄ him Paul. c/o Insomnia — goes out looking for drugs; weight — ↓ 4 stone in 12/12 Appetite — ↓ since moving out of family home.

PTO...

Fig. 5.1.   Record of consultation.

c/o habits of counting recin o rus to give (sleep) a nasd. Denied
Schneiderian FRS of thought alienation + perception. He thinks he
can control other people's thoughts, but they can't read his mind.
Patient requested detention:-

Mental state Examination:-

Appearance: Short young man dressed ü green T-shirt, shorts ±
thongs. Tattoos on both lower arms, scar on ® knee from a
cartilege op 10 years ago following a MVA.

Behaviour:- Co-operative but anxious at being recorded on a
tape recorder.

Conversation:- No clear cut evidence of FTD. Denied
Schneiderian FRS of thought alienation. Content related mainly
to drug abuse which he felt unable to control + requested
admission under detention as a means of stopping his drug
taking. Some evidence of circumstantiality. ʸᵒ Paranoi ʸ
ideation of persecutory nature.

Perception:- Occasional auditory hallucination of a voice
calling his name. Has seen car lights on during day and
off at night (? significance)

Affect:- Some flattening at times but reactive at others.

Cognition:- Appeared intact

Insight:- Aware of drug abuse on his part and mentioned
that he felt they were used therapeutically to assist in
interpersonal relationships, give him a lift + make him feel mellow.

Diagnosis :- (1) Drug abuse - Avil, marihuana, LSD + Serepax
               (2) Schizophrenia - currently controlled ü
                                    Moderate.

DUTY DOCTOR'S OPINION :-

Mother anxious re Paul's drug abuse ü recent o/D ü serepax +
her 2nd husband's non-acceptance of her son's illness +
behaviour. He had no accomodation + step-father won't have
him home unless he receives treatment. Paul requesting
help + detention. H/o absconding in past admission.

Plan:-

① Admit under 3/1 detention to Heathfield House
② R Moderate 25 mgm 3/52 - give dose on admission.
③ Social work assessment - ? accomodation
④ Dr. McCusker may want to see this patient.
⑤ ? Referral to Drug + Alcohol board on F/U
                                    A. George.
                         _____
                         DUTY DOCTOR'S SIGNATURE

ADMITTED TO:_____

NOT ADMITTED— REFERRED TO—   *Outpatients   *Own Doctor }
                             *Own Care   *Other Agency } _____

U4873

Fig. 5.1.   (*cont.*)

a clinical instrument through which to view the patient. Student doctors and nurses were even more reliant on written records. When a batch of new students arrived on the ward they could be seen with their heads buried in the case records before plucking up courage to actually talk to the patients. Even new patients arrived at the hospital accompanied by written documents. The path to the psychiatric hospital was lined with medical practitioners, police officers, and social workers, each generating referral letters, reports, and other documents as the patient passed through their hands.

From interview to document

Interview with Paul's mother

Before seeing Paul, Dr George interviewed his mother, Mrs James, who was anxious to return to her home in the country. A portion of this interview is transcribed below (beginning after the formal introduction).[4] *D* = Dr George; *M* = Mrs James. The numbers (008–028) indicate the lines of transcription.

   008 *D*: Okay . . . . . Uh. Mrs James is your son living home with you?
   009 *M*: Well he did last night.
   010 *D*: Yes.
   011 *M*: I brought him home. He was living on his own.
   012 *D*: Was he?
   013 *M*: Unfortunately he doesn't, his stepfather and him don't get on →
   014 *D*: Mm.
   015 *M*: and, er, they can't live under the same roof →
   016 *D*: I see.
   017 *M*: because my husband's very impatient with this kind of
   018   illness. He thinks he's putting it over all the time you know. He lives →
   019 *D*: Mm hm.
   020 *M*: he's been living on his own.
   021 *D*: Mm. I see. . . . . What . . how long has he been living on his own now?

---

[4] Transcription notation follows conventions set out by Tannen (1982:10). Pauses are indicated by periods (.), each of which represents half a second. An arrow (→) indicates that the utterance continues, transcribed on the next line but one, without pause or break in rhythm.

022 *M*: Um . . . . that's a good question. About three or four
     months I suppose.
023 *D*: Mm. . . . . . . And that's—is that because of conflict with
     his stepfather?
024 *M*: Mm. Yes. [During this seven second pause Dr George
025 began writing.] Yes it's making me ill. I want to have
026 him home to look after him and I can't do it. So →
027 ['Beep, beep'—the electronic paging device.]
028 it tears me inside. . . .

Dr George interrupted the interview to talk on the telephone
in response to his paging device. The first call was from a
general practitioner who wanted to admit a ninety-year-old
man to the hospital. Dr George explained that, in keeping
with hospital policy, he was reluctant to accept such patients.
A second call informed Dr George that another 'troublesome'
patient urgently awaited assessment. Dr George turned his attention back to Mrs James.

064 *D*: Um, Mrs James you said that you sort of would have
065 very much have liked your son to be home with you.
066 *M*: I'm a nurse and it goes against my grain to . .
067 *D*: Are you? It must be very hard for you.
068 *M*: *I'll bet!* Mm. Its *shocking.* I've been *hysterical* a few times
     this week →
069 *D*: Have you?
070 *M*: and um, our doctor is away, not that he could help. He
071 knows what I'm going through . . and the other doctor
072 in the clinic says to more or less . . . . discard him and
     live my own life, but I can't do that.

Finally, Dr George enquired about Paul's drug use and psychotic symptoms and then entered this information into the
record.

Reducing the written account to intermediate typifications

When comparing the transcript with the case record, there
was a striking reduction from the rich detail of the spoken

interaction to the terse entries in the record.[5] Clinicians wrote
while they talked and listened. This led to a telegraphic style
of writing and a liberal use of short-hand notations: Ref:, ?,
no., crying + +, →, 3–4/12, H.P.C., I-P problems, 2nd Hb, or
4/52. They sought to record what they interpreted as the essential nub of the conversation, and in doing so the nuances
and ambiguity of meaning were largely eliminated.

Abbreviation was also accomplished by the use of intermediate typifications. Drawing on Schutz and Luckman (1973:
231), Handelman (1978:17) defines these as 'intermediate
constructions of reality, often uncodified, which mediate between the "stock of knowledge" . . . of protagonists'. In psychiatric work, they mediated between practical and theoretical
knowledge, between lay and scientific terminology, and enabled a shift from the particulars of a case to the abstract notion
of psychiatric illness. One such typification was 'conflict'. Discussing Paul's relation to his stepfather [013–022], Mrs James
employed lay terms such as 'don't get on', 'can't live under
the same roof', and 'thinks he's putting it over', which Dr
George interpreted as 'conflict' [023]. He offered this definition to Mrs James, who concurred, and the word 'conflict'
was entered in the record [025]. Though slightly different
from what she had said, 'conflict' made sense to Mrs James.
At the same time, this term connoted a range of more abstract
meanings within theoretical psychiatry and would not be out
of place on the pages of the *British Journal of Psychiatry* or
Schizophrenia Bulletin. Psychiatric case histories were replete
with intermediate typifications: 'interpersonal problems',
'peer group', and 'stress'. Writing in a purely lay idiom was
discouraged. Perpetrators were chastised at peer review meetings. Where patients' words were included, especially obscen-
ities, the correct procedure was to use quotation marks,
thereby maintaining the professional style of the case history.
On the other hand, clinicians were discouraged from writing
in a conspicuously theoretical style. Those who did so, usually
novices, were gently chided by more experienced colleagues
for having their 'heads in their books' and not being in touch

---

[5] See Cicourel (1968:318, 332; 1974:64–65) on the production of truncated written accounts in medical and legal settings.

with the practical problems of the patient (c.f. Daniels 1975: 322).

Rendering the common-sense framework invisible

In the process of documenting an interview in intermediate typifications, the common-sense understandings which had underpinned the interview were not recorded. The dialogue between Dr George and Mrs James, for example, was based on a common-sense notion of mental illness—a loosely defined, uncodified ensemble of ideas that included madness and craziness as well as marginality, the strange, the unusual, and the bizarre. It could also refer to danger, violence, and loss of control, particularly emotional control. Illogical thinking, unpredictability, and irrationality were also closely related. Agreement between doctor and patient, or in this instance the patient's mother, was made possible by this tacit framework of shared meanings. It was clearly evident in the transcript but not in the corresponding entry in the case record, which is illustrated in the following sequence. Dr George had asked three questions: if Paul had been talking to himself, if he had been different, and if he had been making sense. Each question was framed by common-sense understandings of mental illness. At first Mrs James hesitated, as if she did not understand the point of the questions; but when she grasped that Dr George was asking about 'madness' her replies flowed freely. They canvassed irrationality [223–224], irresponsibility [231], danger [209–210], fear of Paul [226], and 'strange' behaviour [229].

205 *M*: . . . . . . Mmmm. What happened . . . .
206 *D*: Do you understand?
207 *M*: What happened, I went down to clean the house. He's
208   been thrown out of the house of course now, because,
209   er, he left the oven going, and it's a very old stove
210   and it's a sort of stove that would blow up if it got
         too hot.
211 *D*: Mm.
212 *M*: And he was very upset, the owner. I don't blame him.
         And he's got a

213   little pup, and it shouldn't have been inside. Paul was
214   out, and the owner got in the window, turned
215   everything off and he said, 'This is *it*,' and gave me the
216   keys and he said, 'Lock up! And he's not to come
       back.' That's why Paul spent the night at our place.
217 *D*: Uhuh.
218 *M*: But my husband wasn't too bad. He didn't mind him
219   there so long as he came and had treatment.
220 *D*: Uhuh.
221 *M*: He'll do anything within reason. And he came home
222   and slept. I went back this morning to clean up, and
223   I found a cup of coffee in the oven . . a cup of coffee
224   in a saucepan in the oven if you know what I mean?
       [Spoken in a laughing tone that conveyed her
       amazement.]
225 *D*: Uhuh.
226 *M*: That sort of frightened me a little bit . .
227 *D*: Mm hm.
228 *M*: and when I questioned him about it he said he didn't
229   remember. And what else has been strange?
230 *D*: And the oven had been left . . left . . left . . on?
231 *M*: Mm. Mm. And then he'd gone out. He's very
232   irresponsible about all these things. He forgets to feed
       the dog, all these things.
233 *D*: Mm . . . . [writing]. Yes.
234 *M*: And some men would want him to cart some lucerne
235   and Paul wouldn't turn up. He would forget. And then
236   he had to go to court for a driving charge that
237   occurred here in the city a few weeks back and he just
238   forgot to turn up and he left the solicitor and I there.
       I was just so *furious* with him [sigh].

In Dr George's notes there was no trace of the common-sense
ideas of mental illness that provided the underlying sense of
his questions and her answers. The process of documentation

had rendered them invisible. Instead, the documented version had a 'factual' quality. It was written to be read as a primary observation that was neither based on interpretation nor generated by negotiation between Dr George and Mrs James. Through the processes of documentation, 'much if not every trace of what has gone into the making of that account is obliterated and what remains is only the text, which aims at being read as "what actually happened" ' (Smith 1974:260).

Characterizing the interview participants

The transition from interview dialogue to written notes thus required an active process of selection and omission. The extent of this 'editorial' work is illustrated by the way in which I, the observer, was excluded from the record. At the interview my presence was large, seeking permission, taking notes, and smiling empathically at Mrs James when she sighed. My dual relationship with Dr George of ethnographer to doctor and psychiatrist to trainee psychiatrist constrained him to produce a 'model interview'. Yet these influences were not evident in the case record.

An important area in which editorial control was exercised was in the characterization of the main figures. Characterization refers to the way in which a writer portrays the identity of each participant in terms of a limited number of salient features. In psychiatric hospital work, this process of selecting certain features and playing down others was directed toward the immediate practical task at hand—for Dr George the task of admitting Paul. Within the interview, Mrs James was highly emotional. She used such phrases as: 'it's been making me ill', 'it tears me inside', 'shocking', 'hysterical', 'I nearly went berserk', '*furious* with him,' and '*frantic*'. She sighed repeatedly and deeply. The transcripts of the conversation (which are themselves a documentary construction) convey little of the emotional intensity in the room. The case record conveyed even less, merely that she was 'upset' and 'anxious'. Instead, Dr George characterized Mrs James as a mother, a nurse, and a woman who could never 'discard' Paul. By portraying her so positively as a caring figure, he gave authority to her version of Paul and his situation.

'Caring mother' raised the possibility of a negative counter-part: the 'rejecting mother'. At Ridgehaven Hospital the mo-tives of family members were routinely treated with scepticism. They could be viewed as trying to 'dump' a 'problem patient' into the hospital.[6] In an era of deinstitutionalization, where one task of the Duty Medical Officer was to 'fight off' undes-erving admissions, such a patient would often be refused en-try. This issue was pertinent for Mrs James. Paul had previously been refused admission to Ridgehaven, and during the inter-view she had heard Dr George speaking on the telephone about the hospital's policy of not admitting certain patients. She worked hard to avoid being characterized negatively, stressing that she had cared for Paul to the very limits of her endurance despite the difficulties posed by her husband. The need to provide a positive definition of herself perhaps ex-plained her repeated statements that she was not in any way to blame for, or even aware of, Paul's drug taking. Ultimately, it was this definition that Dr George selected for the record by writing: 'Mo. never suspected drugs—supplied by shop-keeper'. A different characterization was equally possible. Dr George could have chosen to write of her, using her own words, as berserk, frantic, shocked, hysterical, and furious; but his practical objective was to admit Paul, as had been arranged by his supervisor Dr McCusker. To render Mrs James a 'caring mother' served this objective.

Dr George was also one of the characters in the record. Within the interview he was subject to the mundane contin-gencies of psychiatric work, notably the pressure to process cases quickly and balance several commitments at once. He answered his electronic paging device and exclaimed '*Mamma Mia!*' on learning that another patient had arrived. These con-tingencies were omitted from the record, as were his ques-tions, reflections, and most of all the ubiquitous 'mm hm's' and 'uhuh's' by means of which he directed the dialogue. The document emphasized his official medical identity as a guar-antee that the same facts would be produced by any other

[6] See Sharrock and Turner (1978) for a comparable analysis of how police main-tain a sceptical attitude when dealing with complaints by members of the public against a third party. It is possible that they will view the complainant, rather than the person complained against, as malicious.

competent doctor who followed the same routine procedure. However, the personal identity of the author was not altogether eliminated, at least for readers within the hospital, where he could be identified by his signature, handwriting, and individual case note style. His entries would be read by other staff members in the light of what they knew of his reputation, professional competence, and idiosyncrasies. Case records were routinely read for what they revealed about the author as much as for what they revealed about the patient. Hospital staff cultivated the skill of remembering signatures and handwriting. Even those who had never met Dr George would have developed an impression of him by reading his case notes. Like patients, many members of staff were initially known through the written word before they were encountered face to face. The document thus depicted the clinician within wider contexts of readership as a model professional and within the local hospital context as an individual with distinctive personal and professional qualities.

The characterization of Paul was initially formed in the dialogue between Dr George and Mrs James. The version of this dialogue Dr George recorded sought to emphasize Paul's schizophrenia, and therefore made no reference to the possibility of him being rational and in control of himself despite evidence in the dialogue that he was. For example, his mother indicated that he was able to control his emotional expression in order to get his own way:

```
156  D: . . . . . . . . . . How? . . what else did you notice?
157  M: Oh up one minute and down the next. But of course
158      I'm used to that. Hhhh [resigned laugh]. He can be
159      very abusive one minute and sweet the next, when he
         wants his own way.
160  D: Mm hm. So he appeared drunk and he's been abusive.
161  M: Yes.
```

Mrs James' statement conveyed the idea that Paul exhibited a range of emotional expressions, which he could control in order to manipulate those around him. In reply, Dr George focused on his abusiveness and reflected it back to Mrs James. When she agreed, the word 'abusive' was entered, underlined, in the record. Dr George could have said, 'So he appeared drunk and he's been sweet' and then entered 'sweet' into the record. However, because it implied emotional control and friendliness, 'sweet' was not relevant to the task of documenting Paul's schizophrenia and drug abuse. There were other examples. His stepfather thought that he was 'putting it over all the time' [018], and when Paul had sought to be admitted to hospital on a previous occasion a staff member had reputedly told him that he was just 'looking for a bed'. These interpretations implied that he was purposefully exaggerating his symptoms for ulterior gain. The final record, however, characterized Paul as lacking self-control, desiring but unable to get off drugs, influenced by a 'poor peer group', and 'irresponsible'. This rendered him an appropriate case for hospital admission.

Admission assessment: separating schizophrenia from the patient

Interview with Paul

In the following interview, *D* = Dr George and *P* = Paul Lawrence.

    007 *D*: Um, Dr McCusker has been looking after you in the
               past?
    008 *P*: Yeah.
    009 *D*: Um . . . . [Paul looked at the tape recorder.]
    010   It's alright. You look at me and talk to me.
               How have you been feeling, Paul?
    011 *P*: Well, feeling pretty good because I've been taking
               drugs, that's why.
    012 *D*: You have been taking drugs? For how long now?
    013 *P*: I have been taking Serepax for about four weeks.
    014 *D*: Four weeks?
    015 *P*: Yeah.
    016 *D*: Uhuh. . . . . . . Can you . . . .
    017 *P*: And Avils car sickness tablets, and Mogadon.
    018 *D*: Mm hm. . . . . [writing] that's er, what drugs have
    019   you been taking? Avil?
    020 *P*: Evil?

021 *D*: Mm hm.
022 *P*: Evil tablets? . . Avil tablets →
023 *D*: Avil tablets.
024 *P*: car sickness tablets.
025 *D*: Yes I know that.
026 *P*: Mogadon.
027 *D*: Mogadon, yes.
028 *P*: And Serepax.
029 *D*: . . . . [writing] And Serepax.
030 *P*: And Serepax.
031 *D*: Anything else?
032 *P*: No.
033 *D*: LSD? Or?
034 *P*: Yeah. LSD
035 *D*: You have. Anything else, Paul?
036 *P*: No. Marijuana.
037 *D*: Mm hm.
038 *P*: That's all.
039 *D*: That's all over this last four weeks.
040 *P*: I've been using Serepax for four weeks. I've been on
041   marijuana since about sixteen
042 *D*: Mm. Any, and what about the other drugs?
043 *P*: No.
044 *D*: No what?
045 *P*: I haven't been taking them for years—the others. I've
046   been taking marijuana for, for years but I've, the
047   other ones I've been taking for about four weeks.
048 *D*: Right. All those you've been taking for about four
         weeks.
049 *P*: Yeah, apart from marijuana.
050 *D*: Except for marijuana. Okay. How much marijuana have
051   you been smoking?
052 *P*: About $60 a week.
053 *D*: Pardon?
054 *P*: About two ounces a week.
055 *D*: . . . . . . [writing]. Two ounces. A week. Has that been
056   sort of a regular thing?
057 *P*: Yeah.
058 *D*: . . . . [writing]. And that's been since the age of
         sixteen?

059 *P*: Yeah.
060 *D*: . . . . [writing]. So that's the drugs you've been us-
061   ing. And what about alcohol?
062 *P*: Yeah. I don't drink any more.
063 *D*: When did you stop?
064 *P*: About two months ago, a few months ago. . . . . . [Paul
065   pauses while Dr George writes]. I have an occasional
          beer but I don't get drunk.
066 *D*: Mm hm. Except for an occasional beer.
067 *P*: Yeah. Social drink.
068 *D*: . . . . [writing]. Okay, Paul can you tell me a bit
069   more? How have you been feeling?

Cycle of talking and writing

I have shown how the clinical staff approached a case by reading the record prior to conducting an interview, as illustrated
by the way Dr George initially gathered background information on Paul. This process entailed a movement from the
written to the spoken word. The interview with Paul's mother
demonstrated the editorial work involved in making notes of
a conversation. This entailed a movement from the spoken
word to the written word. These two processes—from case
record to dialogue and from dialogue back to case record—
formed a cycle that had important implications for the way
case records were constructed and for the way patients were
defined within these records.

When questioning Paul, Dr George chiefly worked in a
reading–talking–writing mode. He was seated so he could
look back and forth between the case record and the patient.
Paul adjusted the pace of his conversation to the doctor's writing speed [064]. Experienced patients often spoke at dictation
pace and might enquire, 'Am I going too fast for you?' Writing
was an important nonverbal means by which clinicians directed patients when to talk and what topics were relevant.[7]

Paul was aware that he was being questioned in light of the
record. The question, 'Um, Dr McCusker has been looking

---

[7] Compare with 'meta-actions' in speech (Labov and Fanshel 1977:60) 'which
have to do with the regulation of the speech itself'.

after you in the past?' [007] did not elicit any new information from Paul, but it did establish that Dr George was in command of the case record and the considerable body of information that it contained about Paul. Although there were routine, open-ended questions [010, 069] that did not stem from the record, most of the enquiry was based on the previously documented evidence of his drug-taking and schizophrenia. When Paul said that he had been taking no other drugs, Dr George continued, 'LSD? Or . . . ?' [033], because there was a record of LSD use in the past. The enquiry [012–068] ceased when the doctor had validated the information that had already been recorded. Similarly, in reference to Paul's well documented history of schizophrenia, Dr George asked him some standard, textbook questions, focusing on the symptoms that he had read in the summaries of Paul's previous hospital admissions. They included questions concerning hallucinated voices heard outside his head, questions concerning his thoughts not being his own, his thoughts stopping, people reading his thoughts, his thoughts leaving him, other thoughts being put into his head, and finally questions about being controlled by an external agent (Schneider 1974). As a result of this enquiry, Dr George recorded: 'C/O [complains of] hearing a voice occasionally call him Paul', and 'Denied Schneiderian FRS [first rank symptoms] of thought alienation and perception'. Clinicians formulated a question from the record, put it to the patient so as to encourage the patient to talk, then recorded an interpretation of what was said back into the record. This was the basic interpretive cycle of clinical interaction.

As a consequence of this cycle, individual entries became embedded within the case record as a whole. Each entry was oriented retrospectively to what had previously been written about Paul's schizophrenia, and also prospectively, anticipating subsequent documentation that would again confirm the diagnosis. What was already written in the record became reinforced when fed through this cycle from documentation to dialogue to documentation. A direct implication of the cycle for patients was that they were providing an account of themselves in response to a version that was already well established in the record. It compelled them to disclose personal details,

either because they knew that these details were already recorded or in an attempt to set the record straight.[8] Resistance
to disclosing personal information was rare. Though patients
sometimes tried, they found it difficult to maintain secrets.
Deception was rapidly uncovered by comparing the patient's
account with that in the record, which included statements
from family members or others who had a close knowledge of
the patient. As with Paul, patients tended to cooperate with
the process of documentation because it was the most tangible
aspect of their treatment. They became active participants in
producing a written account of themselves.

Writing was an expression of power.[9] The clinical staff retained authorship, and the hospital retained ownership of the
case record. It was largely by controlling what was written in
the record that clinicians exercised the power to define cases.
Patients were enlisted to this task or, if they were reluctant to
disclose personal information, were coerced by the imperative
to document their case. Erikson and Gilbertson (1969:411)
have noted that in hospitals where patients are given direct
access to their official case records the staff experience diminished control over patients. However, they usually regain control by developing a second, informal file that they withhold
from the patients. Some staff members who had reflected on
the power associated with writing, reported to me that they
sometimes used it in a deliberate way to quell potential violence. One strategy, they said, to deal with a patient who had
become extremely angry or threatening was to approach him
or her with case records and a pen in hand, asking the patient
to explain what had caused the anger, so it could be properly
recorded. The potential crisis could thus be averted by involving the patient in making an accurate record of their perception of the problem. The patient was tamed by the ordering
processes of documentation. The full extent of the relationship between writing and power was evident in the rare instances in which patients attempted to control the recording

[8] See Goffman (1968:32, 73–75, 143–8) on the role of the psychiatric dossier in
effecting disclosure of informational preserves that constitute the private self.
[9] Wheeler (1969: 20) examines the relationship between control of the dossier
and the exercise of power within modern organizations. Foucault (1977:189–90)
briefly discusses disciplinary power in terms of the accumulation of detailed documentary data on individuals.

process themselves. During my study I collected a number of these instances: an assessment interview seriously disrupted when the patient began to take notes on the psychiatrist; the medical records department in crisis when a patient managed to borrow his own case records; a psychiatric panel discussion temporarily suspended because the patient's father, who was angry about the way his son had been treated, started to tape record what the clinicians were saying.

Divisions in the record and the segmented case

The Record of Consultation was divided into parts, each with a separate heading: Referral, History from Mother, History of Presenting Complaint, Presenting Complaint, Mental State Examination, Diagnosis, Duty Doctor's Opinion, and Plan. The interview was oriented to producing such a segmented account and was achieved, in the first instance, by two strategies of enquiry: questions aiming to establish the duration of symptoms and 'forced choice' questions.

The interview was pervaded by questions that rendered the patient's account into time segments: 'How long. . . ?', 'When did you. . . ?' The previous four weeks was a period of time which, introduced initially by Paul [013], came to assume special prominence. Dr George asked a series of 'four week' questions in order to compare Paul's behaviour on drugs with his behaviour prior to taking drugs. Entered in the record, '4/52' [four weeks] circumscribed the Presenting Complaint, separating it from the background information on Paul and his family. It was a temporal division that established a disjunction between the illness and the patient.

Dr George also structured the patient's account by the use of 'forced choice' questions, which offered two alternatives. For example, he attempted to define Paul's experiences as hallucinatory or nonhallucinatory, delusional or nondelusional. Hallucinations, in turn, were forced into mutually exclusive categories: inside the head or outside the head. Paul was asked to choose between two possibilities: that his experiences were owned by him and located in his mind, or that they were not owned by him and located outside his mind. The more that experiences could be located externally, the more evidence there was for the existence of schizophrenia. By these methods of enquiry, the account was divided along the lines of a self/nonself dichotomy.

148 *D*: Mm hm. Maybe I can ask you a few questions Paul?
149   Um, have you been having any sort of hallucinatory experiences at all?
150 *P*: I have been hearing voices. I'm walking along the
151   street, and car lights go on and off. At night time they go off, and they come on again.
152 *D*: Mm hm. What kind of voices are you hearing?
153 *P*: People I don't know. Any voices. The people I know, I
154   don't hear any of their voices. They say, um, 'Do this!'
155   'Do that!' and 'Try not get into this situation', and
156   especially in bed when I'm lying awake, 'cause I have
157   trouble sleeping. I lie awake and I think. I get a
158   headache and can't sleep and I get up, have a drink of
159   coffee, or walk down the park or take my dog for a
160   walk in the middle of the night, then I come back and
161   manage to sleep about three or four o'clock at night in
162   the morning. I wake up about seven and get very active
          and got to move. I've got to keep on the move. I go to
          Yarrami, or I go to Forbes or Nelson or Gloucester and
          I look for drugs. I want to get off the drugs you know
          it's. . . . [deep sigh].
163 *D*: Mm. These voices. What, can you tell me a bit more
164   about them? Are they actually, are they more thoughts in your head?
165 *P*: Well I don't know what. . . .
166 *D*: Or is it coming from outside?
167 *P*: No I think it is thoughts in me head.
168 *D*: Mm hm. You don't hear the voices talking to you like
169   I'm talking to you at the moment, from outside you?
170 *P*: No. Sometimes I hear some of them say, 'Paul', and I
171   look around and there is no one there.
172 *D*: Mm hm. They just, you just hear a voice call your name?

173 *P*: Yeah.

174 *D*: And that's . .

175 *P*: That's all. That's all. That's apart from the imaginary
ones.

176 *D*: Mm hm. The ones in your head you mean?

177 *P*: Yeah. The ones I can talk to. Like me mate Bronco. He
178   died a week before I had me breakdown. I can talk to
179   him spiritually when I'm lying in bed. I can say, 'How
180   are you going Bronco?' and I can say, I can think
he says, 'Really good, how are you?' You know?

181 *D*: Mm.

182 *P*: I can imagine him saying that.

183 *D*: But that's sort of more thought communication.

184 *P*: Yeah. Communication with the spiritually dead.

185 *D*: Yes. Right. But you don't actually hear the
186   voices talking?

187 *P*: No, only when the one says, 'Paul!'

188 *D*: Mm hm.

189 *P*: . . . . [pauses while doctor writes] And I get paranoid
190   when I'm straight, about how, like when I'm walking
191   down the street and I think there's a car coming
behind me or, I don't trust anybody.

192 *D*: Mm. . . . . Tell me more about these
thoughts, in your head.

193 *P*: Well there's nothing. I've told you about as much as I
can about that.

194 *D*: But . . . . are those thoughts your own thoughts?

195 *P*: They could be, I don't know. I can't understand 'em.

196 *D*: Or are they thoughts that are put into your head but
don't belong to you?

197 *P*: I wouldn't say they don't belong to me. I'd say they're
198   trying to contact me. The dead people, the spiritually
dead.

199 *D*: Mm. Mm hm.

200 *P*: They are trying to contact me and help me.

201 *D*: Mm hm.

203 *P*: Like Bronco says, 'Get help! Get help! Help yourself!
204   Behave yourself!' Because he died of an overdose
of LSD.

205 *D*: Did he?

206 *P*: Yeah.

207 *D*: How long ago was that?

208 *P*: Just about two years ago.

209 *D*: Mm.

210 *P*: There was one . . because you know when I found out

211   he died, you know how you get shivers up and down

212   your backbone, well I had that for about two minutes.

213 *D*: Mm.

214 *P*: Usually people only have that for a few seconds. I had

215   it for two minutes and that's when I started drinking
          beer and taking sleeping pills.

216 *D*: I see. How has your appetite been, Paul?

Questions that sought to establish the duration of symptoms or force a choice between two alternative answers had the effect of interrupting and truncating the patient's account. For example, Paul reported that he could talk with his dead mate, Bronco. For Dr George, this did not appear to fit any standard psychiatric category. Was it thought communication [183]? Was it an hallucination [185–186]? Was it thought insertion [196]? Paul was not able to categorize his experience of Bronco within the framework of the options provided by Dr George. Perhaps it was 'communication with the spiritually dead' [184]. More important to Paul was the help he received from Bronco [200–203], as well as the special meaning of Bronco's death [204–214] and its relevance to his own drug use [215]. Dr George's question, 'How long ago was that?' [207] interrupted these themes, for it required a numerical answer. Although Paul tried to persist, a question concerning his appetite and then another about weight loss finally led him to abandon this topic. Such questions cut across the subtleties of meaning, which for Paul established a continuity between the experience of hearing voices and his drug taking. Bronco, because he could not be categorized as an hallucination, an abnormal thought, or a spiritual experience, did not appear in the written record. By excising ambiguous meanings in the patient's account, the doctor's questions rearranged it into a shape that fitted the categories of the case record, leading to 'a stripping away of the lifeworld contexts of patient problems' (Mishler 1984:128).

Dr George's immediate purpose was to record an entry entitled Mental State Examination, but Paul was not familiar with describing his experiences in terms of mental events. He used a range of alternative idioms, including spiritual ones [178–184, 198]. As a result, an impasse developed between him and the doctor [192–195]. Paul felt that he had said as much as he could about the thoughts in his head, and that he did not know whether they were his thoughts or not. He mainly talked about his relationships with his mother, sister, Bronco, friends, stepfather, and biological father. In the record, the extent of these relationships and their interactional richness was missing. Instead there was a description of his mental state, with its seven subdivisions: Appearance, Behaviour, Conversation, Perception, Affect, Cognition, and Insight. The case record thus depicted Paul as if he could be divided into segments. The segments were located at different depths because the Mental State Examination contained a progression from outside to inside—from surface expressions (appearance, behaviour, conversation) to inner mental events (perception, affect, cognition). This reflected psychiatry's aim to fill out the depth dimension of the case. It implied that the more deeply located parts had causal effects on the surface parts. The way patients spoke or behaved was determined by the thoughts or feelings that lay deep within them. Thus in the record Paul was segmented—divided into sections that exerted causal influences on each other.

Separating the illness from the patient

The most striking effect of segmentation was to create a division between the psychiatric illness and the patient. The first step in this process was to record the symptoms of the illness using conventions of writing that established a professional distance from what the patient said. Dr George's questions had an empathic tone in the interview [010, 069], yet the record resembled the results of an interrogation. When Dr George wrote: 'Denied Schneiderian FRS [first rank symptoms] of thought disorder and perception', it was as if he had accused Paul of these experiences or at least suspected him of concealing them. Similarly, 'He thinks he can control and read other people's thoughts' betrayed the sceptical stance of the clinician. Quotation marks and indirect speech were used to this end, as in the following examples from other case records (with emphasis added):

Believes that he is being talked about on TV and radio.
Claimed that mother was poisoning her soup in some way.
Only *admits* to occasional social drinking.
States that he has not taken marijuana for a year.

Thus the empathic closeness of the interview was translated into a sceptical distance in the record (c.f. Cicourel 1968:123). Empathy involved the patient in the production of the record; scepticism allowed clinicians to distance themselves from what the patients said, especially with respect to their psychiatric illness. Their empathy with the patient but distance from the illness began the process of separating illness from patient.

Another method of accomplishing a separation between the illness and the patient was the use of technical idioms. Within the Record of Consultation the language of each division and subdivision progressed toward increasingly technical language. The History was written in intermediate typifications, as if it represented the patient's or family member's 'own words'. 'Examination' was written in a more technical idiom. The same points were rewritten, first in one idiom and then in the next. For example, under 'History' Dr George wrote: 'C/O [complains of] hearing ~~voices~~ a voice occasionally call him "Paul" '. Under 'Examination' it was rewritten as: 'occasional auditory hallucinations of a voice calling his name'. In the transition from intermediate typification to technical term and then to diagnosis—from 'voice' to 'hallucination' to 'schizophrenia'—the patient became separated from his psychiatric illness. The illness was rendered into a language that was remote from the way Paul articulated his experience and that did not allow him to control how it was defined.[10] On the page, 'Paul Lawrence' was written into a box in the top left hand corner, diametrically opposed to the Diagnosis and separated from it by the intervening text.

[10] Compare with Geertz (1983:57) who, following Kohut, distinguishes between 'experience-near' concepts and 'experience-distant' concepts: 'love' versus 'cathexis', 'fear' versus 'phobia'.

This separation of patients from the written account of their illness was ultimately made tangible in the physical distance maintained between patients and their case records. Patients could clearly see their record being read from and added to but could not read it themselves, nor could they contribute directly by writing into it. It was a breach of etiquette for patients to 'peek', and clinicians developed techniques of moving the record along the desk or shielding the page with a hand to deal with this possibility. The document of their illness was visible but inaccessible: it was about them but was kept separate from them.

Passive versus active

In the process of dividing the account into segments, the patient was characterized as passive, in contradistinction to his illness. Schizophrenia and drug abuse were depicted as controlling him and causing his admission to hospital. Psychiatric illness was attributed agency. There was no place in the format of the Record of Consultation to describe Paul as a person who could exert control over his behaviour and those around him. As has been demonstrated, he was defined as an ensemble of parts located in the different subdivisions of the record but with no coherent volition of his own. Thus Paul was rendered a suitable object for psychiatric work and a suitable case for admission.

This characterization of Paul contrasts with the characterization of Dr George who, as the author, appeared in the record as active, in control, and the source of decisions. The record was structured such that the doctor's conclusions (Diagnosis and Opinion) be read as a logical sequitur of the interview data, as if derived by induction. However, I have demonstrated that the transition from data to conclusions was not a process of induction but one of rewriting in increasingly abstract and technical idioms. Dr George started, not ended, the assessment with the confirmed diagnosis of schizophrenia and the suspected diagnosis of drug abuse, which he garnered from his reading of the log book and the case notes, as well as from his discussion with Dr McCusker. Yet these diagnoses

were portrayed as the culmination of his logic. Irrespective of
the contingencies of individual interviews, the record always
portrayed this ideal of inductive logic. In most interviews the
relation between data and conclusions was an interpretive circle, one set of symptoms suggesting a diagnostic pattern that
in turn led to the search for more symptoms and so on. What
was circular in interaction was always portrayed as linear in
writing. The treatment plan was similarly portrayed as flowing
logically from the diagnosis. In the case of Paul Lawrence, the
decision to admit the patient came first, and the diagnosis
legitimated this decision. The sources of this decision were
probably located in the negotiations between Paul, his mother,
and Dr McCusker. His stepfather, who accepted him into the
house on the condition that he go to hospital the next day,
was also a party to this process. In the record it was rewritten
as the DMO's decision and a logical consequence of his diagnostic formulation. The case record was a principal means
whereby clinicians distinguished themselves from patients. In
the record, the clinician was active, was rational, and pursued
a coherent, linear logic,[11] whereas the patient was irrational,
fragmented, and passive.

Shaping the patient's account of schizophrenia by repetition

Written assessments were repeated many times for an individual patient by different members of the team. Repetition focused the patient's attention on aspects of the illness that were
considered clinically relevant. After Dr George had completed
the assessment to admit Paul to hospital, a psychiatric nurse,
Jean Potter, carried out a second assessment to admit him to
the acute ward in Heathfield House. She glanced through the
record until she came to Dr George's notes, then questioned
Paul on the basis of these notes, concentrating on the diagnostic features of schizophrenia (his disordered thinking, the
voices, his paranoid ideas) and his drug abuse. Paul's responses to her questions were smoother and more practised
during this second assessment. By now he was able to list the

---

[11] Goody (1980, 1982) argues that Western logic is a distinctively literate form of
rationality.

drugs he was taking efficiently without the need for an extended sequence of questions and answers, as in the previous interview. In this dialogue, N = Nurse Jean Potter and P = Paul.

106 *N*: And what sort of things were happening?
107 *P*: Oh, I was taking some downers, barbi . . barbs . . barbiturates.
108 *N*: Mmm.
109 *P*: Serepax, Avil car sickness tablets, Mogadon, marijuana, I don't drink.

In contrast to the protracted negotiations with Dr George, Paul succinctly summarized the key attributes of his hallucinations for the nurse.

286 *N*: . . . . Have you experienced hearing voices at all?
287 *P*: Oh a little bit yeah. I don't . . .
288 *N*: Is that just recently?
289 *P*: No I had them before. I don't hear them much any
290   more. I can control them. I tell them to fuck off.
291 *N*: Mm. What, do they speak to you directly or?
292 *P*: No they just tell me, speak to me, imaginary voices.
293 *N*: Mm. . . . . And when was the last time you had them?
294 *P*: I think it was a couple of days ago. Someone yelled out
295   'Paul', and I looked behind me there was no one there.
296 *N*: Mm.
297 *P*: That was the only time. The last time. It was a strong
298   'Paul' too. Like a yell, '*PAUL!*' . . . . . . And I walked up
299   two streets and I nearly got hit by a car.

The responses to Jean's questions began to converge with Dr George's written account. Paul did not raise many of his former concerns with Jean. He did not even mention Bronco. Paul thus learned to abbreviate his account, bring it to a focus on the clinically relevant features of schizophrenia, and omit what he knew the clinicians would find to be extraneous or ambiguous.

Paul had already been admitted to Ridgehaven on three previous occasions and therefore was practised at producing accounts that were relevant to the assessment procedures of the Schizophrenia Team. The encounters with Dr George, Nurse Potter, and subsequent writer-clinicians continued to shape his mode of accounting for his illness. As a consequence of this shaping process, dimensions of patients' experiences that were not captured in the standard definitions of schizophrenia were often ignored.[12] Schizophrenia became a matter of hallucinations, delusions, and thought disorder because these clinical features were the easiest to identify and record (Strauss 1969).

The transformation of the patient's verbal account toward the written account was ensured by the sheer frequency of repetition. During the course of an admission, patients would describe their illness to the Duty Medical Officer, to the trainee psychiatrist who treated them on the ward, and perhaps to a psychiatrist. They could repeat the history of their illness to other members of the Mini Team, including the social worker and several psychiatric nurses, and to medical students as well. Staff rotation and the tendency for brief, frequent hospital admissions accentuated these repetitions. Patients who resisted psychiatric treatment often became angered by this. They would dismissively tell the next enquirer that they had no intention of going over their story yet again, and that if the enquirer really wished to know what the problems were, he or she should go and read about them in the case records. On the other hand, some patients were only too eager to tell the story of their illness. It was through contact with clinician after clinician, each of whom read from the record and solicited responses to be written back into the record, that patients came to know about their psychiatric illness. This knowledge came from rehearsing its salient features in a language that was relevant to the record. Through the cycle of reading, talking, and writing, patients encountered their illness as an object that was separate from them, and they learned how to account for it in a well defined way.

This circular process was particularly relevant to the definition of schizophrenia. Many patients, such as Paul, were not sure which aspects of their experience were caused by schizo-

---

[12] See Chapman (1966) for a study of early symptoms of schizophrenia that are not included in the standard diagnostic criteria for this disorder.

phrenia and which were not. They were not able to establish a boundary between themselves and their illness. When fed through the cycle of reading, talking, and writing, however, they learned that it was chiefly hallucinations, delusions, and disordered thinking—and that it was an entity separate from them. They learned that they were a person who 'suffered' from schizophrenia. Even those patients who did not believe that they suffered from schizophrenia at least knew and could discuss what, according to the record, this schizophrenia was. The cycle of talking and writing provided all patients with a language with which to represent this illness to themselves and others.

There was a counterpoint between repetition and innovation in clinical work. Sometimes nurses felt that their assessments were mere carbon copies of the trainee psychiatrist's assessment. At other times, when asserting the autonomy of their profession, they stated that they were able to throw a new and distinctive light on a case because they approached it from a unique nursing perspective. Jean Potter produced an account of Paul Lawrence that built on what Dr George had written but at the same time contained crucial differences. Her approach was one of intimacy and informality— 'call me Jean'—a strategy the nurses used to encourage patients to confide in them about matters they might not discuss with their psychiatrist. By this relaxed approach she was able to elicit information Dr George had missed, that alcohol consumption was another significant factor. She was also able to relate Paul's use of drugs and alcohol to his feelings of anger and frustration at not being able to find regular employment or maintain a stable relationship with a girlfriend. She elicited from Paul that drug-taking, in turn, had led to feelings of unworthiness. Her written entry did not challenge the diagnosis but added to it. Again she wrote 'schizophrenia' and 'drug abuse' but augmented these entries by noting the issue of alcohol dependence and the relationship between Paul's drug-taking and his personal problems. Thus patients did not hear exactly the same version of their illness over and over. They were exposed to a dynamic version that gradually changed and extended as each clinician added his or her opinion.

'Full work-up': reintegrating schizophrenia and the person

After these admission assessments, patients underwent a more comprehensive form of assessment known as a 'full work-up', which I described in Chapter 4 as the joint enterprise of the Mini Team. Encompassing a person's background, personality, family situation, early development, and biological status, the full work-up aimed to produce a 'fully documented' case. It was carried out on all newly diagnosed patients and those who were admitted for the first time to the Schizophrenia Team. On subsequent admissions to hospital, the intensity of documentation diminished, the exception being those patients for whom a case review was deemed necessary because of their unremitting psychosis or uncontrolled violence. The full work-up had important implications for the way in which schizophrenia was conceptualized. Unlike the admission assessment, which constructed schizophrenia as separate from the person, the full work-up reintegrated schizophrenia and the person.

The respective contribution of each profession to the full work-up is outlined in Chapter 3. The psychiatric component included a full 'organic work-up', consisting of a thorough physical examination, biochemical and haematological screening tests, computed tomography, and electroencephalography. Psychiatry's focus on the inner body extended the reach of schizophrenia into the person's biological core, reflecting contemporary theories of schizophrenia as having a strong biological basis. Similarly, the uncovering of a family history of mental illness located schizophrenia in the person's genetic code, thus pre-existing his or her birth. These biological concepts tended to anchor schizophrenia as a permanent, essential part of the person's identity as a physical being, persisting throughout life, even if only as a potential to relapse. The developmental history was psychiatry's other major contribution to the full work-up. There was some disquiet among psychiatrists that it focused too much on a person's psychopathology rather than his or her successes or achievements. As a consequence, it frequently reconstructed the person as an epic of failures that anticipated the subsequent evolution of schizophrenia. Furthermore, the developmental history some-

times suggested that the person had shown signs of schizophrenia for much longer than was first recognized (Frank
1979:82; Movahedi 1975). Careful history-taking commonly
uncovered earlier, attenuated manifestations of the disorder.
Patients were discovered to have 'schizoid' traits that had manifested in earlier years, having been loners or quiet at school
with few friends. Patients with paranoid delusions were often
recorded as being generally suspicious for many years prior to
the onset of overt delusions. Schizophrenia was present, in
nascent form, from the beginning. According to Burke
(1969a:13): 'the logical idea of a thing's essence can be translated into a temporal or narrative equivalent by statements
. . . of the thing's source or beginnings'. The psychiatric life
history located schizophrenia at the very beginning of case
time and therefore within the very essence of the person.

By means of their capacity to carry out extended observations in a variety of hospital settings, nurses were able to demonstrate how schizophrenia could pervade many aspects of a
patient's daily life on the ward: a tendency toward isolation, a
degree of suspiciousness, aggression toward another patient,
or a loss of motivation. Furthermore, they discriminated between patients who were 'really' psychotic and those who put
on a façade, where the symptoms were seen to be purposefully
enacted. In the latter instance these symptoms were described
as 'largely behavioural', thereby locating them within the domain of voluntary action. Here schizophrenia was not just an
illness from which the person was suffering but an instrument
that he or she could use strategically to manipulate others.

Social workers contributed to the full work-up by investigat-
ing the context of the patient's illness. Beginning with a definition of schizophrenia as a discrete entity located within a
person, the social worker explored its ramifications throughout the person's family and social network. The term 'identified patient' conveyed the idea that the person was merely
representative of an entire system that was malfunctioning.
Links were made between schizophrenia and elements within
this wider system. The 'strange' mother, the 'schizoid' father,
the 'enmeshed' family, or the family with a high level of 'expressed emotion' became factors that were relevant to understanding the schizophrenic illness. Social circumstances, such

as unemployment or poor living conditions, played a part in the overall picture of the illness. Cultural background was often invoked, especially if it was an exotic one, such as 'Vietnamese refugee' or 'Hungarian immigrant family'. By taking these broader factors into account, social workers often broke down the distinction between a person's psychotic symptoms and his or her everyday reality. In particular, delusions were seen to make sense if viewed from the perspective of the person's religious beliefs, cultural style, or idiosyncratic ideas held by the family. By contextualizing schizophrenia in this way, it was accorded a much broader scope and was shown to extend into the person's lived world.

The full work-up thus produced an all-encompassing definition of the case. It explored every facet of the case in space and time. When applied to schizophrenia, this work-up produced a definition of the illness that was similarly all-pervasive. Schizophrenia permeated each dimension of the case. It was located in the person's inner mental state. It arose from the biological and genetic core. It was manifested in behaviour and could be consciously used for ulterior gain. More broadly, it ramified through the person's family and social networks. Schizophrenia also pervaded the temporal dimension of the case, arising from the person's biographical origins and anticipated to be present in the long-term future. Through this bio-psycho-social approach, schizophrenia was equated with the 'whole person'. The total identity of the person was subsumed by the illness. The 'whole person' became a 'schizophrenic'.

The repository of this schizophrenic identity was the case record. The person became a 'fully worked-up case' with a 'well documented history of schizophrenia'. Such extensive documentation stood as a reference point for any clinical staff who might subsequently become involved in the case, even many years later.

Records grew over the years, some extending into multiple volumes. The treating staff tended to conflate the identify of persons with their case records, especially those treated in the hospital for a long time. Some people were described in terms of the quantity and weight of their records, for example, as a 'five-volume case' or a 'fork-lift job'; that is, it would take a fork-lift truck to move the records. Those patients who embraced the schizophrenic identity developed a special investment in their records. They expected new doctors to have read the contents and to know all about them. Some became distressed on learning that their case records had been misplaced. One patient told me with immense pride that she had eight volumes, 'All of it on me!'

Contrasting versions of schizophrenia

The core of this chapter has examined the interpretive processes through which clinical staff at Ridgehaven Hospital constructed a written account of psychiatric illness in the case record. It has demonstrated how the verbal accounts provided by the patient and family were truncated and translated from intermediate typification, to technical terms, and then to diagnosis. The common-sense understandings that underpinned the assessment interviews were excluded, as were the concerns of the patient that were judged extraneous to the written definition of the illness. There were major divisions in the case record, and the patient's account was rearranged to fit these categories and divisions, thereby generating a segmented case. There was no place in this version to describe the patient's behaviour as the result of conscious volition. Instead, it was represented as the consequences of the interactions between the different segments. Clinical writing separated patients from their psychiatric illness. In the written definition of the case the patient was passive, and the illness was active. The patient no longer caused his or her own behaviour; the illness now caused it. Hence there was a parallel between the process of writing and what was written. The patient did not control what was written down, and what was written down construed the patient as lacking control. During the repeated interactions with different members of the team, patients practised this version of their illness. On the Schizophrenia Team, they learned that they had a schizophrenic illness, that this illness was separate from them, and that it controlled them.

The full work-up produced a contrasting version in which there was no longer a separation between schizophrenia and the person. Schizophrenia pervaded all dimensions of the case. Because the team defined the case as a 'whole person', this person's entire identity became pervaded by schizophrenia. Again, through repeated interactions with their treating clinicians, patients learned that they had an illness that had become synonymous with themselves.

Hence the cycle of talking and writing produced two possible versions of schizophrenia that the hospital staff and the patients could use. In the first, illustrated in the analysis of admission assessments, schizophrenia was distinct from the patient. In the second, illustrated in the discussion of the full work-up, schizophrenia was refashioned into a more general principle that pervaded all aspects of the person. In one version the person was defined as a patient who *suffered from schizophrenia,* and in the other the person was *a schizophrenic.*

6

Moral trajectories: from acute psychosis to 'chronic schizophrenic'

When a person was rendered into a written case format, there was little suggestion that he or she was capable of rational, consciously motivated action. Instead, behaviour was explained in terms of antecedent causes, or what Schutz (1972: 91–96) has called 'because' motives: the person acted in this way because of prior developmental influences or stressful life events. A case was a segmented version of a person in which behaviour was portrayed as the product of interactions between family dynamics, genetic predisposition, intrapsychic factors, and biological disturbances. Responsibility for behaviour was not attributed to the person because it was influenced by forces that lay beyond voluntary control. The schizophrenic illness was the most potent of these forces, either controlling the actions of a patient or pervading his or her entire personal identity. This was a deterministic construction that rendered the person a passive object.

When members of the Schizophrenia Team *talked* among themselves about a patient, however, they also drew on a voluntaristic construction that accorded volition to that person.[1] In these accounts the person was perceived as unified rather than segmented—a single source of consciously motivated action. He or she was understood from within a subjective framework rather than treated as an object. Actions were understood in terms of the future outcome that this person sought

---

[1] Deterministic accounts are grounded in the philosophical tradition of materialism, in which, as Burke (1969b:127) shows, action is reduced to laws of matter and motion, and consciousness is reduced to causal forces. Voluntaristic accounts, by contrast, arise from the tradition of idealism, with its emphasis on 'consciousness', 'will', 'the subject', 'mind', and 'spirit' (Burke 1969b:181–227). See Karp (1992) for a more recent discussion of the difference between these two ways of accounting for the person.

to bring about, or what Schutz (1972:28–31, 86–90) called 'in-order-to' motives. For example, in Chapter 4 Miss Treloar was said to have pretended to forget her shoes in order to trick Margaret into driving her home again. She was regarded as capable of exerting control over her own behaviour, over her schizophrenic illness, and over other people. Endowed with the capacity for rational, purposive action, such patients were able to engage in strategic manipulation of others for self-interest. Schizophrenia was no longer a causal force determining their behaviour; it was an instrument they employed to influence the staff or their relatives.

Within this voluntaristic construction, the person became a moral being who was deemed capable of deciding between right and wrong, acting on this choice, knowing what the consequences of that choice would be, and being held responsible for those consequences.[2] Holding people to account in this way entailed subjecting them and their actions to moral evaluation. It created the possibility of 'good' and 'bad' people who behaved 'appropriately' or 'inappropriately'.

The moral evaluation of patients by staff has been the subject of a number of studies in general hospital settings[3] and psychiatric hospitals,[4] but they have tended to regard value judgements as regrettable and antithetical to proper treatment or as evidence of 'institutional pathology' and the failure of psychiatry. By contrast, I argue that the practice of moral evaluation is, in fact, central to hospital treatment. Although technical aspects of this treatment (pharmacotherapy, psychotherapy, or rehabilitation) are important and have received appropriate emphasis in the professional literature, I contend that the central objective of treatment at Ridgehaven was to transform a case of schizophrenia into a person who could be held responsible for his or her actions.

[2] This explanation accords with McHugh's (1970) criterion of 'theoreticity' in the common-sense ascription of deviance, whereby the actor is 'said to have known what he was doing by having acted in consideration of a rule; that is, he will be held responsible because he intends to do what he does' (1970:78).

[3] See Roth (1972) on moral evaluation and its relation to the control of hospital clientele. Studies addressing this issue have been carried out by Glaser and Strauss (1964, 1965), Duff and Hollingshead (1968), Lorber (1975), Jeffrey (1979), Dingwall and Murray (1983), Mizrahi (1985), and Liederman and Grisso (1985).

[4] See Stanton and Schwartz (1954:280–300), Belknap (1956:163–92), Strauss *et al.* (1964: chapters 5 and 12), and Goffman (1968:117–55).

In this chapter I examine how the staff of the Schizophrenia Team sought to effect the transformation from a deterministic to a voluntaristic construction, from a case to a morally competent person. I show how this transformation, of necessity, involved assigning motive, responsibility, and value. I suggest that the discussions that took place among the staff about their patients were vital to the processes of evaluation that brought about this transformation. Whereas clinical writing was the medium of case construction, clinical talk was the medium of moral evaluation. This analysis is thus developed in counterpoint to my analysis in Chapter 5 of how the clinical staff wrote about patients in the case records.

Moral trajectories and clinical talk

The idea of a trajectory was implicit in the way members of the team evaluated a patient's progress and recovery. I have used the term 'trajectory' in preference to 'career' because the latter concept has been associated in the sociological literature with the progressive passage of a group of people through a series of clearly demarcated stages and statuses to a more or less definitive endpoint (Goffman 1968:119ff; Roth 1963:94). However, for patients with schizophrenia the stages of recovery were never clearly defined, and the endpoint was indeterminate. The concept of a trajectory enables an analysis of the more fundamental movements on which the career concept is based. By trajectory I refer first to a movement through time. The patient was defined in terms of a time frame that took into account when the illness started, how many relapses had occurred since then, and what the anticipated future outcome might be. The trajectory was also a passage through space. The patient moved through the physical spaces of the hospital with their graduated levels of surveillance—from closed ward to open ward, to half-way house, to independent living in the community. At Ridgehaven, spatial metaphors were employed to locate psychotic patients out of their mind or away from mundane reality. The trajectory of recovery also involved a return journey through this metaphoric space.

Although the physiological unfolding of a patient's schizophrenic illness made a significant contribution to his or her
trajectory, my focus is on the 'trajectory work' (Glaser and
Strauss 1968; Strauss 1982:257) carried out by team members:
monitoring a patient's progress, encouraging the patient toward independence, making sense of a relapse, or lowering
expectations of recovery. There were two typical trajectories.
A normal, valorized trajectory was one in which the patient
complied with the treatment and worked toward recovery. An
abnormal, devalued trajectory was one in which the patient
did not make the expected recovery and came into conflict
with the treating staff. Chronic patients were anomalous because they lay outside the normal or abnormal trajectories and
the moral values implied.

Assigning moral value to patients was difficult for the hospital staff, especially when it involved devaluing them, because
it was incompatible with the professional injunction to be
'nonjudgemental'. On the other hand, to describe patients in
technical terms risked objectifying them to the extent of de-
nying their human qualities. Both extremes were avoided in
the case record because it was constrained by peer review and
judicial scrutiny to a style that was neither conspicuously theoretical nor judgemental. By contrast with writing, talk was
subject to less constraint because it lacked permanence and
accountability. Hence it was through discussions with one another that members of the Schizophrenia Team could objectify or devalue patients using terminology that would have
seemed outrageous to them had it been written in the record.

The staff categorized their spoken language as either 'professional' or 'unprofessional'. They likened the language of
professional talk to that of the case record, whereas unprofessional language contained words and phrases that could never
be written. The professional mode was more formal and was
used in situations where there was a marked social distance
between the speakers. The unprofessional mode was informal
and would be used among staff members who saw their relationship in terms of equality and solidarity. It was used between friends or team members. Professional talk consisted of
technical terms such as schizophrenia, whereas unprofessional
talk included lay terms such as 'crazy'. Objective versus sub-

jective was another contrasting pair employed by staff to distinguish these modes. By objective, they meant a clinically accurate description of the patient, uninfluenced by the staff member's own emotions or attitudes. By subjective, they referred to their 'true feelings' about the patient. The staff regarded the professional mode as nonjudgemental, and the unprofessional mode as judgemental.

I observed and recorded this unprofessional talk as it occurred, interspersed with professional language, in clinical discussions that took place out of earshot of patients: at team meetings, at case conferences, and in the staff tea room. My analysis is not directly concerned with therapeutic talk between clinicians and their patients but with those discussions among clinicians about their patients which formed a backdrop to individual therapeutic interactions. Whereas there were efforts made to teach professional concepts of illness to patients, a similar attempt to teach them the unprofessional concepts would have been inconceivable and regarded by the staff as absurd. To be overheard by a patient while engaged in unprofessional talk was one of the extremes of embarrassment for a clinician. Evaluative language was withheld from patients, but I demonstrate in a subsequent chapter how the staff conveyed to them the underlying values of responsibility, self-control, and self-worth.

Normal trajectory and work

From 'off' to 'settled'

When describing a person with schizophrenia who was judged to be extremely psychotic, members of the Schizophrenia Team employed a constellation of spatial metaphors that located the person away from the self and away from the mundane world of the hospital. A person might be described as 'not with it', 'out of it', 'out of his tree', 'away with the birds', 'away with the fairies', 'off in her own little world', 'off the air' or 'off the planet'. Some were described as 'climbing up the walls' which was understood to mean that they were pacing the floor in an agitated manner. These phrases were applied to patients who, in a more professional mode, would be termed 'acutely psychotic', 'grossly thought disordered', 'overtly delusional', or having a 'florid schizophrenic illness'. When a person by the name of Luke was first admitted to the Schizophrenia Team the staff described him as 'completely spaced out' and they nicknamed him Luke Skywalker, in joking reference to a character in the film *Star Wars*. The terms 'high' or 'high as a kite' were used for people with a manic aspect to their illness, but when the diagnosis was one of schizophrenia the person was simply located 'away' rather than above. Many technical terms take root from this spatial metaphor. Thus 'paranoia' is etymologically based on the idea of a person being beside, beyond, or out of his or her mind, 'hallucination' is derived from the Latin, to wander in thought or speech, and 'delirium' means going off the track or out of the furrow (*OED*).

The expression 'off' most succinctly conveyed the idea that the person was spatially away, as in the following observation made by a nurse to another nurse about Trevor, a person who was extremely psychotic:

> Trevor is really off at the moment. He's just sitting in the TV room alone, laughing and giggling at something to himself.

The expression was ubiquitous, woven into clinical discussions in all settings, formal and informal. When I drew attention to it by asking members of the team what 'off' meant, they would characteristically reply they had not stopped to think about it. When they did reflect on the various instances in which they used it, they were able to provide the following contextual rules for its use. First, it was employed to convey a sense of gradual deterioration culminating in florid psychosis, as exemplified by the way a social worker informed a trainee psychiatrist about the worsening condition of a mutual patient, a fifty-six-year-old woman with a diagnosis of schizophrenia:

> Mary's been gradually going off over the last two to three months, and now she's right off. She's wearing a hat with corks dangling from it and says she's joined a comedy troupe! I really think we should do something about it.

Second, 'off' connoted a cluster of idioms that centred on a lay notion of madness. A person who was 'off' could equally be described as 'mad', 'crazy', 'mad, mad, mad', 'mad as a cut snake', 'silly as a wheel' or commonly, 'He's so mad he's just beautiful'. Many of these idioms cast the person as a non-human object. One configuration depicted the acutely psychotic person in food imagery, such as 'bananas', 'crackers', 'nuts', 'a real fruitcake', or 'as nutty as a fruitcake'. Animal metaphors were employed, as in the term 'batty' (and its extended version, 'bats in the belfry') or the above example of the snake. The term 'snake pit' has often been used to refer to a ward for the containment of severely psychotic patients, but at Ridgehaven Hospital, this ward was referred to as the 'wombat farm', thereby invoking an Australian image of a dull, slow, yet potentially dangerous creature. With all these terms the person was assigned a lowly position on a Darwinian gradient from primitive to developed, from lower plant or animal species to a higher human species, from nature to culture. Not only was the person away in a spatial sense, they were dehumanized by being likened to members of other species.

Like 'mad', 'off' also referred to the possibility of violence and danger. With this usage, the patient who was going 'off' was likely to attack the staff or other patients. When building up to this point, the patient was said to be 'escalating', a term that combined a concept of intensification with an ascending image. If escalation culminated in uncontrolled violence, the patient was described as having 'gone off', connoting a cataclysm. Patients who were building up to this state were also likened to an impending explosion that would unleash uncontrollable mechanical or natural forces: 'She's like a time bomb about to go off at any moment' or 'He's like a volcano about to erupt'.

A sudden change from balance to imbalance was implied by variants such as 'gone off his rocker', 'gone off the deep end', or 'gone over the edge'. The image of a person becoming unbalanced informed a range of related terms such as 'tipping up', 'tipping over', 'flipping over' and 'falling out of his tree'.

All of this terminology evoked extravagant and vivid imagery, which reflected the often bizarre quality of the psychotic behaviour that team members were trying to describe. These patients did not simply exhibit the most severe schizophrenic illnesses on a spectrum from mild to severe; rather, they appeared to lie beyond the spectrum altogether. This notion of excess could not be conveyed using the sober language of illness. Instead, it was captured by the use of superlatives such as 'mad, mad, mad', ecstatic expressions such as 'beautiful', and eruptive, explosive imagery. Even when professional phrases were used, they were qualified by the extravagant adverbs 'acutely', 'grossly' and 'floridly'. All hyperboles posited that the person was so unpredictable, uncontrolled, dangerous, and bizarre that he or she inhabited a realm beyond illness and beyond clinical description.

The term 'off' always had pragmatic implications. It was used to activate fellow team members to intensify their surveillance, treatment and control of this out-of-control patient. In the first example cited, the nursing staff observed Trevor more carefully and administered additional antipsychotic medication. In the second, the trainee psychiatrist admitted Mary to hospital for observation and stabilization. At times of immediate danger, when nurses found it necessary to galvanize a concerted response within seconds, it was this terminology—'he's gone right off'—rather than professional language that was employed exclusively. Unprofessional terminology was an index of solidarity among staff members, as in these circumstances all faced the same risk of injury irrespective of rank or profession. Here this language achieved the common, urgent, practical purpose of confining the patient to a locked ward and controlling the danger.

The converse of 'off' was 'settled', as exemplified in the following discussion between three members of a Mini Team: the psychiatrist Elaine, the trainee psychiatrist Chris, and the nurse June. They were discussing Geoffrey, a patient who had been admitted to hospital two weeks previously.

> *Elaine*: I've put Geoff back on his Modecate, 25 milligrams, and ... um ... some chlorpromazine. He's only ever had fluphenazine before so I thought I'd try something different. He *is* settling down isn't he?
> *Chris*: He's still as delusional, but he's not presenting it.
> *June*: No he's not as angry or as pushy.
> *Elaine*: I think just some time to settle down a bit. That's what he needs.

Whereas 'off' referred to madness, imbalance and explosiveness, 'settled' meant sanity, stability and calmness. Anger and the risk of violence could 'settle', as could hallucinations, delusions and thought disorder. The patient who was 'settled' might be described as 'quiet', 'compliant', 'approachable', 'interacting well on the ward' or 'comfortable', these words and phrases describing cooperation with nursing ward authority, or what Goffman (1968:137) called the 'ward system' of control. Antipsychotic medication was given in part to help patients settle; conversely, compliance with this medication was an important indicator that they were settling. Sedatives, as the word implies, were given to help the patient settle at night.

Within metaphorical space, patients were depicted as having returned to themselves and to the mundane world. Thus such a person would be described as 'much more settled within himself', 'with it', 'back to reality' or 'facing reality issues'. It usually implied a descent, for they settled down rather than up. When patients were being treated for mania this was made explicit in the expression 'coming down from a high'.

The pragmatic significance of the continuum from 'off' to 'settled' was related to the nursing practice of applying 'pressure'—placing increasing expectation on a patient to conform to the rules of the ward, to participate in the programme of organized activities, to take increasing responsibility for the management of day-to-day tasks such as washing clothes, and to face those problems in his or her life known as 'reality issues'. 'Pressure' forced the person back to the mundane world which, according to the particular nursing version of reality, involved him or her in dealing with interpersonal conflicts and problems of daily living. The application of pressure was titrated against the position of that patient on the range between 'off' and 'settled'. As patients began to settle, pressure was applied gently at first and later with increasing intensity. Fine distinctions were often made during the early phase of settling, when a patient might be described as 'settled but fragile'. It was commonly said of a patient at this stage, 'If you put too much pressure on him and talk to him about reality issues, he immediately tips up'.

Planning to move the patient from one ward to another or to discharge the patient from hospital was chiefly predicated

on the extent to which he or she had settled. This criterion
was more important than any of the more formal criteria such
as the presence of hallucinations, delusions or thought disorder. Even if these clinical features were still present, a patient
who was settled would be moved from higher to lower zones
of surveillance and confinement: from locked to open ward,
from acute to subacute ward, from hospital to home. One
patient, for example, was permitted to take weekend leave
from the hospital because he was 'settled, though still quietly
mad'.[5] Another patient was discharged 'silly as a wheel but
compliant'. Placing pressure on patients to settle reflected the
policy of brief admissions and early discharge that aimed to
prevent institutionalization. The ideology of progress that pervaded Ridgehaven was applied to patients as well as the institution, propelling them toward rapid improvement and early
discharge.

'Settling appropriately', as the proper passage from 'off' to
'settled', was perceived by members of the Schizophrenia
Team as a normal trajectory. This trajectory referred to progressive recovery through time. The first phase required induction into a recognized sick role and, in the case of those
who appeared to be so 'off' they were beyond illness, the unprofessional language of the Schizophrenia Team members
captured them and drew them into this sick role. That is,
where the professional terminology of 'illness' and 'schizophrenia' was too moderate to describe a patient, it was backed
up by an extravagant unprofessional language of 'madness'
and 'craziness'. In the process of adopting a sick role, patients
began to comply with the staff view that they did indeed suffer
from a severe illness that was undesirable, and that they should
cooperate in its treatment, as classically described by Parsons
(1952:436–7). For patients with schizophrenia, becoming a
unified person was an important aspect of recovery: they were
said to be 'reintegrating'. Demonstrating rationality was another: they were deemed capable of rational choice, having
recovered sufficiently to make 'reality based decisions' about
their lives. As patients recovered, they were attributed responsibility and the capacity to bring themselves, their illness, and

---

[5] Compare with the category *loco tranquillo* (Rogler and Hollingshead 1965:216).

their propensity for unpredictable violence, under control. At the beginning, they were described using deterministic language, but as they progressed along the trajectory they were increasingly described using voluntaristic terminology. Within the spatial metaphors that I have identified, the trajectory described a movement from 'elsewhere' to 'here'. On the evolutionary scale, it was a progression from subhuman to human. Finally, the trajectory referred to a patient's movement across the hospital space from closed ward to community. Thus the principle of a trajectory organized and amalgamated concepts of recovery from psychosis, the imagery of a return through metaphoric space, and a progressive movement through the hospital into a single temporal framework. In figure 6.1, this normal trajectory is represented by the dotted line.

Work and the positive evaluation of patients

Patients who followed this trajectory were highly regarded by the staff because they were a testament to the value of the Schizophrenia Team and its work. At the beginning of the

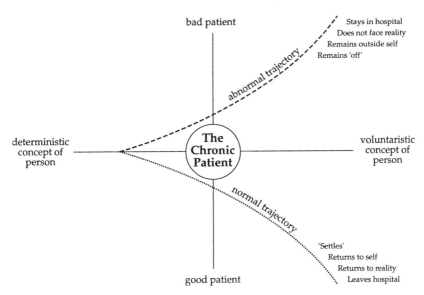

Fig. 6.1. Normal and abnormal trajectories from psychosis to recovery.

trajectory, when manifesting florid thought disorder and obvious hallucinations, these patients exemplified the accuracy
and validity of diagnostic work and were accordingly designated 'fascinating', 'interesting', 'classic' or 'textbook' cases.
In reference to one such patient, a trainee psychiatrist in-
structed a medical student: 'If you ever doubted the existence
of schizophrenia, go and talk to her for a few minutes'. Some
were so highly valued they were referred to as 'good teaching
material'. As they began to settle appropriately, these patients
were valued by the nursing staff because they conformed to
the ward routines, participated in the various treatment programmes, and did not interfere in the day-to-day organization
of work. They cooperated with the plan of management and
were described in the nurses' hand-over meetings as 'using
the ward appropriately' or 'no management problem'.[6] Recovering patients had a special value as the ones who 'made
it all worthwhile' and 'restored your faith in psychiatry', as
there were many patients whom members of the Team believed they were unable to help significantly, especially those
who were repeatedly readmitted to Ridgehaven Hospital. In
sum, patients were valued to the extent that they proved the
worth of the team and its work.

Patients were also evaluated in terms of their own ability to
work, by which I refer to the performance of psychological
work on themselves and their schizophrenia; 'working on her
problems' or 'working on his illness' were phrases characteristically applied to good patients. Using an idiom derived from
psychoanalysis, the staff often said that such patients were
'working through' their problems. There was a closely related
expectation that they should suffer from their illness and its
symptoms. Treatment itself could also cause suffering, as in
the idea of making painful decisions in order to get better.
The idea of a 'struggle' combined notions of hard work and
suffering. Patients who 'struggled' against their illness and
who 'fought hard' to recover were portrayed as entering into
battle with their schizophrenia. In this version, schizophrenia

---

[6] Compare with Lorber's (1975) study on good patients and problem patients.
For the staff of a general hospital, good patients were those who were uncom-
plaining and cooperative, and who did not disrupt ward routines or unduly absorb staff time.

retained its status as a separate entity and causal force, and it was cast as a foe that could be vanquished by the allied struggle of patient and staff. Finally, work could also refer literally to wage labour, for the most prized patient of all was the one who managed to re-enter the work force. When this happened, the staff who had been involved in the treatment would proudly announce the patient's achievement to their colleagues. Thus patients were reincorporated into the dominant value system of work.

The value of a patient was independent of the severity of the psychosis, as illustrated by the following discussion about an outpatient, Rex. The discussion took place at the end of a case conference between Elaine, Chris, and Alan, the social worker on the Mini Team.

> *Elaine*: As far as the outpatients go, the only person we're having problems with is Rex. He's very very psychotic. He seems to be managing as an outpatient, but only just. With sort of little crises every now and then.
>
> *Chris*: I saw him this morning. He's a bit off beam [said with ironic understatement]. What do you do with someone like that anyway?
>
> *Elaine*: Have a look what medication he's on . . .
>
> *Chris*: I mean there are people in this unit that aren't as bad as what he is.
>
> *Elaine*: No, but he's . . . he's hanging in out there, which is worth preserving. His prognosis isn't really that good, so I think if we can keep him out of hospital that's better. But no, what we need to do is . . . um . . . sort of do a decent case review of his past management and his present management and see if we can organize something a bit more satisfactory.
>
> *Alan*: There's a lot of, um, um, friction going on within the family because his brother is bringing a girlfriend home who is not very polite towards Rex, and it means very much to him that somebody says hello to him and talks to him and does not ignore him completely. I think because he doesn't like his . . . this present girlfriend he really gets very very angry. And then of course it upsets the whole family. He's rather a capable person I think, and interested in various things, knows phrases from various languages, and generally I feel, interested in cars especially, and wants to get a driver's licence. But he does express a lot of anger.

> *Elaine*: You can see why. He lives a fairly miserable kind of an
> existence at the moment.
>
> *Alan*: And he was brought up properly by his family. He's
> fairly well mannered, and then he sees people who just
> aren't polite. That really really upsets him. I like Rex, I
> think he's a nice man.
>
> *Chris*: Is he prone to aggressive outbursts?
>
> *Elaine*: Yeah. He doesn't actually hit people though, he just
> bumps the wall or kicks things. He's actually quite con-
> trolled . . . considering.

In this discussion, the team built up a picture of a worthwhile person who, in despite his unremitting psychosis, was making an effort to manage his illness outside the hospital and to control his potential for violence. He was a patient who suffered a miserable existence because of his schizophrenia and as a result of other people's prejudicial behaviour. He was characterized as well mannered and properly brought up, a capable person with a range of interests and a specific project (to get a driver's licence). Rex was worth the extra work of a decent case review in order to preserve his ability to live outside the hospital. Even though he was unlikely to make a significant recovery, he affirmed the values of suffering, work, and progress.

The trajectory I have described was thus a moral trajectory because it rested on a set of values—suffering, work and progress—and was the principal conceptual scheme through which the staff attributed worth to patients. It was a normative trajectory for the patients because it entailed obligations to conform. It was a normal trajectory for the staff insofar as it provided them with a template of the typical manner in which psychotic patients recovered, and the typical characteristics of the person who demonstrated this recovery (c.f. Sudnow 1965: 255).

Abnormal trajectories and play

'Settling too quickly' and 'not settling'

The staff of the Schizophrenia Team were alert to deviations from the normal trajectory (illustrated by the broken line in

Figure 6.1). These variations in the time frame of expected recovery were known, respectively, as 'settling too quickly' and 'not settling'. When patients were described as settling too quickly it was implied that they must have been 'putting on' symptoms in order to gain admission to hospital and, having achieved this objective, no longer needed to maintain a pretence of illness. According to the nursing staff, these patients quickly became 'too comfortable' and 'too settled'. They 'fitted in too well'. Within the spatial metaphor, they had descended too far. One was described as 'digging himself in' and of another it was said, 'He's beginning to put down roots; we'll have to put a bomb under him and get him mobile'.

When a patient was not settling, it was possible that the antipsychotic medication was not yet effective and the schizophrenic illness was still actively causing symptoms. Yet if this failure to settle persisted, the more common explanation was that the patient was purposely 'using' his or her symptoms to remain in hospital and thereby avoid facing problems in the outside world.[7]

In either instance, settling too quickly or not settling, these patients' trajectory across the hospital was the reverse of the expected steady outward movement from the locked ward to the open ward and then home. They actively sought to remain in hospital, and some even appeared to behave violently to make sure they were confined in a locked ward. They divested the staff of the power to confine them because they themselves sought confinement.

Irrespective of whether the rate of settling was too fast or too slow, patients were attributed the same capacity for voluntary intentional action as they were in the normal trajectory. As can be seen in Figure 6.1, both trajectories signified a passage from determinism to voluntarism. However, unlike those who conformed to a normal trajectory, these patients were conceived as engaging in what Goffman (1970:85–145)

---

[7] Compare with Braginsky, Braginsky, and Ring (1969:49–76, 160–2) who studied how patients voluntarily controlled the expression of their symptoms in order to pursue rational outcomes such as achieving or avoiding discharge. Their research presupposes a model of the patient as a rational, resourceful individual capable of manipulating others and controlling his or her fate. However, this model is just one among several that emerge from the culture of the hospital itself.

calls 'strategic interaction'.[8] They were attributed a scheming form of rationality that they used to oppose the work of team members, as epitomized by the phrases 'using his delusions', 'using his illness as a weapon' or 'sabotaging treatment'. They seemed to exert an improper influence over their own trajectory, slowing it down or reversing it. They were typified as 'controlling', 'manipulating', or 'using', and it was often commented, 'There is method in his madness'[9] or 'He may be mad but he's not stupid!'

There was a stock of typical motives that staff attributed to these patients (c.f. Jehenson 1973) because a psychiatric hospital was not, at face value, a desirable place to seek admission. For example, 'peripatetic schizophrenics'—patients who travelled from state to state within Australia—were frequently construed as 'putting on a few timely delusions and hallucinations' in order to secure free accommodation in the hospital while awaiting the arrival of their next welfare payment. A social worker might relate how the patient had previously feigned illness until the very day on which the welfare cheque arrived, only to suddenly leave the hospital. The following excerpt from a newspaper report illustrates this cynical view:

> Young men with schizophrenia are using psychiatric hospitals as hotels, a senior New South Wales doctor says. Lismore Base Hospital Medical Superintendent Dr Rob Griffin said doctors were aware of many young schizophrenics who travelled between Melbourne and Cape York. When their pension cheques ran out, they checked into the nearest mental health service for accommodation.

Patients who lived in unpleasant boarding houses or hostels were also interpreted as 'playing on their illness' to secure the more convivial accommodation of the hospital or to take advantage of the forty-day period of free lodging in order to save their rent, perhaps to buy a small luxury item such as a radio.

[8] See Ditton (1980) for discussions of Goffman's 'strategic' model of the person and its relation to the idea of 'homo economicus'. This model 'emerged from economics and gives in explicit form the economic actor as a rational, calculating, egoistic individual, matched against other individuals in competitive and bargaining situations' (Collins 1980:192).

[9] See also *Hamlet* Act II, scene ii:375 and Act III, scene iv:187 (Shakespeare 1951: 1028–73).

When the patient was viewed as strategic or manipulative, the staff adopted a tactical response rather than a therapeutic one. Instead of assessing symptoms with a view to treatment, they assessed them in terms of the patient's imputed aims, resourcefulness, and credibility. A patient might be admitted directly to a 'paying' ward and thus be charged for the cost of accommodation from the first day in order to dissuade him or her from using the illness for monetary gain.

The concept of time that underlay a normal trajectory was not explicitly defined by the staff. Broadly speaking, there was an expectation that patients should settle in weeks rather than days or months; but within these parameters there was considerable flexibility in deciding whether a patient was pursuing a normal or abnormal trajectory. A patient, three weeks after admission to hospital, might be viewed as settling appropriately, with the positive value that state implied; another, who had been in hospital for the same period, might be viewed as 'not settling'. The underlying temporal framework of each trajectory contained sufficient latitude that time could be used in a flexible way to assign positive or negative value to the patient. Thus by locating a patient between 'off' and 'settled', members of the Schizophrenia Team were not only recording the 'natural' evolution of their schizophrenic illness; they were also beginning the process of reconstituting the case as a person and investing him or her with moral value.

There were additional nuances and permutations of this terminology. For example, 'settling too quickly' could be viewed as an instance of the patient 'not settling' if he or she were judged to be 'covering up' underlying delusions and hallucinations in order to gain early release from hospital. Here the patient was also seen as operating strategically, but in this instance to escape from the hospital and the appropriate commitment to treatment.

Play and the negative evaluation of patients

Compared to the restricted range of terms that attached positive value to patients, there was a rich diversity of colourful idioms that carried a strong negative value. This disparity did not mean that members of the Schizophrenia Team spent a

disproportionate amount of time devaluing patients but reflected a striking elaboration of cultural meanings to deal with
those patients and situations that were highly problematic.

Whereas the ideas of work, suffering, and struggle formed
a framework of understanding patients who trod the normal
trajectory, patients whose trajectories deviated from normal
were understood in terms of play and pleasure. There were
several senses in which the term 'play' was used (see Ehrmann
1968:31–57). First was a dramaturgical sense in which patients
were viewed as play-acting. The nurses, with their capacity for
extensive and systematic observation, were in the best position
to contrast the rational behaviour of such a patient with his
or her ability to enact illness in order to 'impress' the psychiatrist. The patient was typified as 'playing on her delusions',
'performing for his doctor', 'putting on crazy talk', 'playing
mad', or 'putting on theatricals'. Other patients were observed
to be 'quite sane' for most of the day but 'acting crazy' when
in the company of family members who had come to visit
them. Nurses would joke about nominating these patients for
an Oscar, or holding a competition for the best actor of the
month.

In the strategic model, 'play' referred to a competitive or
adversarial idea of making moves to maximize rewards (Goffman 1970:101). The patient was described as 'playing games',
the games in question being those of 'beat the system' or 'use
the system'. The 'system' referred to the hospital as an organization for the delivery of professional care to the deserving
sick. Patients who played games were construed as 'con artists'
who purposely exploited this care and thereby gained an advantage over the hospital staff. Because the game involved
skill, they were commonly referred to as 'skilled manipulators'.

In a third sense of 'play', the patient was compared to a
mischievous child who was 'playing up'. This usage referred
to the purposeful but minimal infringement of ward rules
known as 'niggling', 'stirring', or 'getting a rise' out of the
staff, the imputed purpose being to goad staff into reacting
unprofessionally by getting angry. In Oakley House, the closed
ward, nurses made finely tuned distinctions between 'tipping
up' and 'playing up'. Tipping up was beyond the patient's
control and required emergency physical constraint and major

tranquillizers. Playing up lay within the patient's conscious control and required sanctions such as limit setting, ignoring, or discharge from the ward. When violence was judged to be playing up, the patient would be held responsible and a monetary charge levelled if there was damage to property such as a broken window.

Just as work involved suffering, play implied pleasure and self-indulgence.[10] Some patients appeared to relish their illness and were thought to resist treatment because they enjoyed their hallucinations and delusions. To define schizophrenia in terms of pleasure was threatening for the team members, as it undermined the idea that illness involved suffering. They faced the additional problem of patients enjoying aspects of their treatment. Psychiatrists and trainee psychiatrists were cautious about prescribing minor tranquillizers because some of them could have euphoric effects. Among young patients there was a brisk trade in these tablets. They were referred to as 'uppers', a term that drew on the implicit spatial metaphor. The patients used them to get high rather than pursue the desired downward trajectory to reality and recovery. Not only were the patients perverting drugs of therapy by redefining them as drugs of pleasure, but they were also using them to make money. Furthermore, they were starting to exert control over the distribution of psycho-pharmacological agents, one of the principal sources of psychiatric and nursing power. The prescription of anticholinergic agents was also a significant problem because they too enjoyed a reputation as 'uppers'. They were used to treat the side effects of antipsychotic medication, one such side effect being an acute dystonic reaction, a sustained involuntary extension of the neck and elevation of the eyes. When a patient was observed with neck extended or eyes elevated, it was necessary to evaluate whether this represented a genuine, involuntary acute dystonic reaction or a voluntary enactment of side effects (known as 'putting on the look ups') in order to obtain these drugs.

It was thought that some patients redefined the hospital itself in terms of pleasure. They regarded it as a place of residence rather than a place to work on their treatment. They

[10] See Estroff (1981:233) on patients who 'enjoyed their craziness'.

seemed to 'move in' and 'make themselves at home', and were characterized as 'liking the hospital too much', 'using the place as a motel', 'coming in for a holiday' or, in joking reference to a chain of holiday resorts, 'joining the Club Schiz'. This attitude undermined the basic assumption held by the staff that the hospital was a work space, a place where professional people worked together with psychiatric patients to treat their schizophrenia.

The patients who were characterized as having a trajectory that deviated from normal were those who exhibited active and knowing resistance to professional power (c.f. Wright & Morgan 1990). They undermined the psychiatric definition of schizophrenia by redefining its symptoms as enjoyable. Instead of working on their illness they played with it. Treatment was pursued for pleasure not for the alleviation of symptoms, and they appeared to treat Ridgehaven itself as if it were a resort rather than a hospital. They were regarded as abusing scarce professional resources for personal gratification, and they were therefore treated as undeserving of care. In failing to show any improvement and in actively working against recovery, they were a testament to the ineffectiveness of the Schizophrenia Team and its therapeutic work. Professional power was exercised in part by controlling the gateways of the hospital—the admission and discharge of patients and their movement from ward to ward. Yet these patients were thought capable of wresting this control away from the staff. Instead of suffering from their schizophrenia they artfully used its symptoms to manipulate the staff and to exert control over admission and discharge decisions.

A patient stereotype that epitomized resistance to psychiatric authority was the 'professional patient'. Professional patients were characterized as 'manipulative' and 'controlling', as 'skilled', 'consummate' and 'resourceful', and as 'survivors'. They accrued too much 'book knowledge' of schizophrenic symptoms from the patient education programme. They knew, for example, the Schneiderian first rank symptoms of schizophrenia and were said to 'cotton on' to these symptoms very quickly, then 'trot them out' when seeking admission. They were, to use a hospital cliché, 'bad not mad'. Professional patients also accrued a detailed knowledge of the hospital staff.

They were reputed to be familiar with the personalities of staff members and even the details of rosters. They knew 'the system'. They had 'been around too long'. They were said to know when kind-hearted or inexperienced doctors were on duty and use this information to choose the right time to manipulate admission to hospital. A nurse described one man as follows:

> He's very well educated in this sort of field; he knows the ropes almost too well. He's picked out roles for all of us. He's been here before.

A handful of patients at Ridgehaven so epitomized these 'professional' attributes that they came to serve as negative stereotypes. One of these, David Morrison, became a classificatory category within the hospital in his own right, such that when other patients showed minor degrees of resistance or play-acting they were regularly described as a 'budding Davey Morrison'.

The danger represented by professional patients was that they wrested power from the staff, especially the power to define their illness and control their location within the hospital. Calling them 'professional' acknowledged this status because it attributed to them qualities ordinarily associated with clinicians: rationality, specialized knowledge of schizophrenia, familiarity with routine hospital procedure, control over admission and discharge. However, to use the term 'professional patient' was itself regarded by the staff as unprofessional because it was sarcastic. It devalued those patients to whom it was applied. By denigrating them it neutralized their power, redefined the distinction between staff and patient, and reasserted professional power.

These patients could be described in the formal diagnostic language of psychiatric illness,[11] but such a description was insufficient to control the danger they posed. They had already coopted this language, played with it, and used it to manipulate the hospital staff. The only recourse available to the staff was to move outside their professional language al-

---

[11] The formal diagnoses of 'malingering' and 'factitious disorder' addressed the possibility of conscious deception, but their use was discouraged because they had a pejorative tone (Hay 1983).

together and describe patients in an unprofessional way. It was only in this mode that they could construe patients as deliberately and consciously employing their schizophrenia for ulterior and, as far as the staff were concerned, nefarious purposes.[12] Earlier in this chapter I showed that unprofessional language ('off', 'crazy') was used to capture patients who were too extreme and too 'mad' to be defined simply as sick using sober professional terms. Likewise, in this instance, unprofessional language ('skilled manipulator', 'professional patient') served as a backup to professional terminology, as it captured patients whose deviance and resistance placed them outside the sick role. It was also linked to the pragmatic task of disengaging the team from such a patient. This could range from withdrawing sympathy and therapeutic effort to actively bringing sanctions to bear on the patient. Defining someone as a professional patient activated a 'strict limit-setting' approach and was a prelude to discharge (c.f. Mizrahi 1985).

Members of the Schizophrenia Team were conscious of these explicitly unprofessional terms that openly devalued patients. Their use was characteristically framed by laughter or accompanied by justifications such as, 'I know we're taught not to use these words, but he can only be described as crazy'. Laughter and justification indicated that the usual demeanour of professional concern and empathy was temporarily suspended, but that this was unavoidable. Thus an unprofessional description of the patient was usually followed by a comment on the illegitimacy of the terminology and then a final justification of its use. These three steps might be paraphrased as follows:

1. This patient is quite crazy.
2. As a professional, I should not say things like that.
3. But it is excusable, given the stress of working with schizophrenics.

Justifications were commonly couched in terms of stress. It was an understandable 'release of tension' or 'coping mechanism'

---

[12] In a professional mode it was legitimate to analyze symptoms in terms of their 'secondary gain' or in terms of the 'defensive functions' they served, but such formulations implied that the patient was not consciously aware of the gain, nor deliberately making use of schizophrenia.

for those working with 'schizophrenics' because they were regarded as notoriously difficult to treat: 'If we did not let our
feelings out from time to time, we would end up crazy like
them'. Again, unprofessional language and its justification acknowledged the danger of category confusion, where instead
of patients becoming professional the staff went 'crazy'. The
paradigm of 'stress' and 'coping' also legitimated unprofessional language by redefining its use as a necessary part of
clinical work: 'If we did not vent our feelings, we would not
be able to go on treating them'. Such explanations further
devalued the patients because they argued that no person
could be expected to deal continually with acutely psychotic
'schizophrenics' and survive unscathed. At the same time, they
pointed to the essentially human qualities of the staff members, as in the commonly stated rider, 'We have feelings too
—we are only human'. Thus the contrast was enhanced between the staff as quintessentially human, and the patients as
something else.

Moral evaluation as a reflection of context

Apart from the few patients who served a stereotypical function, it was not possible to identify and count the number of
'professional patients' at Ridgehaven. To attempt such an exercise would be to misunderstand the processes of moral evaluation. Most patients had an ambiguous mixture of positive
and negative qualities. Moreover, the same patient might be
described as 'settling appropriately' by some staff and 'not settling' by others. The trajectories and their associated stereotypical characters were employed to ascribe value to patients
in a way that was dependent on context.

Contexts of consensus

The staff tea room in Heathfield House was one context in
which moral judgements of patients were initiated and stabilized. It was a room in which team members relaxed momen-
tarily between episodes of work and suspended their clinical
demeanour to talk about what they had been doing outside

working hours. Yet the tea room, despite its apparent casualness, was also recognized as an important work site: a good place to find a fellow team member, make her a cup of coffee, and talk over a problem patient with her. The informality of the setting gave licence to talk in an unprofessional mode for which the speaker could not be held accountable. It was thus used to introduce statements that explicitly devalued patients. The communal and relaxed atmosphere of the setting facilitated the development of a consensus among the staff about the moral worth of these patients. Once initiated and stabilized in the tea room, this view of the patient could then spread to other contexts and be inserted, for example, into a case conference, but using less judgemental language. In this way, what was first mooted in an informal setting could achieve definition in a more formal setting.

Evaluative terminology reflected on the staff who used it as much as it described the patient. Whereas academics published papers decrying the use of unprofessional language (see Papper 1970), practising clinicians were not such purists. For them, its use could be a marker of experience and astuteness. To employ terms such as 'professional' or 'manipulative' was a signal to fellow staff members that one was not about to be taken in. It also served as a signal of hard work and efficiency. Those who employed such language were demonstrating their ability to move patients through the hospital, to target the deserving ones, and not to waste valuable resources on those who could not be expected to benefit. These staff members were admired for 'getting in there', 'sorting the patients out', and 'getting them moving'. Conversely, the use of unprofessional language could be seen as a symptom of 'burnout' and the development of a cynical attitude toward patients. The skilled use of unprofessional language thus identified the speaker as efficient rather than wasteful, caring rather than dismissive, canny rather than naive.

When establishing solidarity with one another across boundaries of profession and rank, staff members frequently used evaluative terminology. They might portray patients as skilled manipulators who knew how to play the system. The Chief Executive Officer, for example, began to work in the back wards of Ridgehaven as part of a project to discharge long-staying patients into community accommodation. He was appreciated by the nurses because he took time away from administrative responsibilities to work closely with those patients who had the most severe and chronic forms of psychiatric disorder. An alliance was developed with the ward nurses around the idea that some of the patients were using their illness to control the staff. He fostered this alliance by distributing an article, 'The Weapons of Insanity' (Ludwig and Farrelly 1967), which described the various techniques that patients could use to this end.

As a medium of solidarity, unprofessional language was a key to induction into team membership. When a new member (for example, a trainee psychiatrist) joined a Mini Team, there was an expectation that case discussions were conducted in a professional mode. Established team members indicated their acceptance of that novice when they began to talk to him or her about patients using judgemental statements, calling one patient 'an absolute pain in the neck' or another a 'real little sociopath'. It was a licence for the trainee to describe patients in the same way. Thus socialization into clinical psychiatry through team work involved the acquisition of competence in the judicious and timely devaluation of patients.

Moral definitions of patients were fragile and subject to change. Effecting that change was an important aspect of psychiatric work. Moral rescue was a recognized form of work that involved selecting a patient with a long-standing reputation of diminished social worth and making an intensive effort to improve the patient's functioning. This usually implied a criticism of other staff members for having underestimated and discarded the patient. The value of the patient was thereby transformed from negative to positive, and he or she was reassigned to a trajectory of progress and improvement.

Ambiguity and conflict

Conflicting evaluations were frequent.[13] When there was conflict between professions, perspectives polarized, with psychi-

---

[13] Compare with Stanton and Schwartz's (1954:197, 363) discussion of apparent consensus in the context of polarized views of a patient.

atrists usually taking the view that the patient was suffering
from schizophrenia, and nurses or social workers arguing that
the patient was using the illness for personal gain. Conflict
within professions, too, was fought out on this polarity, as illustrated by the following example. Two nurses became engaged in a protracted conflict over the control of a Day Patient
Centre. The first nurse, Jim, had been associated with the Centre for several years and was regarded by most of his colleagues
as integral to the running of its programmes. He was treated
as the nurse in charge though he was not officially designated
so. The second nurse, Sue, was a newcomer to the Schizophrenia Team. Shortly after her arrival, the relationship between Jim and Sue became openly discordant. Jim argued that
Sue lacked a professional approach, and Sue said that Jim was
too authoritarian. Their conflict was viewed by others as a
'clash of personalities'. Sue did not accept the authority of Jim
and regarded herself as an equal. Eventually Jim, unable to
tolerate the situation any longer, arranged with the nursing
administration for a transfer to the acute ward in Heathfield
House. Sue became the unofficial charge nurse of the Day
Centre. This outcome was not a resolution but a 'standoff',
and each continued to be critical of the other.

During the period of this new arrangement, they shared
responsibility for a patient who spent part of his day in the
acute ward and the other part in the Day Centre. This patient,
whom I have called Kosol Vong, was a young man, originally
from Cambodia, who was unable to speak English. His diagnosis was unclear, although it was thought that he was probably suffering from a schizophrenic illness. The possibility of
temporal lobe epilepsy had also been raised, though the results of electroencephalography were equivocal. Frequent attempts to interview him employing a Cambodian interpreter
failed to clarify the diagnosis. He had become a long-standing
management problem for the team. He walked about constantly during the day with an unusual loping gait and would
sometimes walk backward. He was considered a danger to himself because he was at risk of walking backward onto a nearby
road where he could easily be injured by passing cars. It was
difficult for the nurses to engage Kosol in any programmed
activity.

The definition of this problem patient, whose diagnosis was already unclear, became the arena in which the conflict between the two nurses was played out. Was his behaviour caused by schizophrenia? Was it unconscious? Was it put on? Was he just playing up, trying to annoy the staff? Did he want to avoid leaving hospital? Jim argued that although Kosol was clearly ill the main problem was that he was 'playing on his illness'. According to Jim, he was responsible for his actions, and the appropriate management was to set strict limits on his behaviour. By contrast, Sue was convinced that the patient was not responsible for his behaviour, which she considered might be due to epilepsy. The appropriate management, according to Sue, was to tolerate his behaviour and pursue the investigation and treatment of the epilepsy. Kosol Vong became suspended between polarized definitions. While in the Day Centre his behaviour was tolerated, and while in the ward it was not. Little resolution was achieved in this standoff, and there was little resolution in his condition. Though Sue and Jim lobbied for support among fellow team members, neither was successful in having their definition of Kosol Vong accepted as the consensus view of the team. Their colleagues came to regard their respective opinions more as a reflection of their interpersonal difficulties than as a valid definition of the patient.

As with many patients whose illness was ambiguous and who became the focus of active dissent, the problem of Kosol Vong was addressed by means of humour and mimicry. Another member of staff could mimic his loping gait with uncanny accuracy and periodically amused fellow staff by 'doing Kosol Vong.' There were two interpretations of the patient combined in this performance. In one (a deterministic construction), he was represented as driven by forces outside of his conscious control, as if he were a puppet or a wind-up doll. The other voluntaristic construction represented him as an artful manipulator whose facial expressions betrayed the fact that he purposely 'just missed' bumping into objects and was 'putting on' this display for the benefit of staff. Usually the performance was followed by further discussion of the difficulty of knowing what was wrong with Kosol Vong, how to treat him, and the general problem of uncertainty in the construction of patients with schizophrenia. When patients were construed as enacting symptoms, staff members countered it by enacting the patients.

Anomaly and the 'chronic schizophrenic'

Deterministic and voluntaristic constructs

The ambiguity thrown into relief by Kosol Vong, dramatized by the team humorists, and disputed by antagonists within the team was contained within all chronic patients, though it was not so conspicuously displayed and debated. The deterministic construction of the passive sufferer and the voluntaristic construction of the calculating strategist were interwoven in most formulations of chronic patients. A case discussion of one such patient, Gloria, exemplified this composite definition. The discussion involved Elaine, the psychiatrist, Chris, the trainee psychiatrist, June, the nurse, and Alan, the social worker.

> *Elaine*: Right. What about Gloria?
> *Alan*: Gloria doesn't actually want to return to her, er, to the hostel. She's never liked it there and she's had a run-in with the manager. But she may change her mind so we'll allow her a few days before we start doing anything.
> *Elaine*: I don't want her in hospital too long if we can avoid it because she gets too dependent on it, and then she starts worrying that when she goes out things will get worse. What seems to have happened is that she got the 'flu and got quite ill and then her hallucinations got worse and she never quite picked up. And like a good girl she got herself [admitted] . . . you know, presented herself to hospital. What medication is she on now?

A number of possible changes to her medication were canvassed and the discussion then continued.

> *Elaine*: We'll have to sort all that medication out and try to come up with something. How long has she been at the hostel?
> *Alan*: About a year now. The main thing that's keeping her there is that it's near the beach. When her family come to visit her there the children enjoy going to the beach.
> *Elaine*: That's the other thing. Her son hasn't been visiting her so much.
> *June*: Yes, his child is still in hospital.

> *Elaine*: Do you think she would be better somewhere else?
> *Alan*: We'll try something else perhaps. I think it's worth a try.

Plans were made for her discharge that week lest she become too comfortable in the hospital, but two weeks later she was still there and her case again came up for discussion.

> *Elaine*: Well what about Gloria? What's happening to Gloria?
> *Chris*: Well she's still the same, from her mental state point of view. And we're just waiting for a bed to come up in a hostel on the sea front.
> *Alan*: It should be some time this week.
> *Elaine*: [addressing two medical students]: She's a lady with a very chronic schizophrenic illness who's still suffering from a lot of hallucinations despite the medication that she's on. She describes the voices and what they say to her very clearly. The voices say very unusual things, and it's a challenge to keep a straight face.

The team approached Gloria as a strong-willed person who could decide for herself where she would live and who had the ability to act effectively on these decisions. Disliking the hostel, she had organized her own admission to hospital; and if not guarded against, she was capable of engineering a long stay because she would not want to leave. She had a mind of her own and the potential to change it, so much so that the team members waited on her firm decision before proceeding. On the other hand, she had a chronic schizophrenic illness and suffered from prominent hallucinations, which had become worse as a result of a viral illness and the reduced contact with her family, both factors being beyond her control. She was both suffering and willful—controlled by her schizophrenia and in control of her situation. Her management involved reviewing the antipsychotic medication to treat the hallucinations more effectively while taking into account her wishes and her potential to take control over the discharge decision.

Outside time and trajectory

Gloria epitomized chronicity insofar as she was 'still the same' week after week, and the discharge plans appeared to have fallen into a void. When patients and their schizophrenic illness were categorized in terms of normal and abnormal trajectories, emphasis was placed on the passage of time as an indicator of change, progress, and movement, be it too fast or too slow. For chronic patients such as Gloria, however, the passage of time no longer marked change. They were neither positively evaluated as 'settling appropriately', nor were they evaluated as 'not settling' with its implied resistance to treatment. The notion of a trajectory was inappropriate in such cases because they had come to a standstill.[14] There was no evolution toward independent living, as chronic patients were permanently established in a family home, a boarding house, or a psychiatric hostel. The most severely ill were 'stuck' in the hospital back wards, unable to be discharged. In the spatial sense of a trajectory, these patients had no clear track or destination.[15] Any change in their circumstances took place between two alternatives at the same level (for Gloria, from one hostel to another) and did not represent progress. If there was any sense of trajectory preserved for the chronic patient, it was either one of gradual deterioration or, in the light of Bleuler's (1974) follow-up studies, gradual amelioration over the years; but these long-term predictions were vague, and there was no definitive endpoint.[16] For the chronic patient, the passage of time signified stasis and indeterminacy rather than change.

A subgroup of chronic patients who were repeatedly admitted and discharged were known as 'revolving door' patients. They gave the superficial appearance of change as they came and went, but in fact they were going round in circles and making no progress. Revolving door patients were often depicted as rebounding mechanical objects. They were described as 'yo yos' or as 'bouncing back' into hospital as soon as they were discharged. They might go to a hostel only to be

[14] The idea of coming to a standstill was also applied to staff whose careers had ceased to progress. The shared image was that of 'burn-out', because it was equally possible to speak of a 'burnt-out' staff member as it was to speak of a 'burnt-out schizophrenic'.

[15] Compare with Roth's (1963:20–21) study of tuberculosis hospitals during the 1950s, where the chronic patients were classified as separate from the numerical system of graded privileges and progress toward discharge. They were conceptually outside the timetable and were described in spatial metaphors of stasis ('dead end', 'side track') and banishment ('tubercular Siberia').

[16] Compare with Comaroff and Maguire (1981:117) on childhood leukaemia, where unpredictability of outcome leads to a pervasive uncertainty, and the child becomes an 'ambiguous blend of "illness" and "normality"'.

'bounced back' to Ridgehaven as if they were a ball. Indeed, treatment of these patients could be referred to as 'playing ping-pong'. The exact number of admissions to hospital was not counted, nor was the total time spent in hospital calculated; rather, the patient was loosely characterized as having had 'multiple admissions' or having spent 'the last ten years in and out of hospital'. This lack of arithmetical precision was not evidence of poor accounting, as the data were readily available in the case records. Such vagueness was essential to defining patients as chronic because it enabled team members to invoke the image of an object oscillating back and forth but 'going nowhere'.

Because chronicity did not refer solely to the duration of illness, it took on other meanings. When a schizophrenic illness was severe, it was described as chronic. An illness of similar duration but less severe in nature was more likely to be described as a 'long-standing schizophrenic illness'. By contrast, an illness would be categorized as chronic within months of its onset if the symptoms were unremittingly severe and refractory to treatment. More important than its reference to the passage of calendar time, chronic was thus a synonym for severity.[17]

In Chapter 5 it was demonstrated that schizophrenia could stand separate from the patient as an illness from which they suffered, or it could pervade their personal identity so they became a 'schizophrenic'. Chronicity was, strictly speaking, a quality of the schizophrenic illness. Yet in the same way it often came to qualify the person as a whole, usually when the time frame of the schizophrenia became so indeterminate that it merged with the life-span of the person. A person could become a 'chronic patient', a 'chronic case', a 'chronic schizophrenic', or just a 'chronic'. Like the illness, the patient as a whole was suspended in an indeterminate position outside time and trajectory. The failure to demonstrate recovery and progress was thereby located in the person rather than the

---

[17] Harding, Zubin, and Strauss (1992) commented on how the meaning of 'chronic' has diverged from its Greek root *chronos*, showing that it primarily conveys an expectation of deterioration and deficit when paired with schizophrenia, despite substantial evidence to the contrary from a number of long-term studies. See also Jimenez (1988).

illness. The following type of interchange was frequently heard when one staff member asked another about the progress of a chronic patient:

> How is George Thompson going?
> George Thompson is . . . George Thompson.

Anomaly and value

The 'chronic schizophrenic' was an anomaly. This category partook both of a deterministic model of the patient as a passive sufferer and a voluntaristic model of a person as an active controller. In Figure 6.1 the category is represented at the midpoint of the horizontal axis. I have also argued that 'chronic schizophrenics' were not conceptualized in terms of normal or abnormal trajectories and therefore were not morally evaluated on the basis of compliance or resistance to treatment, or on their capacity for work or play. They were not necessarily valued positively or negatively; they were neither model patients nor professional patients. Accordingly, in Figure 6.1 the category is located at the midpoint of the vertical axis. The 'chronic schizophrenic' was quintessentially interstitial, located conceptually between the normal and abnormal trajectories and at the intersection of the moral axis and the axis linking models of the person. Patients were partly exempt from responsibility for their schizophrenia and partly responsible for its ongoing severity; they were motivated to comply with treatment and control their illness, yet they also appeared to use their illness to secure the ongoing privileges of being served by the hospital staff. It was not possible to understand the 'chronic schizophrenic' in terms of a sick role because this category of person was located in an interstitial position between roles.[18]

The values attributed to chronic patients differed from those I discussed in relation to the moral trajectories. They were often described in diminutive and patronizing terms as 'a real favourite of mine', 'a sweetie', 'a pet', 'a harmless old

---

[18] Parsons (1952:438) himself implied that the sick role did not apply to chronic illness when he wrote that exemption from social obligations was temporary. Following Freidson (1970:234), many have subsequently argued that the sick role is an inappropriate concept for understanding chronic illness.

thing', 'a dear', 'a gem', 'an absolute delight' or, as with Gloria, a 'girl'. Unlike first admissions, chronic cases were of less interest to clinicians because they had already been worked up by others, sometimes many years previously. Like a well worked mine, the 'chronic' had nothing new to offer the staff and added precious little to their accumulated clinical experience. Instead of striving to elicit symptoms by chipping away or prising them out, the staff watched as these symptoms flowed out unchecked. The therapeutic task changed to one of helping the chronic patient hold in their hallucinations and delusions. No longer the prize of diagnostic discovery, symptoms could become a source of amusement: when Gloria spoke about her voices it was difficult to keep a straight face. In many instances, symptoms were redefined from valued objects to rubbish, from 'material' to 'stuff'. Patients who remained actively psychotic over years were described as 'coming out with all that delusional rubbish', 'carrying on all the time with psychotic gibber', or 'going on with ratty talk all day long'. They were often depicted as having a 'head full of rubbish'. These were the same symptoms that earlier in the patient's career might have excited clinical interest and been described as 'fascinating'. In Elder House, the main back ward of the Schizophrenia Team, the nurses regularly made pleas for 'better quality patients'. They believed the staff from other areas of the hospital were using Elder House as a 'dumping ground' for the hospital's 'rubbish', and complained of having a 'ward full of grots'.[19] (The term 'grot' was derived from the word 'grotesque' [*OED*] and at Ridgehaven referred to 'chronics' who made a mess of the the ward by spilling food or by incontinence of urine or faeces.)[20] Just as the chronic illness was depicted in metaphors of rubbish, so the person also became rubbish.

People with chronic schizophrenia were not devalued as bad patients; they were devalued and diminished as uninteresting and polluting because they were anomalous. Treating them with disinterest, patronizing them as mildly amusing, or taint-

[19] Compare with Dingwall and Murray's (1983) discussion of 'rubbish' in hospital accident departments.
[20] Equivalent categories in American general hospitals include 'gork', 'crock', and 'gomer' (George and Dundes 1978).

ing them as rubbish, served to reinforce the basic categories with which the staff worked: the trajectories, their values, and the moral order of the hospital. According to Douglas (1966: 39), 'avoiding anomalous things affirms and strengthens the definitions to which they do not conform'.

This analysis is relevant to psychiatric disorders other than chronic schizophrenia and may be compared to the work of Arney and Bergen (1983) on alcoholism and chronic pain, Karp (1992) on affective disorder, Pollock (1992) on adjustment disorder, and Tiller, Schmidt and Treasure (1993:679) on anorexia nervosa. In 'Patient Role and Social Uncertainty—A Dilemma of the Mentally Ill', Erikson (1957) showed how the person with long-term mental illness became trapped between the pull of opposing expectations: on the one hand to enter into a voluntary contractual agreement with staff and on the other to be incompetent to enter into such agreements. 'In the grip of these discrepant expectations, his behaviour was likely to be a curious mixture of the active and the passive, a mosaic of acts which tended to confirm his competence and acts which tended to dramatize his helplessness' (Erikson 1957:265).

Time, space, and chronicity

In this chapter I have examined the working models of person and illness used by the clinical staff when they talked about their patients at case conferences, in corridors, and during coffee breaks. I have argued that the moral evaluation of patients was not epiphenomenal; it was central to the therapeutic work of monitoring progress and effecting a transformation from a case of schizophrenia to a person who was in control of the illness and who could be held responsible for his or her actions.

To this end, the major organizing concept used by the staff was the trajectory, and my analysis has demonstrated the system of values in which normal and abnormal trajectories were embedded. In contrast to the static idea of the role, the trajectory is a dynamic concept that has enabled me to to examine the central importance of time in the evaluation of patients. A remarkable feature of the way trajectories were applied in practice was the flexible rendering of time. There was significant latitude in determining when a patient had settled and a characteristic indeterminacy of time in the description of chronic patients. Time was not used as an absolute chronological measure but was moulded to the purpose of evaluating patients. As a malleable resource, time could accrue different values according to the practical task at hand. It signified progress and recovery (or relapse and resistance) for patients located on trajectories. However, for patients who were outside these trajectories, it signified stasis, severity, indeterminacy, and aimlessness. In psychiatric work, time was never absolute; it always carried value.

The focus on trajectories has pointed to the salience of spatial metaphors in the understanding and description of acute psychosis. It was as a state in which the person was located metaphorically outside the mundane world and outside the self. Though bodily present, he or she was 'away with the fairies', and the process of recovery involved returning to mundane reality and reentry into the self.

The focus on trajectories has also thrown light on the importance of temporal metaphors in the definition of chronic schizophrenia. It was understood as a state of severe illness and stasis in which the person was located beyond the passage of time, as it normally signified change and progress. Whereas acute psychosis was located outside social space, chronic schizophrenia lay outside social time. The meanings associated with chronicity spread from the schizophrenic illness to the person. The 'chronic schizophrenic', I argued, was constituted in the interstices between voluntaristic and deterministic constructs, partaking of elements from both the normal and abnormal trajectories. The 'chronic schizophrenic' was an anomalous category of person.

7

Historical formulations of schizophrenia: degeneration and disintegration

With its university affiliation, Ridgehaven exemplified a modern psychiatric hospital. It was a site for the accumulation and treatment of patients with mental illness as well as a site for the production of knowledge about mental illness. Between episodes of treating patients, practitioners read journals, undertook research projects, and wrote scientific papers and books about schizophrenia.

The template for institutions such as Ridgehaven, which combined treatment with university teaching and research, was developed in Europe over the course of the previous century. In this chapter I trace the rise of the modern psychiatric hospital from its origins during the late eighteenth century to its subsequent encounter with the university in the late nineteenth century. From this evolving infrastructure, a new moral and scientific discourse on mental illness arose, and schizophrenia was among the most important diagnostic categories to emerge from this discourse. My purpose here is to gain an understanding of the core ideas that comprise schizophrenia by exploring the institutional milieu and intellectual climate within which such ideas first became conceivable. I identify two themes within nineteenth century thought that made it possible for a concept of schizophrenia to emerge. One is a literary-clinical concern with the individual and its obverse, the disintegrated person; the other is a politico-clinical preoccupation with progress and its obverse, degeneration.

This chapter is not intended to be an exhaustive treatment of the origins of psychiatry. Rather, it is a sketch for a history of the present: its focus is limited to the core elements of schizophrenia that have maintained currency, and I conclude the chapter by showing their ongoing relevance for the clinicians and patients of Ridgehaven.[1]

When specifying the historical and cultural underpinnings of schizophrenia, I am not debasing or diminishing the category, nor seeking to reduce it to the status of artifice or fiction. Here I distinguish my approach sharply from Szasz's polemics of schizophrenia as 'myth' (Szasz 1973;1976), which rests on a misunderstanding of myth as falsehood and tends to negate the experience of patients by implying that they are lying. By contrast, my approach assumes that patients who report psychotic experiences are not lying. Schizophrenia is not a fabrication. It is a historically constructed category that captures, constitutes, and shapes reality.

The person

The concept of the 'person' is one focus of this analysis. Psychiatric thinking about schizophrenia is structured within a framework of Western thought about what it is to be a person. The 'schizophrenic' becomes the antithesis of the idealized person or, more characteristically, is thought of as part person, part nonperson.

Following an essay in 1938 by Marcel Mauss (1985), this topic has been a focus of anthropological inquiry, based on ethnographic observations that in various cultures entities other than living humans are considered persons (for example, deities, ancestors, spirits, animals). Furthermore, a person is not always an individual (for example twins or descent groups), and not all living humans are necessarily considered persons (slaves or embryos). The comparative literature identifies several attributes or capacities that are universal and fundamental to the concept of person. The capacity for interpretation is the most fundamental of all and is closely tied to the ability to use language (Taylor 1985:271). A person is an entity capable of interpreting the actions of others and, as a corollary, can be interpreted by others as engaging in meaningful

---

[1] By 'history of the present' I refer to the method of 'isolating the central components of political technology today and tracing them back in time' (Dreyfus and Rabinow 1982:118–25).

action (Pollock 1985:7). By using interpretation as the primary criterion, we have a definition grounded in social interaction. That is, a person is, *ipso facto*, located in the social order. Fortes asserts that 'the notion of the person in the Maussian sense is intrinsic to the very nature and structure of human society and human social behaviour everywhere' (Fortes 1981:288). To be located in the social order is also to be located in a moral order. Hence a person is an entity that can be held morally responsible for its actions, be subject to sanction, and be attributed moral value by others.

The ideology of individualism, though not unique to the West, has played a major role in shaping the concept of the person in modern Western society. It is necessary to distinguish between the *individual* as a human organism and *individualism* as an ensemble of cultural values (La Fontaine 1985: 126). By individualism I refer to ideas and policies that sanctify uniqueness, independence, freedom, privacy, self-reliance, and self-development (Lukes 1973) and that are promoted by institutions of the modern state: private enterprise, political parties, organized religion, and medicine. The individualistic person is autonomous, with a distinct boundary that separates him or her from society and from nature (Strathern 1981: 168–9). Internally, the individualistic person is indivisible, as suggested by the derivation of the word. This is an atomistic concept of the person as a unified centre of conscious experience (Hirst and Woolley 1982:105) and a unified centre of moral responsibility (Clay 1986:3).

The origins of individualism have been variously traced to capitalism,[2] German Romanticism, the Enlightenment, the Reformation, the Renaissance, mediaeval mysticism, early Christianity, and even Epicurianism.[3] Idealist historians have stressed the importance of Christian thought, especially since the Reformation, when the individual was attributed the capacity for direct communication with God and therefore defined in terms of subjective consciousness. Foucault (1977: 135–228) takes a total departure from this subject-centred rea-

[2] See Marx and Engels (1975:120), Kolakowski (1978:163–71), and Pashukanis (1978) on the idea of the 'egoistic individual' defined in terms of consent and contract between autonomous economic units.

[3] See Dumont (1986), Lukes (973:40–5) and Macfarlane (1978:196).

soning as the apex of Western thought on the essential features of humanity. Instead, he seeks to identify the conditions within which the individual is constituted as a subject, and he finds these conditions within 'disciplinary society'. The various institutions of 'discipline'—prisons, schools, barracks, hospitals, asylums—are administered by experts whose function is to discriminate between normal and abnormal persons. Individualizing the person by such means as the examination, report, case record, and life history becomes central to the execution of this function. Foucault asserts that these institutions, their ideas and practices, are integral to advanced capitalism: they are sites for the production of individuals who can be deployed usefully as labour.

The importance of individualism, however, is often overestimated. It is easy to assume that individualism is uniformly embraced by all subcultures and classes and by both genders, thus failing to recognize that it is a specific ideology promulgated by specific institutions within Western society. There is an alternative and equally pervasive concept of the person as an ensemble of parts.[4] This concept is exemplified by the common-sense notion that a person is made up of various component roles, for example, mother, wife, and working woman, and that in an ideal situation the person can balance competing obligations:[5]

> We carry on a whole series of different relationships to different people. We are one thing to one man and another thing to another. There are parts of the self which exist only for the self in relationship to itself. We divide ourselves up in all sorts of different selves with reference to our acquaintances. . . . A multiple personality is in a certain sense normal. (Mead 1934:142)

These ideas have their biological counterpart in scientific and popular beliefs about heredity, according to which a person is seen as a composite of nature and nurture, or a combination of characteristics inherited from maternal and paternal genes.

---

[4] Compare with Marriot (1976:111) on the 'dividual' concept of person, based on ethnographic work in an Indian context dominated by Hindu thought.
[5] This common-sense idea is reflected in anthropological formulations of the person as 'a complex of social relations' (Radcliffe-Brown 1952:194) and sociological formulations of the person as a 'role set' (Merton 1957).

When put together, the individual and the ensemble form a concept of the person as a tension between whole and parts.[6] A spatial metaphor is invoked, as if the person could be represented by a circle or a sphere, with a clearly demarcated external boundary and an interior that can be divided into sections.

Harris (1989:604) has argued that our idea of what a person is also contains an implicit time dimension—a trajectory or a biography—that is crucial to the ascription of moral value,[7] because only when there is continuity of identity through time can someone be held responsible for past actions. As a broad generalization, the ideal person in Western culture is frequently characterized in linear terms of development, evolution, progress, or career—from young to old, from simple to complex, from lower to higher. It is not always an ascent, as society not only invests but also divests, as Fox and Willis (1983:129–30) have shown in the case of the terminally ill, the demented, the comatose, and the 'brain dead'.

A whole–part spatial image and an ascending, linear temporal image are two ideas that underpin our common-sense notions of what it is to be a person. Furthermore, they are reproduced by the professional person-definers of modern Western society: philosophers, psychologists, and social scientists among others. Psychiatrists have played no small part in the definition of the ideal modern person by their focus on its obverse, the mad person. Thus in temporal terms the 'schizophrenic' is characterized by deterioration rather than progress. In spatial terms, instead of being a unified whole the 'schizophrenic' becomes a disintegrated person or, where disintegration involves a division into just two fragments, a split person.

---

[6] 'But we know today', writes Durkheim, 'that the unity of the person is also made up of parts, and that it, too, is capable of dividing and decomposing' (1965:305 fn). See also Hawthorn (1990) on the Western person as both unified and fragmented. He associates indivisibility with romanticism and fragmentation with post-modernism, whereas I argue that both have always been implicit in modern Western concepts of the person. See also Ewing (1990) on whole–part conceptions of the person in contemporary anthropology and psychoanalytic theory.

[7] This point was first made in Fortes' (1981) classical account of how personhood is attained by degrees over the course of a lifetime; only after death can a Tallensi become a full person.

Nineteenth century psychiatric institutions and ideas

Nineteenth century institutions and a new discourse on mental illness

The birth of modern psychiatry took place during the last years of the eighteenth century, although the institutional conditions that made it possible, notably the 'Great Confinement' of vagrants, paupers, the insane, beggars, and idlers began in Europe two centuries before (Foucault 1967:38–84). Administrative and legislative attempts had already been made to sort out this miscellany—to distinguish between the criminal, the lunatic, and the pauper—mainly driven by the need to discriminate between the incapacitated and the able-bodied. It was a preoccupation of the rising bourgeoisie to maintain the stability of the labour market, and this meant ensuring that those capable of work did not receive poor relief (Scull 1979: 37–9). The asylum emerged during the late eighteenth century as a reform of these earlier institutions. Because of historical and political differences, it took different forms in France, Germany, England, and North America. Yet in all four countries the blueprints for the state management of the insane were drawn up during the Enlightenment, the first institutions started to appear during the last three decades of the eighteenth century, and the final consolidation of the asylum system occurred between the 1820s and 1850s. These developments were part of the wider emergence of modern state institutions. For example, they occurred in parallel with the evolution of the modern hospital as a new locus of medical practice in Paris, Vienna, London, and Dublin (Ackerknecht 1982:145–56).

'Moral therapy' was the specific reform movement that created asylums out of the older institutions. Its intellectual roots lay in the ideas of John Locke and the empiricist tradition, which held that man is essentially malleable. If knowledge is derived from experience (which largely comprises sensations that have their origin in the external world), it follows that a person may be modified through such experience (Miller 1980:76). The movement developed in England, promoted at first by William Battie[8] and then by Francis Willis,[9] who used this form of treatment on King George III. It drew on Protestant thought, especially that of Methodists such as John Wesley and Quakers such as Samuel Tuke, who established the Retreat near York as a model institution of moral therapy. Moral therapy also drew on the Romantic movement, with its concern for sensation, passion, and the idea of over-excitement as a cause of madness. It took hold in France well before the Revolution, but it was Pinel,[10] drawing mainly on English sources,[11] who grafted it into the revolutionary spirit of egalitarian humaneness and gave it the effusive sentimentality of French Romanticism (Goldstein 1987:119). Pinel's influence was quickly felt in the German-speaking countries, a translation of his work being made in 1801, the year it was first published (Peters 1991:60). Moral therapy became an American enthusiasm during the first half of the nineteenth century, and by mid-century it swept full circle back to England as the nonrestraint movement championed by John Conolly.

Moral therapy replaced physical treatments such as purging, bleeding, spurts of cold water, ducking, and rotating, with treatments that worked more selectively on the intellect and emotions. The first step was isolation from society to harness the curative power of 'nature' and to protect the individual from disordering and exciting sensations, especially those of modern civilization, which were regarded as pathogenic. The patient was then exposed to philanthropic humaneness, a model of patriarchal family authority, a strict regimen of emotional self-control, and farming work, which connoted the virtue, integrity, and bucolic simplicity of a bygone age. External restraints were replaced with internal self-restraint. The model

---

[8] Battie was a Governor of Bethlem Royal Hospital from 1742, the proprietor of a madhouse opened in 1754, the author of *Treatise on Madness* published in 1758, and president of the Royal College of Physicians in 1764 (Doerner 1981:39–48).

[9] Willis, the proprietor of a private madhouse in Lincolnshire, was originally a cleric who was persuaded to qualify as a doctor. He became hugely influential throughout Europe after his successful treatment of George III's madness and his subsequent treatment of the Queen of Portugal (Doerner 1981:73–5).

[10] Phillipe Pinel was a confidante of key theoreticians and administrators in the new regime. Among the first to be awarded the Napoleonic *Légion d'Honneur*, he was ultimately appointed Consultant to the Emperor (Goldstein 1987:67–72; Allen and Postel 1992:353).

[11] See Lewis (1967:9–17) for a discussion of Pinel's debt to John Locke, Thomas Sydenham, William Cullen, and the English practitioners of moral therapy.

person, according to moral therapy, was characterized by inner control.

In continental Europe, many of the asylums were converted castles, palaces, monasteries, convents, military barracks, or almshouses—disused monuments of the old order that were selling cheaply.[12] The new building programme was more extensive in England and even more so in America where it was necessary to start from scratch. In these countries asylum design was influenced by the fashion for classical revival in Romantic architecture. Asylums were located in tranquil country settings, in keeping with the Romantic idealization of nature. The main edifices for the superintendent and his administrative functions were set off with neoclassical cupolas, Doric columned porticos, or bell towers. The wings that housed patients were constructed according to classical principles of simplicity and geometric symmetry, allowing for expansion by adding one identical segment after another. Domestic architecture of that era used Hellenic references to serve a nostalgic and evocative function; their purpose was 'to draw sorrowful reflections from the soul' (Janson 1986:575). By contrast, the institutional architecture of asylums used the uniform regularity of neoclassicism to counteract the frenzied emotions of mania, to impose a rational spatial order on the chaos of insanity. This architecture had its counterpart in the punctual daily routine, which imposed a temporal order on the inmates (Rothman 1971:138–40). Asylum design was also influenced by Jeremy Bentham's idea for a panopticon, which he first published in 1791 (Foucault 1978). He employed a geometric principle that enabled a single, centrally located supervisor to exert visual control over a large number of inmates located in peripherally arranged cells. It led to the construction of semi-circular or star-shaped buildings or, in modified form, the characteristic H-shaped ward blocks. Whether they were monasteries and castles from the *ancien régime* or new buildings that sought to recapture classical regularity, asylums expressed a rhetoric of absolute authority. This was an architecture of constraint (Conolly [1850], cited in Donnelly 1983:50). It em-

---

[12] The asylum at Sonnestein in Saxony was formerly a castle, the asylum at Bayreuth was the Palace of the Princesses, the one at Seigburg was a Benedictine Abbey, and Hildesheim was previously a convent.

ployed space to isolate, order, observe, and classify the insane (Miller 1980:73).

The gridwork of asylums that was laid down across each country was the foundation on which professional organizations were established from the 1840s onward (Renvoize 1991), at first comprising asylum doctors but later expanding their constituency to form today's national psychiatric associations. Journals published by these associations, the most important of which arose between 1843 and 1853, created a medium for a new discourse on psychiatric illness. Prior to this time psychiatric knowledge had been distributed by means of treatises and monographs. Journals allowed for a more prolific and rapid communication of psychiatric opinion and enabled the emergence of new genres of psychiatric writing such as the case report. These professional bodies and their publications promoted an international psychiatric culture that was formalized at the first international congress of mental medicine in Paris in 1878 (Bynum 1991:166).

In recent times, technological advances such as magnetic resonance imaging have rapidly generated a flood of new observations on schizophrenia. In the same way, the asylum, as an architectonic breakthrough, immediately made possible a new way of observing the insane both individually and collectively. Three novel techniques were developed for the recording of observations on individuals. The first was the case history. This was a new clinical genre, the fullness of its descriptive style distinguishing it from precursors such as the desultory one line entry in the case book (Donnelly 1983:91). Thus it was Pinel in 1801 and Haslam[13] in 1810 who are credited with the first full clinical descriptions of schizophrenia (Howells 1991:xiii). The second was the life history, which was a narrative genre developed by early German institutional psychiatrists as a way of describing the person and his or her uniqueness in terms of evolving inner experience.[14] The third technique was the questionnaire. When the asylum at Sieg-

---

[13] In *Illustrations of Madness* [1810], John Haslam (1988), the apothecary at Bethlem Royal Hospital, described the 'brain sayings' of John Tilly Matthews, which resemble symptoms of schizophrenia.

[14] Especially Zeller and Binswanger (Verwey 1985:152–4). In England, this method was championed by Sir Henry Maudsley. It was taken to America by Adolph Meyer.

burg was opened in 1824, the director, Jacobi,[15] arranged for new patients to be evaluated by means of a personal history, a family history, and questionnaires that took approximately three weeks to complete, or two to ten days in an emergency (Marx 1991:9). Thus for the first time, mental illness was systematically linked to the person's family background and evolving life history.

For the collective observation of insanity, asylum doctors introduced the practice of reporting all cases coming within the orbit of an institution, whether the treatment was successful or unsuccessful. It entailed two techniques. One was statistical analysis. Pinel was well placed to introduce this method to psychiatry. He had a background in mathematics, had already published on its applications to medicine, and was conversant with Enlightenment probability theory (Lewis 1967:11). Also, he was thrust to prominence at the birth of statistics, when the modern state was first concerned to systematically record every dimension of the population: its demography, its wealth, and its health. Thus Pinel, describing his method as a 'calculus of probabilities', carried out a four year experiment starting in 1800 in which he compared the outcome of two forms of treatment, the old physical methods and a method of expectant observation combined with moral therapy (Goldstein 1987:102–5).

The second technique for the collective study of insanity was to assemble a so-called *Klinisches Bild* (clinical picture). It was a meticulous method of describing a syndrome by layering case description onto case description until a fully formed picture was developed (Peters 1991:60). It was the qualitative handmaiden of statistics in that it informed the raw material for quantitative generalizations, which could then be examined for covariance and causal links.

Because of these techniques, it now became possible to apply a time dimension to the description and classification of psychiatric illness. In retrospective time, the life history enabled a conception of psychiatric illness as unfolding in relation to the patient's evolving biography, and the family history enabled a classification of psychiatric illness according to the

---

[15] Karl Wiegand Maximilian Jacobi (1775–1858) was the director of the asylum at Siegburg when it became a pre-eminent centre of psychiatry in Europe.

presence or absence of inherited traits. Prospectively, for the first time psychiatrists could describe the evolution of an illness over the course of a patient's life, since many patients remained under observation in asylums until they died. As a consequence, the criterion of whether the patient recovered emerged in nineteenth century psychiatry as the paramount criterion on which to base the classification of mental illness. In France the earliest attempt at such a classification was produced by Pinel (Lanzic 1992:53). The work of his disciple Esquirol[16] was more systematic (Jaspers 1963:849), defining such concepts as relapse, remission, and intermission. As psychiatry started to focus on the course of illness a major distinction emerged between circular madness and madness characterized by linear deterioration. In parallel, Neumann[17] in Germany developed a theory about the evolution of mental illness from melancholia to mania to *Verwirrheit* (mental confusion) and ultimately *Blödsinn* (dementia). These ideas foreshadowed Kraepelin's distinction between a linear, progressive illness that was incurable (dementia praecox) and a circular or periodic form of illness that was curable (manic depressive psychosis).

Although created in a climate of optimism, asylums never fulfilled their promise. During the second half of that century they quickly became centres of hopelessness and pessimism, the orderly routines of moral therapy deteriorating into regimens of oppression and deprivation. Parsimonious economizing turned them into overcrowded storehouses for long-term incarceration of the mentally ill. Throughout the nineteenth century there was a progressive increase in the mental hospital population that far outstripped population growth.[18] It was

[16] Jean Étienne Dominique Esquirol (1772–1840) became the director of the asylum at Charenton near Paris.

[17] Heinrich Neumann founded a private mental hospital near Breslau in 1852 and exerted a strong influence over German psychiatric theory.

[18] The situation in England and Wales provides the best illustration because it has been carefully tabulated by Scull (1979:187–253) relying on the Annual Reports of the Commissioners in Lunacy. In 1827 there were nine county and borough asylums, their average size 116 beds. By 1890 there were sixty-six asylums with an average size of 802 beds (Scull 1979:198). During that period the proportion of the population officially designated insane (mostly inmates of these asylums) rose nearly five times, from 0.06% in 1828 to 0.29% in 1890 (Scull 1979: 224). In the United States, there were 8,500 patients in 1860, but by 1890 this figure had multiplied 22 times to 187,000 (Castel, Castel & Lovell 1982:20).

clear to contemporary authorities that this striking increase mainly represented an accumulation of chronic cases. It was equally clear to contemporary critics that these gargantuan institutions caused their inmates to deteriorate into chronic insanity. In 1859 the 'gigantic' asylum was described as 'a manufactory of chronic insanity' (Arlidge, quoted in Scull 1979: 220), and in 1877 it was observed that the practice of treating patients collectively rather than individually produced 'a tendency to make whole classes sink down into a sort of chronic state' (Granville, quoted in Scull 1979:200).

The nineteenth century thus saw the invention of a new and complex machine, the asylum, which for the first time could absorb any number of insane. With its moral equipment, it delivered a form of therapy designed to produce individuals characterized by inner self-control. With its clinical equipment it could produce detailed case histories that included an extensive life history of the patient. Its scientific equipment measured, grouped, and sorted patients in terms of heredity and course of illness. The professional organizations and journals that grew out of the asylum enabled the widespread and prolific distribution of a new discourse about mental illness. The asylum isolated and incarcerated patients and, abetted by government policies that led to overcrowding and deprivation, processed psychiatric illness into an incurable form.

Degeneration

Though a consequence of long-term confinement in asylums, incurability came to be regarded by asylum psychiatrists as an essential feature of insanity, and it was explained in terms of 'degeneration'. The concept of degeneration has a provenance that extends back to Renaissance thought (Boon 1985: 25), but it was during the Enlightenment that it was developed into a major theory within the discipline of natural history. In fact, it became the dominant pre-evolutionary paradigm. The problem that confronted natural historians of that era was how to account for the observed variation among life forms. For Linnaeus,[19] variation was produced by hybridization. This

---

[19] Carl von Linné (1707–1778), the Swedish botanist and physician who originated the binomial system of nomenclature.

explanation allowed him to preserve the idea of species as perpetual, immutable entities and thus retain a religious conception of nature as a changeless order designed by God. Against this, Buffon,[20] doyen of French Enlightenment natural history, proposed the doctrine of 'degeneration'. He argued that the genus, not the Linnaean species, was fixed. Each genus was a perfect original type, members of which migrated to different parts of the globe. There they encountered different climatic conditions and degenerated into various local forms known as species. Buffon claimed to demonstrate that if each species could be returned to its initial environment it would regenerate to an original pure form. Thus the theory of degeneration accounted for the varieties observed throughout the plant and animal kingdoms, including the racial varieties of man. Notwithstanding their differences, Buffon and Linnaeus shared a common starting point—a static view of nature as God's creation, unchanged since the beginning of time—and they both made tentative steps toward a more fluid view of nature. However, by the end of the century their world view was swept aside by a new political, intellectual, and scientific appetite for progress. They were superseded by the evolutionary accounts of Lamarck,[21] with his theory of use-inheritance, and later Darwin with natural selection.

Morel[22] took up the eighteenth century theory of degeneration and refashioned it in the mould of nineteenth century progressivist thought. For Buffon degeneration had been the source of variety; for Morel it became the opposite of progress. A central debate in this age of population growth, urbanization, and industrial expansion turned on the question of whether society, by modernizing, was actually improving or declining (Erksteins 1985:2). Was civilization for good or evil? Why, if progress promised the betterment of humanity, were we surrounded by increasing human misery? Positivists such

[20] Georges-Louis Leclerc comte de Buffon (1707–1788), superintendent of the *Jardin du Roi* in Paris and author of an extensive *Histoire naturelle de l'homme* published from 1749 onward (Bowler 1984:67–72).
[21] Jean Baptiste Pierre Antoine de Monet, chevalier de Lamarck (1744–1829), physician and naturalist appointed in 1794 to the *Muséum d'histoire naturelle* in charge of invertebrates.
[22] Bénédict-Augustin Morel (1809–1873) was the director of Maréville asylum at Nancy and then Saint-Yon asylum near Rouen.

as Auguste Comte argued that the march of civilization advanced mankind from superstition to reason (Nye 1985:52). Against this view, Romantics idealized nature and the savage, regarding civilization as artificial and corrupting and responsible for the creation of large scale human suffering, including mental illness. Morel's formulation preserved an overall commitment to progress but at the same time invoked its obverse, degeneration, to account for social ills.

His theory of degeneration, set out in the 1857 *Traité des dégénérescences physiques, intellectuelles et morales de l'espèce humaine* (Treatise on the Physical, Intellectual and Moral Degeneracy of the Human Species) was an amalgamation of moral and biological reasoning, an attempt to reconcile Roman Catholic theology with natural science (Liégois 1991). Morel argued that degeneration was caused by sin, but it could also be caused by a bad social milieu or physical intoxication. It led to a physiological decline that culminated in extinction, a pessimistic message for the degenerates themselves, who would die off within several generations, but an optimistic message for society as a whole, which would soon be cleansed of these self-limiting strains.

Degeneration theory became influential throughout Europe because it so plausibly explained physical and mental illness (and indeed every form of social pathology) in terms of heredity. Morel himself was concerned about the growing rates of crime and the diminishing number of productive individuals (Huertas 1992:392), especially among the workers and peasants. In France his ideas had particular appeal to the authorities, who were seeking to explain the disconcerting decline in the birth rate and the high rates of alcoholism and syphilis (Nye 1985:60). Applied to different races, degeneration explained the anticipated extinction of the American Indian. Also, it had long been accepted that Negroes, with their compressed craniums and protruding jaws, were the most degraded and primitive of the human races. Now it was argued that they were degenerating more rapidly to a diseased and sexually depraved state because they had been removed from their natural habitat, the tropics, and placed in a temperate climate and an environment that was too intellectually stimulating (Stepan 1985:98). Though Morel himself denounced racism, an influential body of scientific opinion concluded that Negroes were a lower species closer to anthropoid apes than to Caucasians, and that mulattos were more degenerate still, to the point of being sterile, or at least subfertile, as would be expected of hybrids. Racial types provided a model for degenerates of all sorts within European society. Thus in their physiognomy and behaviour, criminals and the insane were likened to primitives. For the followers of Morel, social class was analogous to race. The urban poor, including prostitutes, criminals, and other immoral types, were degenerates, exemplified by their low brain weights, protruding jaws, and misshapen skulls. This theory provided a powerful justification for those who were opposed to the migration of 'inferior' races, who attempted to prevent the mixing of races (miscegenation), and who saw upward social mobility of the working classes as dangerous. Degeneration theory had to do with the proper place of races and classes (Stepan 1985).

Most importantly, it was used to explain the apparent increase in the rates of mental illness and their incurability (Rogler and Hollingshead 1965:3; Scull 1984; Dowbiggin 1985: 200–21). It served as a convenient justification for the asylum in the face of its failure because it located the problems of incurability and deterioration within the patient and his or her genetic endowment, not in the asylum itself. Psychiatric treatment could still be represented as progressive and Utopian, providing the objects of this treatment, the patients, were portrayed as regressive and degenerative. The application of degeneration theory to insanity was delineated in the 1860 *Traité des maladies mentales* (Treatise on Mental Illness). Here Morel linked heredity to degeneration in the *law of progressivity*, according to which inherited traits became worse in each generation:

> Morel gave detailed examples of this process, which appeared disheartening in its inevitability. The first generation was characterized by a nervous temperament and a tendency toward cerebral vascular congestion, accompanied by irritability, a quick temper, and resulting violent behaviour. The second generation ran the risk of illnesses of the central nervous system: cerebral haemorrhages, epilepsy, and the neurotic disorders of hysteria and hypochondriasis. The third generation felt the gathering

malevolent force toward insanity. Its members would appear to be eccentric, disorderly, and dangerous. The accumulated defects reached lethal proportions in the following generation and the family line was, or soon would be, gone. (Carlson 1985: 122)

His classification of hereditary derangements contained four subtypes that corresponded more or less to these four stages of deterioration (Huertas 1992:404).

In his 1852 *Clinical Studies*, Morel had described case reports of young patients who appeared to have a good prognosis.[23] 'But after careful examination,' he wrote, 'one remains convinced that idiotism and dementia are the sad fate that will terminate the course' (Morel, cited in Pichot 1983:19). When in 1860 Morel introduced the term *démence précoce*, he was not referring so much to a disease entity as 'a particular form of evolution or course of mental disease' (Menninger 1963:449). Morel provided a case vignette that epitomized 'heredity in a progressive form'. The patient, who was thirteen or fourteen years of age, had effortlessly topped composition at school. Gradually he became taciturn, withdrawn, and melancholic. He then developed a violent hatred for his father and ultimately had ideas of killing him. His mother was a madwoman and his grandmother eccentric:

> The young patient progressively forgot everything he had learned; his intellectual faculties, formerly so brilliant, underwent a very disturbing period of stoppage. A sort of hebetude-like torpor replaced his former activity, and when I revisited him, I judged that the fatal transition to the state of *démence précoce* was in progress. This desperate prognosis is normally far from the minds of parents—as of doctors—who bestow their care on these children. Such is, nevertheless, in most cases, the dire termination of hereditary madness. (Morel cited in Wender 1963:1147)

By 'dementia' he referred to end-stage mental deterioration. By precocious, he referred to the rapidity of the patient's decline. This single case was paradigmatic. *Démence précoce* was the epitome, the culmination, and the proof of degeneration

---

[23] *Études cliniques: Traité théorique et practique des maladies mentales* (Nancy, Gumblet/ Masson, 1852–1853).

theory. Unlike cretins, imbeciles, or idiots, persons with this illness appeared to develop normally at first, but began to decline before reaching their prime. Unlike the more common forms of dementia that occurred in middle-aged or elderly patients, the age of onset was early enough to prevent reproduction and transmission to the next generation. Dementia praecox was the end of the line.

Morel, it is believed, was unaware of *The Origin of Species* when writing his 1860 treatise, but his successors quickly refashioned degeneration theory into a Darwinian format. As a consequence, degenerates came to be viewed as casualties of natural selection. They had succumbed in the struggle for survival. Darwin's own interest in insanity is evident in the 1872 publication *The Expression of the Emotions in Man and Animals* in which he drew extensively on clinical examples provided by Dr J. Crichton Browne from West Riding Asylum (Darwin 1965:154 *passim*) and by Mr Patrick Nicol from the Sussex Lunatic Asylum (*ibid*:184). He used this material to compare the expression of emotions in animals, infants, the various races of man (especially tribal people and Orientals), and the insane. An atavistic concept of the insane person as a 'throw back' was a consequence of this approach. Darwin endorsed the views of Henry Maudsley[24] that patients with degenerative brain disorders had reverted to a more primitive form, as evidenced by their savage snarls, their wild howling, and their brutish behaviour (Darwin 1965:244).

There was a reciprocal, mutually reinforcing relationship between Darwin's theory of natural selection and prevailing theories about society as a free market economy (Sahlins 1976: 101–3). On the one hand, society was a model for biology. It was Marx and Engels who were the first to point out that Darwin had taken on board the central ethos of *laissez-faire* capitalism—competitive individualism—and unwittingly made it apply to the natural kingdom as a whole (Young 1985:52). On the other hand, biology became a model for society. Once established as an authoritative scientific theory, natural selection was taken up by political theorists to justify their ideas for

[24] Sir Henry Maudsley (1835–1918) was the leading English proponent of degeneration theory (Walk 1976:22). See Lewis (1967:29–48) for a biographical sketch.

a progressive society. Social Darwinists, in the wake of Herbert Spencer, would argue that the improvement of human society depended on the 'survival of the fittest' at the expense of the weak, and the eugenics movement, in the wake of Sir Francis Galton and his pupil Pearson, would agitate for sterilization. The provision of social assistance to degenerates, such as the poor or the insane, it was argued, would enable their survival and reproduction and would thus weaken society as a whole. The person with mental illness became the antithesis of the ideal person in competitive capitalism in having an inherited taint that led to a permanent failure to adapt, compete, or engage in productive labour (Barham 1984:35–36).

During the second half of the nineteenth century this Darwinized form of degeneration theory became the central topic of critical debate in French psychiatry, and it was successively applied to more and more psychiatric conditions (Carlson 1985:129). Magnan[25] championed the theory, notably in his work on *folie dégénerative* and alcoholism (Huertas 1993a:4). In Germany Krafft-Ebing viewed sexual perversions as stigmata of degeneration (Bynum 1984). In America it was applied to the new diagnostic category of neuraesthenia, and in Italy Lombroso came to international prominence with his theory of criminal types based on degenerative stigmata (Tagliavini 1985:188; Huertas 1993b). Degeneration theory ultimately fell into disfavour during the first half of the twentieth century, partly in the wake of World War I, when it became clear that men with no genetic predisposition could develop severe mental illness (Beer 1992:507), and partly in the wake of World War II, when the Nazi programme of exterminating the mentally ill forced geneticists to distance themselves from eugenics.

Nonetheless, the original exemplar, dementia praecox, continued to be understood in terms of Morelian degeneration, chiefly through the influence of Emil Kraepelin. Before examining how important the concept of degeneration was to Kraepelin, it is necessary to trace another constellation of ideas to do with the split person, which he also wove into the concept of dementia praecox.

[25] Jacques J. Valentin Magnan, the director of the Psychiatric Asylum of Sainte Anne.

The split person

The idea of the split person was articulated with greatest clarity in German academic psychiatry, which, in the course of the nineteenth century came to dominate European psychiatric thinking, largely as a result of the rising influence of the German universities. The struggle to form a united German nation out of the various ecclesiastical and secular German-speaking states became a struggle against Napoleon; and it was the German universities, supported and controlled by the aristocracy and the emerging state, that were enlisted to the patriotic task of promoting an ideology of freedom and a spirit of national unity through the study of language, culture, and philosophy. Berlin University, founded in the aftermath of the defeat of the Prussian army at Jena in 1806, was an important focal point around which the nation was built. It soon became a model for other universities in Germany and indeed a model for the rest of Continental Europe. Before long Germany could boast a cohort of full-time professional medical scientists based in universities, many of them pupils of Müller.[26] Under their influence, hospital-based medicine, which had relied on pathological anatomy, gave way to laboratory-based medicine and the new field of pathological physiology. The rising influence of German psychiatry occurred against the backdrop of these broader political and medical changes, which entailed an underlying transition from a religious to a materialist orientation—from romantic medicine to scientific medicine—as power shifted from the asylums to the universities.

German medicine and psychiatry during the first four decades of the nineteenth century has been characterized as romantic, idealist, and anthropological. Romanticism, drawing on Rousseau and the English Romantics, through the *Sturm und Drang* movement, assumed a special intensity in Germany because it became the principal expression of national unity and resistance to French domination. Madness was an obvious focus for this movement, with its aesthetic concerns for passion and irrationality. Romanticism gave to medicine the no-

[26] From Berlin University, Johannes Müller (1801–1858) established modern physiology (in conjunction with Helmholtz), histology (with Schwann and others), and histopathology (continued by Virchow).

tion of a self-reflective 'inner man'—the person as a well-spring of feelings—which was crucial to the development of medical psychology and an important source of the modern psychotherapy movement. The hallmark of this inner man was unity in the face of contradiction, notably in the works of Herder, Schiller, and Goethe, who each explored the theme of integration achieved by reconciliation of contradictory forces (Marx 1990:358).

German idealist philosophy proposed similar ideas about the unity of the self in the face of division. Kant, on the one hand, posited an *a priori* concept of self as a 'transcendental unity of apperception'. This transcendental 'I', he argued, was a necessary and prior condition for the ordering of experience that 'must be presupposed if any recognizable experience can occur at all' (Collins 1985:55). It could be described as a unity of apperception because it was the capacity for synthesis, the ability to join diverse cognitions together by grasping them in one cognition (Kitcher 1984:114; Young 1992: 104). Yet in counterpoint to this unifying, transcendental self that was free, Kant envisaged another self that was not free. It was locked into the natural, or 'phenomenal' world and was subject to its necessary laws (of space, time, and causality). Thus Kant's system of philosophy stressed the unity of self, yet of necessity posited 'two selves', one free and the other determined (Kolakowski 1978:44–50; Wood 1984:74).

The work that most directly influenced psychiatric thinking was his *Anthropology from a Pragmatic Point of View* [1798] (Kant 1974). Based on a lecture series first given during the winter of 1772–1773, it contained an outline for an empirical psychology and a classification of mental disorders.[27] In this work, the inner person was defined as a 'unity of consciousness' (Kant, 1974:9), which was inseparable from freedom of the will. Inspired by Kant, German psychiatry identified itself as anthropological, meaning that it promoted a doctrine of psycho-physical unity and was concerned with the study of man as a union of soul (or mind) and body (Verwey 1985:3).

---

[27] Kant distinguished between disorders of cognition and disorders of emotion, thereby anticipating Kraepelin's distinction between dementia praecox in contrast to manic depressive psychosis (Spitzer 1990).

Thus the medicine and psychiatry of that era was romantic in its inspiration, idealist in its philosophy, and anthropological in its paradigm; and its theoreticians were principally concerned to define the person in terms of unity prevailing over division. Reil[28] for example, in 1795 promoted a view of man as an inseparable unity of soul and body (Crighton 1990:233). He advanced a holistic theory of the brain as an essential unity, in which the differentiated parts were in a state of dynamic tension (Lewis:1967:24–25). Reil wrote at a time when medicine and psychiatry were beginning to divide into separate professions with their separate domains, the general hospital and the asylum. He sought to span this divide by founding psychological medicine. It is not surprising that he promoted a psychosomatic theory of the person in which unity prevailed over division. This particular constellation of ideas about the person also reflected the broader social and political context. While Germany was building itself into a unified nation by reconciling truculent states and principalities, so its institutions, the universities, and its ideologues—novelists, philosophers, academicians, and doctors espousing Romantic medicine—were coining a notion of the person as a unity achieved by reconciliation of contradictory forces.

In Heinroth's[29] *Lehrbuch der Anthropologie*, unity was paramount. Man was indivisible (Marx 1990:375). Heinroth's model of health and illness was hierarchical and Christian. He defined unity, at the human level, in terms of self-consciousness and individuality. At a higher spiritual level there was a kind of ultimate unity that could only be realized in surrender to God. Psychic derangement was essentially a disorder of the soul or psyche, caused by sin and leading to a loss of freedom or enslavement. Heinroth championed the 'psychicist' faction in early German psychiatry, and he was strenuously opposed by Jacobi and the 'somaticists', who argued that the pure mind (characterised by self-consciousness, freedom, and belief in God) could not become ill, as it was dysfunction of the bodily organism that underlay all psychic illness. Disorders of the

---

[28] Johann Christian Reil (1759–1853) was professor of medicine at Halle from 1788 and, like many of the Romantic doctors, a fervent German nationalist.

[29] Johann Christian August Heinroth (1773–1843) occupied the first chair of psychological medicine, which was in Leipzig (Cauwenbergh 1991:365).

mind or soul were mere manifestations of somatic dysfunction. Verwey (1985:22–34) shows how the adherents to the somatic school saw man as divided rather than unified. They posited a dualism of soul and body, enabling them to separate their religious views from their clinical practice, which was to treat their patients' physical disorders. At one level, the psychicists and somaticists were debating the precedence of the soul or the body. At a more fundamental level, it was a debate about whether the modern person was basically a unified whole or a divided duality.[30]

A pivotal figure in Germany at mid-century was Griesinger.[31] Like the early somaticists he regarded diseases of the mind as diseases of the brain. From his teacher, the Christian psychiatrist Zeller, he took the idea that there was just one psychosis. From the anthropological tradition he inherited a belief in man as a psycho-physical unity. At the same time, Griesinger had studied the work of Müller and became a key advocate of the new physiological paradigm in medicine, making his first mark in the area of infectious diseases with a study of hookworm anaemia. As a transitional figure, he embodied the change from the speculative, synthetic, anthropological approach of the first half of the century to the positivist, analytical, natural science of the second half. He campaigned against asylum-based psychiatry, effected a rapprochement of psychiatry with general medicine, and exemplified the rising dominance of the university. As professor of psychiatry in Berlin, he developed the model of the university clinic that combined psychiatry and neurology with a strong outpatient emphasis (Doerner 1981:274). He inherited the great tradition of viewing the person in terms of unity versus division. 'Greisinger was the first to "see" clearly the symptoms of schizophrenia which "existed" conceptually only since the turn of the century, i.e., the "dichotomy of the soul", the schism or "split in the ego," and the permanent mental deficiency' (Doerner 1981:284).

---

[30] See also Johann von Herbart (1776–1841), professor of philosophy at Göttingen, who proposed a model of the person as divided into an aggregate of egos but also unified by means of an undivided soul (Verwey 1985:117–30).

[31] Wilhelm Griesinger (1817–1868) was professor of psychiatry, first at Kiel university in 1849, then in Cairo, and eventually in Berlin from 1864.

At the same time as these themes were emerging in psychiatric theory, they found parallel expression in popular literature. This period was an era when journals, periodicals, and mass circulation magazines were springing up to cater to the newly literate middle classes and when the novel emerged in its modern form. A central figure within German Romantic literature was the double—Jean Paul's[32] *Doppelgänger*. Goethe, who himself reported encountering his double as a phantom riding toward him as he journeyed along the road to Drusenheim (Jaspers 1963:92), developed this theme by internalizing the double so that it came to reside within the person. Goethe's Faust is perhaps the most celebrated literary example of man divided within himself.[33] As he walks outside the city gate, just before noticing that he is being followed by the curious black poodle (Mephistopheles) Faust declares to Wagner, his companion, that he is torn between the sensuous world of passionate desire and a higher spiritual plane—between earth and heaven:

> In me there are two souls, alas, and their
> Division tears my life in two. (Goethe 1987:35–36)

The high point of this genre was Hoffman,[34] who like Goethe located the double within the personality. He advanced a theory of duplicity in which madness became a 'folly that estranges one's own self from one's self' (Peters 1991:61), and he illustrated this with extravagant images, such as that of the two princes whose bodies had grown together but who had different heads. Neither could tell whether the source of his thoughts was himself or his twin. Hoffman referred to this state as 'chronic dualism', by which he meant a split in the person characterized by a failure to recognize that the inner subjective world is different from the outer objective world. In Romantic literature, as in its clinical counterpart, splitting was increasingly portrayed as a sign of abnormality. Miller (1985:

---

[32] Jean Paul Friedrich Richter (1763–1825). See Menhennet (1981:184) for a discussion of dualism within his literary output.

[33] See Jung (1982a:50) and Van den Berg (1977:128) on the recurrent theme of 'two souls' in Goethe.

[34] Ernst Théodor Amadeus Hoffman (1776–1822) the Romantic writer, painter, and operatic composer. Liptzin (1973:260fn) lists a large cast of doubles in Hoffman's output.

47) shows how the subject of the Romantic genre was the stranger, the outcast, the fugitive, or the orphan; and splitting into a double came to be seen as both a product of duplicity and a harbinger of death.

The connection between psychopathology and literature was abstract and thematic, betraying a common concern among the intelligentsia with the inner unity of man. But there were also direct and tangible connections between a handful of philosophers, literary figures, and doctors who taught (or themselves became) the administrators of the new German state. Thus psychiatry was directly shaped by Goethe, both Heinroth and Jacobi being personally influenced by him at Weimar (Verwey 1985:12). Conversely, literature was informed by clinical psychiatry. As a civil servant and judge, Hoffman kept abreast of the contemporary psychiatric literature as part of his forensic reading, and he liberally borrowed case histories with little modification for his tales. Novalis,[35] the paragon of Romanticism, was actually a student of Langermann, the director of St George's asylum at Bayreuth.

The 'craze for duality spread from Germany to the rest of Europe' (Miller 1985:49). It took hold in English literature through the Gothic novel, the exemplar being Mary Shelley's *Frankenstein; or, The Modern Prometheus* (1818), and then through a Gothic strain in mainstream literature, as in Walter Scott's *Redgauntlet* (1824) and Charlotte Brontë's *Villette* (1853).[36] In Russia Dostoevsky struggled with the theme of duality throughout his productive life.[37] In a passage from *A Raw Youth* on duality of the will, he wrote:

> What is a second self exactly? The second self, according to a medical book, written by an expert, which I purposely read afterwards, is nothing else than the first stage of serious mental derangement, which may lead to something very bad. (Dostoevsky 1916:548)

---

[35] Also known as Friedrich von Hardenberg (1772–1801). His 'magical idealism' epitomized the Romantic protest against the Enlightenment and the French Revolution (Menhennet 1981:64–80).

[36] See also the *Doppelgänger* story 'William Wilson' (1839) by Edgar Allan Poe (1872:305–23).

[37] The main example is *The Double*, although the theme is also evident in other works, such as *The Brothers Karamazov* and *The Possessed (The Devils)*. Dostoevsky drew on Gogol, who developed this theme in *Dead Souls* and in his stories, 'Diary of a Madman' and 'The Nose'.

Hawthorn (1983) and Miller (1985) have traced the development of the duality motif in English literature through to its revival at the end of the century in Robert Louis Stevenson's *Deacon Brodie or The Double Life* (1880) and *The Strange Case of Dr Jekyll and Mr Hyde* (1886), which explored the opposition of good and evil, reason and passion. In Oscar Wilde's *Picture of Dorian Gray* (1891) the polarities were youth and age, innocence and debauchery, the true self and the image of self.[38]

The idea of the split person was not restricted to German romantic psychiatry and the Gothic novel. It informed a diverse range of nineteenth century thought on normal and abnormal persons. In the field of neurophysiology, an obscure figure, A. L. Wigan, published *The Duality of the Mind* in 1844 (cited in Hawthorn 1983:51), in which he argued that each person has two separate and conflicting wills, located in the right and left hemispheres, respectively.[39] A later, more influential formulation was developed by Wernicke, in which the division lay between higher and lower brain functions rather than right and left hemispheres. His idea of 'sejunction' referred to a disconnection of neuronal associations, especially between cortical and subcortical areas of the brain, leading to a psychopathological 'disintegration of individuality' (Scharfetter 1975:7).

[38] See James (1908/1957), Conrad (1912/1960), Woolf (1933), and Borges (1970) for examples of this theme in twentieth century literature. Alasdair Gray (1983: 4) begins 'The Spread of Ian Nicol' thus: 'One day Ian Nicol, a riveter by trade, started to split in two down the middle.' During the twentieth century, the cinema has assumed special importance in the portrayal of the split person because one actor can play several roles. There have been numerous remakes of *Dr Jekyll and Mr Hyde* (by Thanhauser in 1912, Paramount in 1920 and 1932, Metro-Goldwyn-Mayer in 1941, American Broadcasting Corporation–TV in 1968, and Amicus in 1970). *Superman* probably achieved the greatest exposure of all through several films, a television serial, cartoons, and comic books. When Thigpen and Cleckley's (1957) clinical study, *The Three Faces of Eve*, was produced as a motion picture, one reviewer commented that 'its box office success was sufficient to start a schizophrenic cycle' (Halliwell 1977). *Sybil* (Schreiber 1975) is another example of this quasiclinical genre that has translated well into film (National Broadcasting Corporation 1976).

[39] These ideas have resurfaced in the work of Flor-Henry, Gruzelier, and others who have postulated left hemispheric (cognitive) dysfunction in schizophrenia as against right hemispheric (emotional) dysfunction in affective disorders (Gruzelier and Manchanda 1982). See also Wexler (1980) on the hypothesis that schizophrenia involves a dissociation between right and left brain leading to emotional functions being disconnected from cognitive functions.

The category of multiple personality was also based on the idea of the split person. The first reports appeared in Europe from 1791 onward (Ellenberger 1970:126–31), but the most celebrated case was the American, Mary Reynolds, with her two distinct personalities. First described by the physician John Kearsly Mitchell, this case came into public prominence when a more complete account was published in 1889 by his son, the neurologist Silas Wier Mitchell, who also wrote popular versions for *Harpers* magazine.

Animal magnetism and hypnotism, which thrived in the borderlands between medicine, spiritualism, and physics, were underpinned by a theory of 'dipsychism'. A popular formulation of this theory, expounded in an 1890 publication *The Double Ego*,[40] proposed that the mind consists of two layers of consciousness, upper and lower. 'Polypsychism', the idea of the personality as a multiplicity within a unity, was a well known elaboration on dipsychism.[41] In France the idea of the split person was expressed in Janet's concept of 'dissociation' or 'double conscience', which resulted from a weakening of the 'integrative' psychic functions.[42] This concept was also one of the fundamental starting points for the development of psychoanalytic theory. In his 1895 *Project for a Scientific Psychology,* Freud (1950:283–398) divided man into two parts: the first a reduction to a series of atoms governed by principles of attraction and repulsion (matter) and the second an 'observing ego' (mind). His thought then underwent a transition from dipsychism to polypsychism and split the person topographically into unconscious, preconscious, and conscious compartments. Later, in a more original contribution, he split the person dynamically into id, ego and superego.[43]

'The entire nineteenth century' writes Ellenberger (1970: 145), 'was preoccupied with the problem of the coexistence of these two minds and of their relationship to each other'.

[40] Max Dessoir, *Das Doppel-Ich*, cited in Ellenberger (1970:145).
[41] See Noll (1985:237–9), for a discussion of the relation between the hypnotists' concepts of polypsychism and the theories of William James, Freud, and Jung.
[42] See Freud (1957a:19–22; 1957b:11) on the concept of 'double conscience' within French psychopathology and its relation to his own concept of splitting.
[43] In Melanie Klein's theory, the child was the archetypal split person, and psychological development was a process of integrating good and bad parts or 'introjects' (Segal 1973). More recently the 'borderline personality' has taken on the mantle of the split person (Akhtar and Byrne 1983).

Degeneration and the split person in Kraepelin and Bleuler

At the end of the nineteenth century, Emil Kraepelin inherited the twin institutions—the psychiatric asylum and the university clinic—that had been evolving over the previous hundred years. Two great traditions—the theory of degeneration and the image of the disintegrating or split person—were also passed on to him. As a pupil of Wundt,[44] he absorbed the paradigm of academic experimental physiology that had been developed by Müller and Helmholtz. Kraepelin amalgamated all this to formulate a new class of disease—dementia praecox.

In 1891 Kraepelin was appointed professor of psychiatry at Heidelberg and director of the Grand Duke of Baden University of Heidelberg Hospital for the Insane. Janzarik has made the point that the conjunction of these two institutions, a university and a hospital housing chronic patients, provided a unique setting in which Kraepelin could carry out an empirical study of deterioration: 'Neither the usual university hospital nor large institution would have afforded the opportunity, as Heidelberg did, to follow up exemplary courses of illness over a long period and discern their common factors' (Janzarik 1992:25). The internecine politics of German psychiatry exerted a crucial influence on this hospital and thence on Kraepelin's clinical practice and scientific findings (Berrios and Hauser 1988:814). A protracted feud between asylum psychiatry and university psychiatry, stemming from the time of Griesinger, had delayed the establishment of this hospital for more than half a century. This dispute continued even after the hospital was opened and led, during Kraepelin's time, to an accumulation of chronic cases. Kraepelin fought unsuccessfully for the right to select his patients and was forced to accept all patients sent to the hospital. Also, he wished to treat voluntary inpatients but could not do so. The process of admission was encumbered by complex legal procedures that could result in patients having to stay in a workhouse cell or a refuge home for months before finally entering the hospital.

---

[44] Wilhelm Wundt (1832–1920), himself a student of Müller and Helmholtz, established a laboratory in Leipzig in 1879 and is regarded as a founder of experimental psychology.

Furthermore, it became increasingly difficult to transfer incurable patients to the already crowded state institutions,
prompting Kraepelin to lobby for the establishment of a long-
stay hospital to take care of them. However, he was effectively
blocked by the asylum lobby and was consequently confronted
with the all too familiar problem of running a hospital
crammed with the most severe and incurable cases. Although
the atmosphere was optimistic at the beginning, the situation
progressively worsened. It was in the context of this deteriorating situation, with patients clogging up his teaching hospital, that Kraepelin gradually came to realize that inexorable
decline was a fundamental characteristic of mental illness:

> It gradually dawned on me that many patients, who initially pre-
> sented a picture of mania, melancholia or amentia showed pro-
> gressive dementia. In spite of individual differences they began
> to resemble one another. It seemed as if the earlier clinical dif-
> ferences had little bearing on the course of the illness. . . .
> Thus, I could not resist concluding that only one illness process
> might be affecting many of the institutionalized patients that
> developed dementia. The process might be slow or quick and
> sometimes accompanied by delusions, hallucinations and excite-
> ment. (Kraepelin, cited in Berrios and Hauser 1988:817)

It was on this patient sample that Kraepelin systematically
studied the longitudinal course of illness and developed his
classifications of psychiatric disorders. Such a project, combining diagnosis with prognosis, had been anticipated from the
beginning of the century. I have mentioned how Pinel, Esquirol, and Neumann had earlier drawn attention to the evolution of psychiatric illness. Kahlbaum,[45] however, with his
particular emphasis on course and prognosis, most directly
influenced Kraepelin (Hoenig 1991:77).

By examining the relevant sections of Kraepelin's successive
diagnostic systems, it is possible to identify the principal concepts that organized his classificatory logic (Table 7.1). Between 1883 and 1915 he produced seven such classifications
by rearranging these concepts into different formulations,
permutations, and levels of abstraction. They were concepts,

---

[45] Karl Ludwig Kahlbaum (1828–1899), though he spent his working life outside
the academy, had a strong influence over academic psychiatry in general and
Kraepelin in particular (Lanzic 1992).

Table 7.1. *Excerpts from Kraepelin's successive classifications*

Date	Category	Subcategory
1883	States of psychological weakness	a. Idiocy, cretinism, feeble-mindedness, homosexuality b. Moral insanity, litiginous insanity c. Neuraesthenic states, obsessions, phobias, impulsions d. Senile dementia e. Secondary weakness states (secondary *Verrücktheit*, secondary *Blödsinn*)
1887	Acquired states of weakness	a. Senile dementia b. Mental weakness resulting from organic brain diseases c. Secondary states of mental weakness
1891	Psychic degeneracy processes	a. Dementia praecox b. Catatonia c. Dementia paranoides
1896	Acquired mental diseases metabolic diseases	a. Myxoedema b. Cretinism c. Dementifying processes i. Dementia praecox ii. Catatonia iii. Dementia paranoides
1899	Dementia Praecox	a. Hebephrenic form b. Catatonic form c. Paranoid form
1909– 1915	Endogenous conditions with evolution toward deterioration dementia praecox	1. Hebephrenia 2. Depressive form 3. Catatonia 4. Paranoid form 5. Schizophasic form

Following Menninger (1963:457–64)

as it were, in search of a disease. In the earliest publication, written at Wundt's instigation, the organizing category was 'psychological weakness'. Kraepelin modelled his work on that of Griesinger and borrowed the latter's concept of 'weakness of the psychic functions' with little modification. In the 1891 edition of his textbook, 'psychic degeneracy processes' had become the organizing idea, bringing Kraepelin's diagnostic system into alignment with the degeneration paradigm and introducing for the first time Morel's illness category, dementia praecox.[46] By 1896 Kraepelin had grouped dementia praecox, catatonia, and dementia paranoides together because all three were degenerative processes (Lewis 1979a:156). The psychiatric century culminated with Kraepelin's 1899 text in which dementia praecox was elevated to the status of a major disease, formed by fusing all these degenerative processes into one category. A succession of related ideas had unfolded over sixteen years—psychological weakness, degeneration, dementia praecox—each idea immanent in its predecessor. Whereas in 1891 dementia praecox had entered Kraepelin's classification as a subspecies alongside catatonia and dementia paranoides, by 1899 it had expanded and engulfed these two. In fact, it had traversed the entire classificatory space of psychiatry, beginning as a paradigmatic case report in 1860 and ending as one of the major classes of psychiatric disease. By 1916 Kraepelin had documented 1,054 cases of this disorder.

Thus degeneration was an implicit framework that organized the definition of dementia praecox. First, there were the deficits inherited from previous generations, observed by Kraepelin in approximately 70 percent of cases. Then there were the 'so-called signs of degeneracy': 'smallness or deformity of the skull, child-like habitus, missing teeth, deformed ears' (Kraepelin 1896/1987:22). More important than these physical features were the psychic manifestations of degeneration: in boys shyness, laziness, a dislike of work, and an inclination to 'nasty tricks'; and in girls excitability, nervousness, and 'a tendency to bigotry' (Kraepelin 1919:236). Although these traits were present from childhood, the patient frequently achieved an average or above average level of ability.

---

[46] Kraepelin continued to be influenced by the degeneration theory until the 1920s (Beer 1992:515 fn).

Then began the decline in intellectual function, which most commonly progressed to end-stage dementia.[47] For Morel, the adjective *précoce* referred to the speed with which the patient progressed to dementia, but for Kraepelin (1919:4) *praecox* signified that the illness began during the patient's youth. He had no doubt that it was associated with serious lesions of the cerebral cortex 'that as a rule can only be regenerated in parts, if at all' (Kraepelin, cited in Peters 1991:63). In sum, it was 'slow deterioration in a constitutionally weak psychic state' (Kraepelin, cited in Roccatagliata 1991:2).

Loss of inner unity was the defining feature of dementia praecox. Kraepelin inherited a century old tradition of German psychiatric theory, which from Kant onward had idealized freedom of the will and unity of consciousness. How could he see this illness as anything other than a weakness of volition that culminated in a 'peculiar destruction of the internal connections of the psychic personality' (Kraepelin 1919:3). By definition, dementia praecox was a '*weakening of those emotional activities which permanently form the mainsprings of volition*' and that leads to a '*a loss of the inner unity* of the activities of intellect, emotion and volition' (Kraepelin 1919:74; original emphasis). Bleuler's pre-eminent contribution was to focus on this 'tearing apart or splitting of psychic functions' (Bleuler 1908/1987:59) and crystallize it into the word 'schizophrenia':[48]

> I call dementia praecox 'schizophrenia', because . . . the 'splitting' of the different psychic functions is one of its most important characteristics. . . . If the disease is marked, the personality loses its unity; at different times different psychic complexes seem to represent the personality . . . . one set of complexes dominates the personality for a time, while other groups of ideas or drives are 'split off' and seem either partly or completely impotent. (Bleuler 1950:9)

[47] There has been a debate over what Kraepelin actually said about recovery. Although he admitted to the possibility of cure (Kraepelin 1919:4), his outcome figures spelled pessimism (ibid:180–4).

[48] During an era when the coining of new disease categories was central to the establishment of eminent reputations, a plethora of new names, proposed by different authorities, competed with one another for this disease. 'Dissociative psychosis', 'dementia dissociativa', 'dementia dessecans', 'dementia sejunctiva' and 'intrapsychic ataxia' all reiterated in different ways the idea of splitting.

The primary, or core, pathology, for Bleuler, was 'associative splitting', a disintegration of the connections between one thought and the next.[49] *Restitutio ad integram* was the term he used to designate recovery.

Modern psychiatry usually honours Kraepelin as having identified the syndrome of dementia praecox, though it takes issue with him for overemphasizing incurability. By contrast, I have demonstrated that incurability was an organizing principle of nineteenth century psychiatry, and it was this principle that resulted in the disease category. Just as Kant had pronounced mental derangement to be incurable, so Kraepelin devised a category that epitomized incurability. Even those who purported to be more optimistic became ensnared in the mutually defining relationship between incurability and dementia praecox. Bleuler (1908/1987:61) stated clearly that *restitutio ad integram* was not possible in schizophrenia. His colleague Jung explained this in a publication intended for the education of the lay public: 'Unfortunately the disease is too often incurable; even in the best cases, in recoveries where the layman would notice no abnormality, one always finds some defect in the patient's emotional life' (Jung 1982b:161). Although Bleuler (1950:9) rejected the theory of degeneration, he had a pessimistic view of the prognosis for schizophrenia and maintained an expectation that patients would slowly deteriorate (Abrahamson 1993).

Psychotic symptoms such as hallucinations, thought disorder, delusions, and motor disturbances were described in hundreds of pages of rich detail by both Kraepelin and Bleuler, yet they did not figure in either's core definition of the disorder. For

---

[49] A full discussion of the origins of Bleuler's 'associative splitting' is beyond the scope of this chapter. It was the culmination of a tradition that had its sources in Locke's empiricist theory of mind and his views on human development, both of which took sense perceptions as their starting point (Locke 1976:33–45). This tradition presupposed a view of the 'self', best expressed by Hume as 'nothing but a bundle or collection of different perceptions, which succeed each other with inconceivable rapidity, and are in a perpetual flux and movement' (Hume, cited in Russell 1961:636). In eighteenth century medicine, these ideas were central to David Hartley's associationist psychology, which viewed the mental functions as chains of association and madness as a breakdown in natural associations (Donnelly 1983:111–12). These ideas were pursued in France by the 'sensualists' and in Germany by Herbart with his theory of 'complexes' (clusters of psychic forces that could induce mental dissociation). Wernicke drew on this tradition with his theory of 'sejunction': 'a break in continuity, a structural loosening of associations' (cited in Berze 1987:55).

Kraepelin (1919:256), 'no single morbid symptom' characterized dementia praecox. The diagnosis depended on a recognition of the 'entire picture'. He did not demonstrate any interrelation between the great variety of symptoms that he described, except that he saw them all as a reflection of dementia and a loss of psychic unity (Wilkinson 1987:242). Similarly, for Bleuler (1950: 95–137) the only primary feature was a loosening of associations; all others were either 'secondary' or 'accessory'.

Kraepelin understood degeneration and loss of unity in terms of weakness because his personal world view was centred on a concept of the will. For Kraepelin, the natural, instinctive urges of the will determined the constitution, expression, and development of every living creature. Adult man,[50] possessed of a strong will that was freely and forcefully expressed through a fighting spirit, represented the evolutionary apex, the touchstone of perfection (Engstrom 1991:112; Kraepelin 1992a:518). The paragon was Bismarck. Kraepelin not only idolized him but published on the similarities between Bismarck's psychological qualities and his own (Berrios and Hauser 1988:814). Kraepelin was a fervent nationalist; he championed the unity and national identity of the German state (Engstrom 1992:255). During World War I he was a prominent member of a civilian lobby that agitated for annexation of parts of France. His international profile was high enough for this sabre-rattling, in the end, to become an embarrassment for an administration that had grasped Germany's impending defeat and that was actively suing for peace to prevent the economic collapse of the nation.

Kraepelin detected a weakness of the will in a range of conditions, classes, and peoples. Soldiers manifesting combat neurosis had 'infirm personalities', and the problem worsened as the army drafted more and more 'morally inferior' recruits. He saw a parallel in 'accident neurosis (that is, the reluctance of weak-willed persons to return to work after suffering an injury) . . . which has been spawned by pension legislation' (Kraepelin 1992b:258). Primitives, children, and women were

---

[50] I have deliberately used the term 'man' throughout this chapter to emphasize that there is a gender bias in these models of the person and psychiatric illness. They were ideas produced by eminent Victorian men who ran eminent Victorian institutions.

likewise susceptible to weakness. Thus symptoms of mental illness could be seen in undeveloped 'wild tribal people' with their demonic and magical beliefs (Kraepelin 1992a:520), in children with their 'spineless submission' (ibid:523), and in women with their propensity for extremes of excitement, their volatile mood, and lack of self-control (ibid:513). For Kraepelin, patients in mental hospitals were the weakest of all. The iron fist of war had exacted its toll on them, many of them having died of starvation and tuberculosis. Although he found this situation disagreeable, he thought it would temporarily ease the economic burden posed by incurable patients (Kraepelin 1992b:260). Ultimately, it was those with dementia praecox, the acme of inferiority, who more than any other group epitomized weakness and degeneration.

Current images of degeneration and disintegration

Many of the distinctive features of Ridgehaven Hospital that I observed during the 1980s had their source in the developments that have been sketched in this chapter. The old H-shaped double-storey wards were copies of nineteenth century English asylum designs. Of all the wards, it was Heathfield House, the most recently built, with its four corridors radiating out from a central information area and its large glass windows for observing patients, that came closest to Bentham's 1791 panopticon. The architect's vision of a natural aesthetic and his assumption that this design would exert a therapeutic effect on patients echoed the 'naturalism' of the early European Romantics. The idea of the psychiatric case, with its detailed clinical observations and extended developmental history, also had its roots in the first decades of the nineteenth century. Like the early adherents of the moral therapy movement, clinicians at Ridgehaven worked with the idea that a person has an interior, emotional core over which he or she should exercise control. The clinicians also worked with an idea of the person as a part-whole duality, where therapy was a matter of putting the parts back together to form a whole person. This approach employed a holistic style of thinking first formulated by the German anthropological psychiatrists with their psychosomatic theories of health and illness.

Degeneration

During the period of this study, the concept of degeneration continued to influence lay and professional understandings of schizophrenia. A Kraepelinian revival was sweeping through psychiatry. The advent of computerized axial tomography (CT) and then magnetic resonance imaging led to a renewed interest in degeneration:[51]

> The early CT findings were regarded as evidence for an underlying degenerative process and focused attention back to Kraepelin's early ideas. Schizophrenia was again viewed as a degenerative process. . . . This view fitted with the correlation between ventricular enlargement and cognitive impairment, a finding to be expected in a neurodegenerative condition. (Roberts 1991: 11)

The clinical definition of schizophrenia at that time placed emphasis on decline. The *Diagnostic and Statistical Manual III (DSM III)* stated that the disorder 'always involves deterioration from a previous level of functioning' (American Psychiatric Association 1980:181–93). When it was difficult to distinguish between schizophrenia and manic depressive disorder, many clinicians relied on this single criterion to discriminate between the two. Not only the staff, but patients and their families, saw schizophrenia as an incurable process of deterioration.

Disintegration and splitting

The spatial image of a disintegrating or split person also persisted as a habitual way of thinking about schizophrenia at Ridgehaven. Educational pamphlets, popular books, and television documentaries about schizophrenia commonly associated it with a 'split personality'. An article in the popular press, which cited a psychiatric authority, stated:

> Schizophrenia was often mistakenly described as a 'split personality' with a Dr Jekyll and Mr Hyde behaviour. Most patients suffering from this illness are passive folk who would not harm anyone and do not have split personalities.

---

[51] Although a neurodevelopmental hypothesis has recently become more popular (Jones and Murray 1991), degeneration is still a subject of active research and debate (Waddington *et al.* 1994).

Though it was by negative example, the very evocation of Jekyll and Hyde implied that schizophrenia *does* have something to do with splitting. A similar press article underscored this point:

> Only seven years ago, when Anne Deveson's son was first diagnosed as having schizophrenia, public knowledge of this common mental illness went little beyond misconceptions about split personalities and horror movies like *The Many Faces of Eve*. (*The National Times*, Sept. 6–14, 1985)

Dominating the page of the newspaper in which this article appeared was a large representation of a human face divided into two halves: one black and the other white, one side smiling and the other grimacing, one side surrounded by rain and the other by fire. By representing several sets of opposite values, this image unwittingly reproduced the very notion of splitting that the article was seeking to dispel.

Conversely, the word 'schizophrenic' in everyday language could be used to refer to inconsistency, contradiction, or being torn between conflicting roles, as in the following newspaper account of a busy Australian comedian:

> No one would blame Garry McDonald if he sometimes feels a little schizophrenic. The man . . . has taken on more roles than a bakery.

By the 1980s, clinical manifestations of disintegration or splitting no longer featured prominently among the formal diagnostic criteria for schizophrenia. The *DSM-III* retained only two such criteria, 'loosening of associations' and 'inappropriate affect', the latter referring to an incongruity between the patient's ideas and his or her emotional expression (American Psychiatric Association 1980:188). The International Classification of Diseases still included Bleuler's notion of 'ambivalence' which refers to an opposition between conscious and unconscious motivation (World Health Organization 1978:27). Despite this lack of emphasis in the official nomenclature, mental health workers continue to reproduce the idea of schizophrenia as a split person, notably in their ongoing use of the word itself, meaning a split mind (*OED*). In Chapter 4 I showed how the Ridgehaven staff used images of fragmentation in their day-to-day practice. They talked about their patients 'cracking up', 'going to pieces', 'falling apart', or undergoing 'psychotic dis-integration'. A pre-psychotic patient could be described as 'a bit loose at the edges' or 'beginning to fragment'. A first epi-sode of schizophrenia could be called a 'first break'.

Splitting also pervaded the visual imagery that accompanied the professional literature. Illustrations on the covers of books or pamphlets regularly split the word schizophrenia into two. For example, on the title page of a book by Neale and Olt-manns (1980), each letter in the word schizophrenia had a horizontal crack running through it; and in Karger's advertis-ing flyer for a book on positive and negative symptoms edited by Nancy Andreasen (1990) the word schizophrenia had each letter divided in half and dislocated, creating an uncomfort-able visual distortion. The patients' art work featured on the covers of *Schizophrenia Bulletin* sometimes employed a faceted or cubist style, with human faces divided into two or frag-mented and dispersed across the page. Similarly, in the adver-tisements carried by psychiatric journals, the pharmaceutical industry frequently employed the image of a split person to persuade psychiatrists to prescribe their antipsychotic medi-cation. For example, Smith, Kline and French advertised Ste-lazine using images that include a broken egg, an abstract representation of a human form with the limbs and head com-ing apart from the torso, and a representation of a human face on fabric, where the face was rent asunder as the fabric was stretched and torn. In an advertisement for Clopixol by Lundbeck there were two images of the same face appearing on two surfaces of a prism, and one of Squibb's advertisements for Modecate relied on an optical illusion: a frowning face that became a smiling face when turned upside down. A disturbing image that was used by McNeil for Orap was of an unsmiling woman whose own smiling face appeared in each pupil, as if there were two of her inside her head.

Weakened boundaries

The counterpart to the concept of internal disintegration was the idea that the patient had a fragile external boundary.[52]

---

[52] Tausk and subsequently Federn (1952:10–14, 230–6) were the earliest to write on the weakened 'ego boundary' in schizophrenia.

Patients who had been acutely psychotic sometimes expressed this quite explicitly, reporting the feeling that they were merging physically or mentally with other people around them, or that they had become confused about which ideas and feelings belonged to them and which belonged to family members or friends. Many of the symptoms of schizophrenia listed by Schneider (1974)—the so-called Schneiderian first rank symptoms—were an expression of this theme of the 'permeability of the ego–world boundary' (Koehler 1979:236). They included the feeling that thoughts were being taken from or inserted into one's mind, that one's own thoughts were being broadcast to those around, or that one's thoughts and impulses were externally controlled. Fabrega (1982) shows how these symptoms are predicated on a Western concept of the bounded individualistic person: 'These symptoms imply to a large extent that persons are independent beings whose bodies and minds are separated from each other and function autonomously' (Fabrega 1982:56–57). For the staff of Ridgehaven, the idea of a 'permeable ego boundary' had important implications for the treatment of schizophrenia. They tended to avoid intense forms of psychotherapy that involved intimate emotional work with patients for fear they might lose their sense of identity, merge with the therapist, and disintegrate. Treating a person at a distance, it was thought, helped him or her to reintegrate and to be restored as a bounded individual.

Schizophrenia and the person

Schizophrenia was the most important new diagnostic concept to emerge during the nineteenth century from the bringing together of the asylum and the university research institute. This chapter has traced two sets of ideas that were integral to the formation of this diagnostic category: one a concept of the divided person, arising from German Protestant thought; the other a concept of degeneration arising from French Roman Catholic thought. These ideas, I suggest, continue to inform psychiatric theory and practice in relation to schizophrenia.

I have argued throughout this chapter that psychiatric theories of schizophrenia are structured within a framework of Western concepts of the person. Inasmuch as we think of the person as *homo economicus*, invested with the values of progress and productivity, the 'schizophrenic' is the quintessential failure to achieve these ideals. Insofar as we conceive of the person as a unified, coherent, bounded whole, then the 'schizophrenic' epitomizes the converse of this conception: a divided, fragmented person without boundaries. The internal divisions within the 'schizophrenic' are not merely those caused by conflicting role demands, they are more deeply penetrating and disruptive divisions between intellect, emotion, and volition. Western concepts of the person draw on a basic metaphor of order, according to which the individual whole encompasses and orders the ensemble of parts. Schizophrenia represents a basic disorder of the person in which the parts disrupt and disorganize the whole.

Put together, progress and unity inform the way we think about the idealized person.[53] Their antitheses, degeneration and disintegration, structure the way we think about schizophrenia. That is, schizophrenia is more than a biological disease or a sick role. It is culturally defined as a basic flaw in the core attributes of personhood. The patient with schizophrenia becomes a fundamentally diminished person. Because these ideas are so deeply embedded in our history, they do not simply melt away in response to the community education programmes that seek to dispel the so-called myths of split personality and incurability. In the popular imagination, as in psychiatric thought, schizophrenia still implies an incurable disintegration of the person.

[53] There is a close affinity between unity and progress in Western thought. Unity is not static: it emerges or is achieved. For example, in the concept of the dialectic, unity progressively evolves from the synthesis of antithetical ideas. Nowhere is this more clearly set out than in the philosophy of Hegel (Forster 1993), whose influence was strongly felt by the early German psychiatrists.

8

Contemporary formulations of schizophrenia: explaining the inexplicable

The definition of schizophrenia changes as psychiatric institutions and practices undergo change and as innovative research techniques produce new knowledge. Already suffused with cultural imagery, schizophrenia is like a sponge that absorbs new meanings with the passage of time. This chapter identifies several of the most important of these meanings by examining the pre-eminent twentieth century causal theories. Aetiological theories have tended to cluster around two poles—biological and psychosocial—which during the first part of the twentieth century were thought to be competing paradigms. In the last thirty years, a bio-psycho-social model of schizophrenia has emerged that encompasses these poles and necessitates a particular characterization of the patient's family in terms of expressed emotion.

I do not intend to provide a comprehensive survey of the causal theories of schizophrenia or seek to adjudicate as to which among these theories are right or wrong. That is the task of psychiatrists, neurophysiologists, psychologists, and social scientists involved in schizophrenia research. My purpose here is to identify the salient theories, explore their institutional and cultural underpinnings, and examine their radiating consequences. This anthropological approach is especially germane to biological theories. There has been a tendency in the social science literature to assume that if an illness has a biological basis cultural factors must be less important and *vice versa,* as if biology and culture were mutually exclusive. A number of social scientists have sought to debunk the biological evidence in order to assert a sociocultural explanation for the illness. Jackson (1960) and Coulter (1973) are good examples. As a consequence, they quickly become entangled in arguments about the validity of particular hypotheses, and the methods of verifying or refuting them: they become trapped within the technicalities of the discourse. I am not concerned to evaluate the scientific merit of genetic and biochemical ideas about schizophrenia; rather, I wish to understand the cultural meanings they carry. Biology does not lie outside culture. Biological theories are developed by scientists and clinicians who work and think with cultural metaphors and images as well as underlying conceptual models of the person. Hence this chapter explores the meanings expressed in genetic and biochemical theories of schizophrenia and examines the consequences of accounting for one's experiences through these idioms.

There are two central arguments I wish to develop. The first concerns the reciprocal relationship between forms of knowledge and psychiatric institutions. Theories of schizophrenia bear the stamp of the institutions that produce them. At the same time, they legitimate the relationships and practices of the people working within these institutions. The second concerns the figure–ground relationship between knowledge of illness and concepts of personhood. Aetiological theories of schizophrenia tacitly presuppose cultural definitions of the person. They imply a defect in the most fundamental attribute of personhood, the capacity to be interpreted as engaging in meaningful action.

Schizophrenia is a diagnostic category used to classify and describe patients. It is also a window through which to view changing psychiatric institutions and cultural definitions of the person.

Beyond understanding: biological theories

Many causal mechanisms have been proposed for schizophrenia, most of them a variation on the theme of an inherited chemical or hormonal abnormality leading to a malfunction of the brain. At first it was tentatively linked to abnormalities in the 'processes of the sexual organs' (Kraepelin 1919:243). This idea reflected psychiatry's focus on sexuality at the turn of the century and its tendency to view sexuality as the polar opposite of rationality. It also explained the onset of this disorder soon after puberty or after childbirth in women. The research of Frederick Mott[1] carried out between 1907 and 1923 is representative of this early phase and has been summarised by Meyer (1973:506):

> There is a genetically conditioned lack of *élan vital* in patients affected by dementia praecox, expressing itself in atrophic change and reduced function of the endocrine glands, especially of testes, ovaries and adrenal cortex. This reduced function would most markedly bear upon . . . the neocortex, and especially its supergranular layer. The Nissle granules disappear; function is first 'suspended' and recoverable, but if the process continues, irreversible 'suppression' supervenes.

Many variants of this idea have since been put forward as each generation of researchers brings its own ideological focus and its particular technological advances to the field of schizophrenia research. In recent decades the most widely accepted version has been the 'dopamine hypothesis', in which it is postulated that schizophrenia is an inherited abnormality involving a neurotransmitter, dopamine, found in certain areas of the central nervous system.

The institutional basis for biological theories of schizophrenia

Biological theories of schizophrenia are the outcome of psychiatry's close relationship with laboratory medicine. In the main, they have been generated by scientists based in research institutes affiliated with universities and hospitals. The prototype for such an institute was the *Forschungsanstalt für Psychiatrie* in Munich, founded by Kraepelin in 1918 to bring all the allied sciences of psychiatry into one building (Peters 1991: 70). Within the English-speaking world, the Maudsley Hospital and its medical school (later to become the Institute of Psychiatry) was the exemplar. It was a neurologist and pathologist, the above-mentioned Frederick Mott who, even more than Maudsley himself, is regarded as responsible for its founding. Not long after his appointment in 1895 as pathol-

---

[1] See Meyer (1973) for a biographical sketch of Sir Frederick Mott (1835–1926).

ogist to the London County Council Asylums and director of the central laboratory at Claybury, Mott began his personal campaign to establish an institute in London. He envisaged a mental hospital in a city location with teaching and research facilities along the lines of Kraepelin's institute, with which he was personally familiar. Its central purpose would be 'the acquisition and spread of knowledge of the causes and treatment of insanity' (Mott, cited in Allderidge 1991:84). Its method of acquiring knowledge was to bring clinical sciences and basic sciences to bear on psychiatric problems, at first neuropathology, endocrinology, and genetics and later biochemistry, neuropharmacology, brain imaging, psychology, and statistics.

The Maudsley Hospital was not built in a day. The major components were put into place, one by one, over a quarter of a century, beginning in 1908 with a bequest of private capital (£30,000 from Sir Henry Maudsley), which was used to secure the financial backing of the London County Council. Then came the acquisition of a city property in 1911, the construction of a building during 1913–1914, the arrival of laboratories in 1916, the admission of patients in 1923, eventual recognition by the University of London in 1924, and liaison with a general hospital (Kings College Hospital) in 1932 (Lewis 1979b). Private capital became crucial from 1935 when the Rockefeller Foundation became the principal donor, thereby enabling the continuation of research through the Depression and World War II. After the war, the sources of research funding broadened to include recurrent university grants as well as grants from the Medical Research Council, (MRC), charitable trusts, and industry.[2] The pharmaceutical industry has increasingly provided financial support for basic neuroscience research to the extent that it is now an important source of intellectual leadership in this field. More recently, community organizations for those who suffer psychiatric illness have begun to sponsor research.

---

[2] See Institute of Psychiatry (1991:14, 29) for a typical breakdown of the sources of research funding. See also Pincus and Fine (1992) for a representative picture of research funding for psychiatric disorders in the United States. In 1988 the major contributors were the various national research institutes ($550 million), the pharmaceutical industry ($145 million), state governments ($66 million), and private nonprofit organizations ($30 million).

The 'ununderstandable' core of schizophrenia

The type of knowledge that is acquired and spread by such institutions asserts that schizophrenia is, in essence, a biological entity. This assertion is based on what Engelhardt (1975) has called an ontological view of disease: the assumption, usually tacit, that it is a real object rather than a logical type. In ontological terms, disease is conceived as having an existence independent of its particular form of expression in individual cases. When looking at schizophrenia from this viewpoint, the patient is regarded as categorically *different* from other people inasmuch as there is a schizophrenic 'thing' within him or her causing an 'extraordinarily unique alteration in the brain' (Snyder 1982a:595).

Using this approach to schizophrenia, symptoms are explained by means of a 'causal' paradigm. Drawing on Dilthey and Weber, Jaspers (1974) has distinguished between meaningful and causal connections. Meaningful connections are those that are established by an empathic process of understanding (*Verstehen*). We understand psychic events in terms of how they emerge from other psychic states or events. An example is an understanding of how the content of a person's thoughts arise from various moods, wishes, or fears. Causal connections, on the other hand, are explained (*Erklären*) rather than understood. Such explanations are expressed as equations or laws, established by the inductive methods of the natural sciences. The examples provided by Jaspers—a hallucination explained in terms of abnormal bodily functioning, a manic syndrome explained in terms of a cerebral process— suggest that in psychopathology physical events are most often posited as causes and mental events as effects. Such causal connections involve neural mechanisms that by definition are beyond consciousness. Consequently, when we are establishing a causal explanation for a mental event, its meaning content is irrelevant to this form of explanation. In theory, any psychic event—a thought, feeling, hallucination—may be subject simultaneously to a meaningful understanding and a causal explanation, but these two modes of comprehension operate independently; they do not help each other in any way. In practice, causal explanations apply to the domain that lies beyond understanding. That is, when we reach the limits of empathic understanding, we turn to causal explanation.

Jaspers' view of schizophrenia is especially pertinent to this discussion in view of the clarity with which he has illuminated (and thereby influenced) twentieth century psychiatric thought. For Jaspers, schizophrenia lies squarely within the domain that is closed to empathy, the domain of the '*ununderstandable*'. He draws a contrast between 'delusion-like ideas', which emerge understandably from preceding mood states, and the 'primary delusions' of schizophrenia:

> If we try to get some closer understanding of these primary experiences of delusion, we soon find we cannot really appreciate these quite alien modes of experience. They remain largely incomprehensible, unreal and beyond our understanding. (Jaspers 1963:98)

When compared to affective illness, which can be understood as an exaggeration of commonly experienced moods, schizophrenia as a whole is defined as beyond understanding. 'The most profound distinction in psychic life seems to be that between what is meaningful and *allows empathy* and what in its particular way is *ununderstandable*, "mad" in the literal sense, schizophrenic psychic life' (Jaspers 1963:577). Because schizophrenia is, at its core, an ununderstandable state, it can only be grasped by causal explanations that invoke extraconscious biological mechanisms.

The mysterious gene

The biological explanation opens with the idea that schizophrenia is an inherited disorder. Systematic research began with a family study carried out in 1916 by Rüdin, who worked in association with Kraepelin. He started with probands, or index cases,[3] who had a diagnosis of dementia praecox and sought to determine the rate at which their siblings were similarly affected. This and many subsequent family studies showed that schizophrenia was more prevalent in blood rela-

---

[3] The proband, or index case, is the person who forms the starting point of a genetic study.

tives of patients with the disorder than it was in the population at large: in general terms, the closer the relationship, the higher the prevalence. For many years the most convincing evidence for a genetic contribution to schizophrenia came from studies of twins, which demonstrated that monozygotic or identical twins of index cases were approximately three times more likely to develop schizophrenia than dizygotic or fraternal twins (McGue and Gottesman 1989). Another strategy was to look at adopted children. A pioneering study was that of Heston (1966), who showed that five of forty-seven adopted children whose biological mothers had schizophrenia subsequently developed the illness, whereas none of fifty adoptees whose biological mothers did not have schizophrenia developed the illness.

The optimistic claims of early researchers to have identified the 'schizophrenia gene' have given way to more circumspect reappraisals as the methodology has become more rigorous. Kallman (1946) found that 85.8 percent of monozygotic twins were concordant for schizophrenia, whereas Kendler and Robinette (1983) found a rate of 30.9 percent. Generally speaking, the greater the rigour in sampling methods and the techniques for determining zygosity, the lower is the concordance rate.[4] In a similar vein, early family studies showed the risk of developing schizophrenia among first-degree relatives to be as high as 12.3 percent. Later studies that used strictly defined diagnostic criteria, prospective selection of probands, and 'blind' independent diagnosis of probands and relatives demonstrated a risk as low as 1.61 percent (Abrams and Taylor 1983) or even no risk at all (Pope *et al.* 1982). These findings were highly controversial (Kendler 1983b; Pope *et al.* 1983), and the pendulum has subsequently swung back. A review by Kendler and Diehl (1993) of seven well designed studies suggested that the aggregate risk for first-degree relatives is 4.8 percent (with a range of 1.4 to 6.5 percent), 9.7 times the risk for relatives of matched controls. With the recent develop-

---

[4] The use of 'pairwise' concordance (the percentage of *twin pairs* in which both twins have a diagnosis of schizophrenia) yields lower rates than 'probandwise' concordance (the percentage of *individuals* who have a twin with schizophrenia) because with the latter method each twin in a pair may be counted separately (Kendler 1983a). In these examples, I have quoted probandwise concordance.

ment of gene mapping and the use of 'linkage' research strategies, which seek to localize a schizophrenia gene by showing its co-inheritance with known DNA gene markers, the cycle of optimism and cautious reappraisal has taken another turn. Sherrington *et al.* (1988) reported that schizophrenia was linked to two markers on an arm of chromosome 5 in two English and five Icelandic families, but in the same volume of *Nature* Kennedy *et al.* (1988) reported no evidence of such linkage in an extended Swedish family with thirty-three affected members. Subsequent studies failed to confirm Sherrington's findings (Hallmayer *et al.* 1992). Thus after a spectacular start for molecular genetics, 'euphoria rapidly turned to disquiet as several failures to replicate this linkage were reported' (Owen 1992).

The method of diagnosis has a profound effect on the findings of genetic studies. Gottesman and Shields (1982:13) first made this point by showing it is difficult to demonstrate that schizophrenia is inherited if the diagnostic criteria are too inclusive or too restrictive. By using criteria that lie midway between these extremes, however, it is possible to demonstrate that genetic factors play a part (McGuffin *et al.* 1984). That is, whether schizophrenia is inherited depends on how it is defined clinically. As a consequence, it has become common research practice to test a range of clinical definitions, from narrow to broad, determine which among these alternatives has the highest heritability, and call this one schizophrenia (Pato, Lander, and Schulz 1989). Instead of taking the illness as a starting point, this innovative method works backward from what appears to be inherited. However, in the area of molecular genetics a number of commentators believe that this practice may lead to spurious evidence in favour of genetic transmission (Owen, Craufurd, and St. Clair 1990). As a consequence, there is a growing consensus that failure to develop a clinical or laboratory method of defining the phenotype (the actual manifestation of the disorder) is now the major stumbling block to identifying the genotype (the abnormal genetic code) (Tsuang 1993:305).

A striking feature of this field of research is the elusiveness of the proposed mode of inheritance and the mysterious nature of what is inherited. There is no simple Mendelian inheritance. Family pedigrees show no consistent pattern. In monozygotic twins there is a high level of discordance (a situation where one twin has schizophrenia and the genetically identical twin does not). Using the pairwise method, Kendler and Robinette (1983) calculated that 81.7 percent of monozygotic twins are discordant for schizophrenia. Perhaps there are two schizophrenia genes, perhaps several. Perhaps the inheritance is heterogenous (different genes in different families), or it may be multifactorial, with the illness declaring itself only when a threshold of genetic and environmental factors is exceeded. Many of these explanations also invoke the idea of 'incomplete penetrance', where the genotype is not necessarily expressed as a phenotype, so family members who do not develop schizophrenia may still carry a genetic loading for the illness.

Geneticists also argue that it is not schizophrenia *per se* that is inherited but a diathesis—a vulnerability or predisposition to the illness—sometimes manifesting as schizophrenia and other times as a spectrum of related disorders. The 'schizophrenia spectrum' concept first appeared in early adoption studies, where it was used to account for the transmission of schizophrenia through blood relatives, even when they could not be diagnosed as having the disorder. For Kety *et al.* (1971) the spectrum encompassed acute schizophrenic reactions ('undifferentiated' type, 'schizo-affective psychosis', 'possible schizophreniform psychosis', 'acute paranoid reaction' and 'homosexual panic'), as well as borderline states ('pseudoneurotic' or 'ambulatory schizophrenia', 'questionable simple schizophrenia', 'psychotic character', and 'severe schizoid individual'). It was further broadened by including cases where the diagnosis was uncertain for lack of information. The final category within the spectrum was 'inadequate personality'. A high prevalence of these schizophrenia-like disorders was found among the biological relatives of adopted persons with schizophrenia. A related study added a 'soft spectrum' to this list, incorporating 'schizophrenic personalities' such as the 'subparanoid' personality (Rosenthal 1975). Heston (1970) had a different idea of what constituted the spectrum. He included 'schizoids', by which he meant 'eccentric, suspicion-ridden recluses', as well as antisocial men designated 'schizoid

psychopaths'. Both groups were lumped together with 'schizophrenics' into a conglomerate 'schizoidia-schizophrenia disease' group. The spectrum concept was rightly criticized for
its vagueness but it has nevertheless survived and has more
recently come to include new *formes frustes*: 'schizotypal personality disorder', 'probable schizotypal personality disorder',
and 'paranoid personality disorder' (Baron *et al.* 1985). Over
the years the spectrum has even come to include people who
are considered colourful, creative, imaginative, or artistic
(Heston 1966). Karlsson (1968) devised a category of 'super-
phrenics': gifted scholars, politicians, and financially successful
officials, who seemed to appear frequently in the pedigrees of
people with schizophrenia. His genealogies included a member of the Icelandic Parliament, a renowned linguist, a wealthy
farmer, a man who emigrated to America where he became
an electrical engineer as well as establishing two newspapers,
and another man who, ahead of his time, developed a plan
for the electrification of Reykjavik.

For geneticists, it is as if what is inherited is the essence of
creativity, strangeness, eccentricity, or difference. Only in some
instances is it expressed as schizophrenia.

The elusive neurotransmitter

As with the search for the genetic defect, there have been
repeated cycles of enthusiasm and disappointment in the
search for a faulty neurotransmitter in the brain. As one substance after another was implicated, investigated, and then ex-
onerated, investigators closed in on the biogenic amines, substances responsible for electrochemical transmission from one
nerve cell to another. Dopamine[5] emerged from a large field
to be the most likely suspect.[6] In 1963 Carlsson and Lindqvist
discovered that antipsychotic drugs (chlorpromazine and

---

[5] The name dopamine is a shortened form of the full chemical name. The initials
DOPA stand for dihydroxyphenylalanine.

[6] See Malek-Ahmadi and Fried (1976) for a review of the many substances that
have been implicated – mostly breakdown products of tryptophan, dopamine, epi-
nephrine, or norepinephrine. Most of the early theories, which have since fallen
by the wayside, postulated an inherited enzyme deficiency leading to the accumulation of metabolites that functioned as 'autotoxins'.

haloperidol) caused an increase in the breakdown products of dopamine in mice brains. They proposed that antipsychotic drugs worked by binding to dopamine receptor sites and blocking the action of this neurotransmitter. The blocking probably stimulated the synthesis and release of more dopamine by means of a feedback mechanism, leading to the observed increase in its breakdown products (Carlsson and Lindqvist 1963). It was speculated that if antipsychotic drugs worked by blocking dopamine, there might be an excess of dopamine in schizophrenia (Carlsson 1977). In support of this idea, the clinical potency of antipsychotic drugs was found to correlate with their affinity for dopamine receptors (Creese, Burt, and Snyder 1976). Thus the dopamine hypothesis, the most widely accepted of the biochemical hypotheses, arose secondarily from the postulated actions of psychotropic drugs. There was further indirect support. Amphetamine, which initially stimulates the release of dopamine, was known to cause a schizophrenia-like psychosis. Direct evidence, however, was lacking. It was not possible to demonstrate convincingly that there was an excess of dopamine or its breakdown products in the cerebrospinal fluid or in the brains of people with schizophrenia. Consequently, secondary elaborations were proposed. Perhaps there was an excess of dopamine in type I schizophrenia[7] and a deficit in type II (Crow 1980; Seeman *et al.* 1984). These alternatives also foundered for lack of experimental support.

After the failure to demonstrate excess dopamine, the focus shifted from neurotransmitters to receptor sites, specialized parts of the nerve cell membrane to which neurotransmitters bind. A new cycle of research began with the proposal that patients with schizophrenia had an increased density of dopamine receptors (Snyder 1976). The attention of the research community concentrated on a subtype of dopamine receptor called D_2 (Seeman *et al.* 1976), and it was considered

---

[7] Type I schizophrenia is characterized by the 'positive' symptoms of hallucinations, delusions, thought disorder, and incongruous affect. It has a good prognosis and is thought to be associated with dopamine hyperactivity. Type II schizophrenia is characterized by 'negative' symptoms, such as poverty of speech, affective flattening, lack of drive, and social withdrawal. It has a poor prognosis and is thought to be associated with structural changes in the brain. For a review of these distinctions, see Crow (1989).

important to study patients who had never been treated with antipsychotic drugs because these were well known to cause proliferation of D_2 receptors. Receptor studies were made possible by the development of a new technique known as positron emission tomography (PET), which enabled the researcher to visualize the location and measure the density of receptors in living humans. (The patient is injected with chemical substances such as 3-N-[^{11}C] methylspiperone or ^{11}C-raclopride, which contain a radioisotope. These substances bind to receptor sites and emit positrons as the isotope within them decays. The positrons, in turn, interact with nearby electrons, causing mutual annihilation and the emission of photons, which can be detected by crystals arranged in a ring around the patient's head (Buchsbaum and Haler 1987). From these data it is possible to reconstruct the location and density of the receptors.) Using PET, a group of researchers at Johns Hopkins Hospital in Baltimore demonstrated that untreated patients with schizophrenia had a two- to threefold increase in receptor density at a particular site within the brain (Wong *et al.* 1986). However, counter-evidence soon appeared in the literature, first from a group at the Karolinska Institute in Stockholm (Farde *et al.* 1987) and then from a group in France (Martinot *et al.* 1990), demonstrating no increase in the density of D_2 receptors.

Since then, the pursuit of the elusive receptor site has taken a number of directions. It is known that the antipsychotic drug clozapine, which is effective in schizophrenia, does not have a marked affinity for the D_2 receptor. It may exert its effects on the D_1 or D_4 receptors (Lieberman 1993), and perhaps these receptors are implicated in schizophrenia. Clozapine is also known to have a potent blocking effect on the receptor of another neurotransmitter, serotonin. Perhaps schizophrenia involves a complex interplay between dopamine and serotonin systems (Kahn and Davidson 1993).

Biochemical models of schizophrenia emanate from the pharmaceutical industry and the psychopharmacology research community (Lieberman 1993). They are by-products of research into the mechanism of antipsychotic drugs; and thus as new antipsychotic drugs are synthesized, so new models of schizophrenia are synthesized.

The inaccessible location

The search for abnormal dopamine receptors was largely concentrated on the extrapyramidal system within the brain, even though this site is unlikely to be implicated in schizophrenia (it is responsible for the coordination of motor functioning). Indeed the only reason for choosing it was that it was large enough for the PET scanner to focus on. A biochemical abnormality in schizophrenia is more likely to be located in nearby mesolimbic pathways because they are responsible for the functions that are impaired in schizophrenia. The latter pathways begin with neurons in an area of the midbrain known as the ventromedial mesencephalic tegmental area.[8] They project forward into the limbic system, a complex central relay station, and they ultimately terminate in areas of the forebrain known as the olfactory tubercle, nucleus accumbens, and central amygdaloid nucleus (Snyder 1982b). Mesolimbic pathways have not yet been amenable to direct study because of the limited resolution of the PET scanner (Martinot *et al.* 1990; List and Cleghorn 1993). There are a number of reasons for continuing to think that the limbic system may be impaired in schizophrenia. At an empirical level, atrophy of some component parts (medial temporal lobe structures, hippocampus, and amygdala) has been observed in a subgroup of patients. At a hypothetical level, one might expect to find a disturbance in the limbic system in schizophrenia because one of its primary functions is the regulation of emotional behaviour.

Neurophysiology has long distinguished between higher and lower centres of the brain. Higher centres are distributed diffusely across the various lobes of the brain cortex and serve complex functions, such as perception, motor coordination, language, and thought. Lower centres serve more basic functions, such as reflex action, hormonal regulation, and sexual appetite. Since the time of Hughlings Jackson,[9] this distinction has been given an evolutionary accent (Berrios 1991). Higher centres represent more recent developments in the evolution

[8] For a description of these pathways, see Wyatt, Kirch, and DeLisi (1989). For a schematic representation, see Cohen and Servan-Schreiber (1993).
[9] See McHenry (1969) for a biographical sketch of John Hughlings Jackson (1835–1911), which includes a discussion of Jackson's intellectual debt to the social evolutionism of Herbert Spenser.

of the animal kingdom. They are conceptualized as layered on top of the lower centres, inhibiting or controlling them. The limbic system is one such lower centre. It is regarded as archaic or primitive in both embryological and phylogenetic terms.[10] A principal function is to relay information coming from higher centres. It receives input from the so-called association areas, which interconnect those adjacent lobes that serve higher functions (Roberts 1991; Tamminga *et al.* 1992). In turn, the limbic system projects into the frontal cortex, which is concerned with higher order functions such as judgement and motivation.

The pursuit of the putative dopamine abnormality has thus led neuroscience into anatomical regions that have their own particular meanings in the discourse of neurophysiology. They are central, lying within the inner recesses of the brain. They are relatively inaccessible to investigation in humans. Of the alternative sites that have been proposed,[11] all are informed by the same idea that schizophrenia must somehow involve a malfunction of central, integrating neural pathways. Because these pathways are located in the lower regions of the brain, schizophrenia can be depicted as a chemical malfunction of the lower, primordial aspects of the person. Because they integrate the higher centres, schizophrenia can also be depicted as a disintegration of the highest, most complex human func-

---

[10] In the human embryo, for example, parts of the limbic system develop at a very early stage from the 'archipallium' and have recognizable counterparts in reptiles and lower vertebrates. By contrast, the 'neopallium' begins to differentiate only after three months. It undergoes a major expansion to form, among other things, the higher sensory and motor centres and association areas, which have no recognizable counterpart in lower vertebrates (Johnston, Davies, and Davies 1958:135–43). In keeping with the archaic image, the areas of the brain cortex implicated in schizophrenia are referred to as the paleocortex in contradistinction to the neocortex. In comparative psychiatry, too, there is a tradition of equating these lower subcortical structures with 'natural' functions of the human (e.g., reflex action), whereas higher cortical functions are associated with human 'culture' (see Al Issa 1982:13).

[11] Cadet (1984) suggested the so-called isodendritic core of the brain stem, extending from the spinal cord to the basal forebrain. Carlsson pointed to the possible involvement of 'corticostriatothalamocortical feedback loops', modulated by 'mesostriatal dopamine pathways' (Crayton 1990). More recently, attention has focused on mesocortical pathways, which project to the prefrontal cortex (Glowinski, Tassin, and Thierry 1984). Functional abnormalities (hypofrontality) in this region of the brain have been observed in schizophrenia (for a collection of papers on this subject see *Archives of General Psychiatry*, Vol. 49, December 1992).

tions. Alternatively, it can be seen as a breakdown in the connections between the higher self and lower self, recalling the nineteenth century language of splitting and Wernicke's notion of 'sejunction' discussed in Chapter 7. Another variant draws on the Jacksonian model of 'dissolution'—the idea that damage to higher cortical levels leads to the release of subcortical functions (Hardie 1991). Schizophrenia is thus seen as a state in which the lower functions escape from higher control. 'Positive symptoms represent aberrations in a primitive (perhaps limbic) substrate that is for some reason no longer monitored by higher cortical functions' (Andreasen 1990:3).

The search for a chemical abnormality in schizophrenia has led to these obscure regions of the brain because it has not been possible to find more obvious and straightforward pathology, as in Alzheimer's or Parkinson's disease. These practical considerations notwithstanding, cultural meanings have set the framework for biological research. From the outset, schizophrenia has been defined as an 'ununderstandable' state, an obscure disease, and a splitting or disintegration of the person. The search for its cause has led neuroscientists to assert that it is an unknown fault in the inaccessible core of the brain where neural pathways are integrated. That is, neuroscientific research reproduces cultural definitions of schizophrenia in its own technical idioms.

Scientific scepticism and optimism

From the outset, scientists at the leading edge of this research have expressed caution and scepticism about the role of dopamine in schizophrenia. Although there is ample evidence that major tranquillizers block dopamine receptors, 'none of this proves that dopamine is the causative "germ" of schizophrenia' (Snyder 1976). Evidence against the hypothesis has been compelling. Antipsychotic drugs have little effect on certain negative symptoms of schizophrenia, especially loss of drive and emotional blunting. Indeed up to thirty percent of patients do not respond to these drugs at all. Whereas the dopamine blocking action of the drugs occurs within hours, it is several weeks before their antipsychotic effects are observed, which raises the possibility that there are other pharmacological mechanisms, as yet unknown, that are more relevant to therapeutic efficacy. Furthermore, the schizophrenia-like psychosis associated with amphetamine does not support the idea that schizophrenia is caused by an excess of dopamine. Amphetamine stimulates dopamine release but ultimately causes dopamine depletion, and the onset of the psychosis coincides with this depletion phase (Alpert and Friedhoff 1980). More fundamental theoretical doubts have been raised. The idea of a defect in a single neurotransmitter is not compatible with contemporary models of neuronal transmission, which emphasize feedback, complexity, the interplay between multiple neurotransmitters, and a dynamic model of the receptor site. The people who opened up this field of research and who continue to lead it have always doubted that dopamine plays an exclusive role in schizophrenia (see reviews by Bowers 1980; Haracz 1982). From the beginning, Carlsson (1978) expressed caution: 'We are dealing with a very complicated interplay of many different systems, and we cannot disregard the other biogenic amines or the amino acid or peptide transmitters'.

News about the dopamine hypothesis comes from the laboratory to the psychiatric community through research reports and then, in summary form, in review articles and textbooks. It also appears in epigrammatic form in pharmaceutical advertisements interspersed between the pages of psychiatric journals. In this medium the hypothesis is portrayed in a more definitive style, which lacks the caution and doubt expressed by the researchers themselves, though drawing indirectly on their authority through the use of images derived from neuroscience and enhanced by means of colour and graphic design. During the early 1970s Janssen Pharmaceutical Limited advertised:

> Delusions, hallucinations, withdrawal, the bizarre symptoms that haunt the schizophrenic are now commonly associated with an excess of cerebral dopamine. Selective blockade of this neurotransmitter by Orap® (pimozide) offers the psychiatrist a new dimension in the treatment of schizophrenia.

In the late 1970s an advertisement for Melleril by Sandoz contained a stylized grey-green illustration of the human brain with the limbic system colored in soft red.

> Melleril, like all effective major tranquillizers, blocks dopamine receptors in the limbic system. Current theory suggests that this may be the site of action of major tranquillizers.

During the same era, an advertisement by Smith Kline and French Laboratories promoted the 'highly selective dopaminergic blocking action' of its product by depicting its chemical structure, the benzene rings, in attractive canary yellow standing out against a sky blue background. More recently, advertisements for antipsychotic drugs with an affinity for 5-HT_2 receptors imply that the role of serotonin is well established, although this idea is still highly speculative. An advertisement by Janssen shows a simplified version of how Risperdal blocks serotonin. The difference before and after administration is displayed using the vivid colour of PET scan images.

When compared to neuroscientists who develop and test such hypotheses, the psychiatrist reading these review articles and advertisements is a lay person; but when it comes to public education, the same psychiatrist becomes an expert. Public education usually conveys two clear messages: one, schizophrenia is caused by an abnormality in the brain; and two, we do not know what this abnormality is. In an interview conducted in 1987 for an Australian current affairs television programme, E. Fuller Torrey stated:

> We know it's a disease now. We know it's a brain disease like . . . multiple sclerosis or Alzheimer's disease or Parkinson's disease. And like these other diseases we don't understand the precise causes. We have theories about viruses, we have theories about the immune system, we have theories about biochemistry, and we have theories about the genetics. We know that in about one-third of people with schizophrenia there will be a family history of the disease. But we don't yet have the precise cause.

In a television documentary widely employed in schizophrenia education (Brightwell 1982), the viewer was taken right into the synaptic cleft, the microscopic space between nerve cells. A wave of dopamine molecules (represented by red balls) surged out of one cell across the synaptic cleft, bouncing onto the cell membrane opposite and landing in the receptor sites (represented by holes). A case of schizophrenia was depicted as an uncontrolled excess of red balls that swamped the synaptic cleft. This picture was followed by a treated case in which antipsychotic medication blocked the receptor sites. This case was represented by green tablets guarding the holes so the red balls could not land, and they eventually bounced away. There was a striking contrast between schizophrenia as a chaotic excess of red balls, connoting danger, and the medication as an orderly assembly of green tablets, connoting safety. The viewer was then informed that this representation was a hypothesis, not a fact, and that the biological causes of this disorder were considerably more complex than such a simplified model might suggest. These causes were still in the process of being unravelled by medical science.

In documentaries about schizophrenia, the dopamine model conveys the hope offered by scientific advance, while at the same time showing the impenetrable complexity and unintelligibility of this illness. Schizophrenia always lies one step beyond the grasp of science.

The inexplicable nature of schizophrenia

Themes of mystery, elusiveness, and inaccessibility are not restricted to genetic and biochemical research. The idea that schizophrenia is caused by a viral infection has a similar stamp. In 'Stalking the Schizovirus', Torrey (1988) reviews the inconclusive evidence for the hypothesis that schizophrenia may be caused by a 'slow virus', a 'latent virus', or a 'crypto-virus'. It is a restatement in a virologist's idiom of the underlying idea that there is something hidden within the brain that is yet to be detected.[12] An imaginative variation is the 'virogene' hypothesis, initiated by Crow (1984), in which it is speculated that a 'retrovirus' inserts its own genetic material into a parent's DNA, which is transmitted to his or her child, in whom it interferes with a gene, as yet unidentified, to cause schizo-

---

[12] See also Eagles (1992), who implicates prenatal polio virus infection, and Sham *et al.* (1992), who examine the relationship between schizophrenia and influenza epidemics.

phrenia. There has been no experimental support for these highly creative ideas (Carrigan and Waltrip 1990).

Some members of the scientific community express the opinion that technological advances such as detailed gene mapping or higher resolution brain imaging will ultimately reveal the true nature and location of schizophrenia:

> This terrible disease of the young will yield many of its secrets to neuroscience in the next few decades if the extraordinary flourishing of research begun in the 1960s and 1970s is not stifled by insufficient support. In the year 2000 an essay such as this might be able to discuss when in the developmental cycle specific genes and their products, in response to specific exogenous insults or stresses, produced various biochemical and electrophysiological abnormalities that, in turn, were the basis for specific abnormal behaviours in the numerous subtypes of schizophrenia. (Meltzer 1982:434)

Such millenarian statements tend to reinforce the elusiveness of schizophrenia because they project a precise understanding of its cause into an uncertain future.

A more significant body of opinion holds that current technology has already outstripped the capacity to define schizophrenia clinically in a way that is relevant or useful to research. Although it is possible to diagnose the condition reliably, it is unlikely that schizophrenia is a single disease entity that is explicable in terms of a single cause. As suggested by Bleuler, who coined the name, it is probably a group of disorders. This perspective locates the elusiveness of schizophrenia firmly in the present because it asserts that we cannot know what causes schizophrenia because we do not know what it is.

In 1896, Kraepelin (1987:23) stated that 'the real nature of dementia praecox is totally obscure', and in 1919 he wrote that 'the causes of dementia praecox are at the present time still wrapped in impenetrable darkness' (Kraepelin 1919:224). Carpenter, McGlashan and Strauss summed up the state of knowledge in 1977:

> We know virtually nothing about the etiology of schizophrenia. Despite evidence for a genetic contribution in some forms of schizophrenia, we know nothing about the nature of this component, how it may contribute to vulnerability, or to what extent it accounts for the variance in manifest schizophrenia. At

> present no factor can be said to be a necessary and sufficient
> cause of schizophrenia, or even a necessary but insufficient
> [cause] . . . Recognition of the paucity of etiological knowledge
> about schizophrenia is important since psychiatrists often as-
> sume that a reasoned understanding of its cause does exist,
> lacking only in detail. In fact, no other disorder in the history
> of psychiatry has had a richer panoply of global claims to its
> cause and cure. (Carpenter, McGlashan and Strauss 1977:14)

Since then, prominent researchers have continued to find different expressions for the perplexing nature of this disorder.
It has been described as a 'puzzle' (Gottesman and Shields
1982), it is 'complex' and 'enigmatic' (Carpenter 1983), 'elusive' (Ludwig 1983), 'baffling' and 'still a mystery' (Bleuler
1984). Schizophrenia is depicted metaphorically as poorly visible, its cause being 'murky' (Paykel 1980), 'obscure' (Roberts
1991) or 'clouded' (List and Cleghorn 1993). Schizophrenia
defies definition. Karno & Norquist (1989) regard it as 'the
classical refractory mental disorder—refractory to consensual
conceptualization, definition and identification of etiology'. In
reference to its convolutions and complexities, Tsuang (1993)
likens schizophrenia to the Gordian knot. Many others see it
as something that requires 'unravelling' or 'untangling'.

Schizophrenia, by definition, refers to actions and speech
that are bizarre, unintelligible, inaccessible to empathy, or 'ununderstandable' (to use Jasper's language), and which therefore demand the sort of causal explanation that can be provided by biological research. To provide such an explanation,
biology first renders patients into objects, ridding them of
their subjectivity. This is evident in the language of research
reports, in which a person with schizophrenia becomes a
'schizophrenic', a 'proband', an 'index case', or a 'schizophrenic brain' (Farde *et al.* 1990). These objects are then scientifically classified, observed, and measured to determine
their cause. However, the end product of this process, the resulting explanation, is that schizophrenia is caused by something unknown. Thus an inexplicable biological fault is employed to account for an incomprehensible state. What is
beyond empathic understanding is beyond scientific explanation. Because scientific research progresses by ongoing falsi-
fication of existing theories and continual modification of ex-

isting definitions, it produces ever changing knowledge and thereby constructs schizophrenia as a receding reality that is always just beyond the limits of science—just beyond the grasp of advancing reason.

Failure does not daunt biological science but spurs it on. Hypotheses that are ultimately proved false are still regarded as having been useful insofar as testing them generates a vast body of knowledge about physiological brain function. In pursuit of schizophrenia, the biological sciences discover the inner workings of the normal human brain.

It has long been recognized that the aspirations of scientific research to be value-free can never be fulfilled because science itself is embedded in the social institutions and culture of its practitioners. Statements about the biological aspects of schizophrenia are far from neutral. In this field, biology itself serves as a cultural metaphor for the unintelligible.

Empathic understanding: psychosocial theories

In contrast to biological theories, psychosocial approaches to schizophrenia seek an understanding of the patient's subjective experience. They come from several perspectives—psychoanalysis, interpersonal psychology, communications theory, social class analysis, labeling theory—some of which are hostile to one another. Whereas the biological theories are mainly coherent, reflecting the international uniformity of the research institutions from which they arise, the psychosocial theories are heterogeneous, reflecting the diversity of their sources. They represent psychiatry's close relationship to psychoanalysis, its long standing interaction with social science, its encounter with existentialism, and its feud with antipsychiatry. A number of the chief proponents of these approaches have been located outside academic psychiatry and the psychiatric hospital. They may be found in private practice or in university departments of sociology and anthropology, although they have made intermittent forays into mental hospitals to develop a critique of psychiatric practice. Their literary style is in stark contrast to the research reports of biological psychiatry. Instead of a statistical computation performed on a large number of patient-objects, there is an intensive analysis of a small number of patient-subjects, using the literary device of frequent quotations from the patient to represent his or her subjectivity. They publish in interdisciplinary journals such as *Psychiatry*, but their appeal has been much broader than this, for the leaders in this field have developed a constituency among professionals, academics, and radical students because their ideas resonate with a middle-class liberal consciousness, and their works have become best-sellers.

Notwithstanding this diversity of perspectives, there has been a common attempt to develop an empathic understanding of the patient by employing a 'physiological' or 'functional', view of illness. Englehardt (1975) shows how this view stems historically from humoral conceptions of disease as a state of imbalance, a reaction of the individual organism to its physical or social environment. For schizophrenia, this physiological approach posits a continuity between normalcy and psychosis rather than a categorical difference between the two. The patient is *similar* to other people. His or her behaviour is essentially meaningful: a logical, albeit severe, reaction to an untenable situation.

However, attempts to render patients' speech and behaviour intelligible were never fully successful because of the obdurate core of unintelligibility, the basis on which schizophrenia was defined in the first place. This unintelligibility could not so easily be rendered meaningful. It had to be displaced onto nearby people and institutions. The differences between the various psychosocial approaches depended on where they relocated this irrational madness: onto the individual's development, the 'crazy' family, the psychiatric profession, the mental hospital, or onto society itself.

Psychosocial theories and the diminished person

As a consequence of Jung's working relationship with Bleuler, psychoanalysis played an early role in attempting to develop an empathic understanding of patients with schizophrenia. Among the early analysts, Adler adopted the most radical position, arguing that schizophrenic symptoms, no matter how bizarre and apparently meaningless, were fully accessible to

psychological understanding (Rattner 1983:173–5). Psychoanalysts attempted to 'understand schizophrenia in terms of
factors common to all human experience' by positing basic
similarities between neurosis and psychosis (London 1973:
169). As with the neurotic patient, the person with schizophrenia had the capacity to form a transference relationship
with an analyst, and the illness could be understood in terms
of conflicts and defences.[13] Neurosis and psychosis were located on the same continuum of regression. Whereas neurosis
involved a mild regression to early childhood, schizophrenia
was a more profound regression to the psychological functioning of the infant, or even the foetus, with the emergence of
primordial or archaic processes (Arieti 1955:35). At these levels of regression 'ego splitting' was said to occur, thus invoking
the nineteenth century idea of the split person. Another consequence of profound regression, according to psychoanalytic
theory, was that the irrational 'primary process' thinking of
the unconscious mind would erupt into consciousness and
dominate rational 'secondary process' thinking. Instinctual
drives would burst out of control as they overwhelmed the
mechanisms that normally kept them repressed.

However, a division arose within the psychoanalytic community. A body of opinion asserted that schizophrenic behaviour was not on a continuum with neurosis but 'unique and
separable from other groups' (London 1973:171). According
to this school, schizophrenia was an 'internal catastrophe', a
severe disruption of the person's internal organization, accompanied by 'withdrawal of libido' from the world. The patient could not enter into a transference relationship and was
thus beyond psychoanalytic understanding and treatment.

Taken as a whole, the psychoanalytic movement characterized the person with schizophrenia as amenable to empathic
understanding on the one hand and requiring causal explanation on the other. A large element of schizophrenic behaviour lay beyond the limits of understanding and therefore required explanation in terms of extra-conscious mechanisms,
such as drives, instincts, and the unconscious. Both schools

---

[13] In a transference relationship, emotions from the patient's past are transferred
to the analyst. Working through this transference relationship is held to be the
essence of psychoanalytic therapy.

within psychoanalysis created analogies with marginal persons: child, infant, foetus, and split person.

Despite superficial differences, there is a fundamental parallel between psychoanalytic and biological constructions of schizophrenia. Both portray it as a disintegration of the person: for neurobiology, a defect in the central integrative neural pathways; for psychoanalysis, an internal catastrophe or split. Both portray the disorder as a state in which primordial aspects of the person overwhelm and dominate the more complex aspects: the primitive dominates the developed, the lower dominates the higher. Biology represents it as a surge of dopamine in the limbic system and psychoanalysis as an upsurge of instinctual drives. Although formal psychoanalytic therapy is no longer used for patients with schizophrenia, phrases such as 'regression', 'primary process thinking', and 'loss of impulse control' continue to be used in psychiatric hospital practice, reiterating the theme of psychosis as an uprising of the 'primitive' within the person.

Growing out of psychoanalysis, there was an attempt to understand schizophrenia as a meaningful reaction to the environment. Psychiatrists looked first to the patient's immediate social group, beginning with the mother. 'Its most primitive, and perhaps its most important, part' wrote Sullivan (1962: 250), 'is contributed by the mother and/or her equivalents, nurses and the like'. For Fromm-Reichmann (1948) the 'schizophrenogenic' mother was one who related to her child in a contradictory way: covertly rejecting but overprotective. It was a short step from the mother to the family. Before long, several theories arose that transposed the irrationality and splitting of schizophrenia to the family system as a whole. Bateson, who followed the long tradition of comparing primitive or non-Western people with people who had schizophrenia,[14] discovered the 'double bind' in the families of patients (Bateson *et al.* 1956). He employed a cybernetic metaphor of the person as an information processing machine and located psychopathology in a 'system' or 'pattern' of communication. This was more than a novel theory of schizophrenia. It became a focus for a new family therapy movement that developed in

[14] The double bind hypothesis of schizophrenia grew directly from the earlier concept of 'schismogenesis', which was derived from ethnographic observations in New Guinea and Bali (Bateson 1958:175; 1973:11).

opposition to biological psychiatry and psychoanalysis and that was taken up by the growing professions of psychiatric social work and clinical psychology. No longer was the patient split, the entire family was split, as is evident in the work of Lidz on family 'schism' (Lidz, Fleck and Cornelison 1965). Irrationality did not come from the patient, it arose in the family and was 'transmitted' to the patient (Singer and Wynne 1965).

Antipsychiatry too was concerned to relocate the core features of schizophrenia away from the patient. Like family therapy, it was a reform movement that made schizophrenia into a *cause celebre* in the process of developing a radical critique of institutional psychiatry and the family.[15] By focusing on the mystificatory structure of the family and the negating practices of institutional psychiatry, Laing reaffirmed the essential rationality of the patient. Symptoms became a 'deliberate use of obscurity and complexity as a smoke-screen to hide behind' (Laing 1965:163). Schizophrenia became a 'special strategy that a person invents in order to live in an unlivable situation' (Laing 1967:95). The patient became a rational, self-acting agent who had the capacity for choice and whose authentic nature was located in subjective consciousness. This resonated with both Goffman's idea of strategic interaction and Szasz's idea of mentally ill behaviour as a calculated means of soliciting help to solve problems of living. Such attempts to render schizophrenia meaningful were only partially successful. In the end, it was possible to sustain the argument that the patient was rational only by dividing him or her in two, thereby resurrecting the old metaphor of the split person. In *The Divided Self*, Laing wrote, 'A certain amount of the incomprehensibility of a schizophrenic's speech and action becomes intelligible if we remember that there is the basic split in his being . . . the individual's being is cleft in two' (Laing 1965:162). By this statement he meant a split in the totality of experience, a split between the self and the world, between self and body, and between 'true' and 'false' selves.

---

[15] Schizophrenia also became the *cause celebre* of a French antipsychiatry movement that evolved from Lacanian psychoanalysis. For Deleuze and Guattari, schizophrenia became a model of therapy known as schizoanalysis or schizophrenization. See Turkle (1981:174–7) for a critique of this movement, its irrelevance to most patients, and its restriction to the radical chic element of the French intellectual community.

The luminaries of the antipsychiatry movement were a left-wing existentialist, a sociologist, and a right-wing psychoanalyst promoting the values of free enterprise capitalism—strange bedfellows by any reckoning. The common ground shared by these disparate figures was an individualistic ideology in which the model person was epitomized by rationality, choice, and self-control. All three were engaged in a search for the meaning of schizophrenia. All eventually rediscovered commonplace Western ideologies of the person. Laing, in particular, embodied the tradition of the sceptical insider who, although ostensibly mounting a critique of psychiatric practice, reproduced the essential ideologies of institutional psychiatry and reaffirmed it as a privileged site for the definition of cultural concepts of the person.

Psychoanalysis, family therapy, and antipsychiatry each sought in a different way to develop an empathic understanding of schizophrenia and to treat the patient as a fully competent person whose speech and behaviour could be interpreted as meaningful. They sought to render understandable someone who was, by definition, 'ununderstandable'. Although schizophrenia was peripheral to the psychoanalytic movement, it was crucial to the development of the family therapy and antipsychiatry movements, becoming a test case or model demonstration of how it was possible to find meaning in people who had been disqualified by society. Thus the very idea of schizophrenia came to serve as a window on an ideal. Each major theorist tried to look at schizophrenia and discover its cause. Instead, they looked through schizophrenia and rediscovered widely available cultural conceptions of the person. It is little wonder that when these attempts to comprehend irrational patients ran into difficulty, they fell back on metaphors of diminished personhood: the primitive, the infant, the split self.

Bio-psycho-social schizophrenia and the 'EE' family

Team processes and the bio-psycho-social model

Since the 1960s there has been an attempt to integrate biological hypotheses and psychosocial perspectives into a comprehensive bio-psycho-social approach. This approach was originally developed in the context of general hospital psychiatric practice and psychosomatic medicine, and was first popularized by Engel (1977) when he worked at the University of Rochester at Strong Memorial Hospital. Strauss and Carpenter (1981) have provided one of the best examples of its application to schizophrenia. The ascendancy of this new approach reflects two important changes within psychiatric institutions. One is the advent of teams. The other is deinstitutionalization, which has led psychiatrists to renew their alliance with the families of patients and with the community organizations that represent these individuals.

At the same time the team approach came to clinical psychiatry it began to appear in psychiatric research. Increasingly, research projects became collaborative ventures undertaken by psychiatrists, psychologists, and social scientists, working together in a group that was reminiscent of a clinical team. A well known early example of this approach was the work of George Brown, a sociologist, who carried out studies in collaboration with a number of psychiatrists, including Morris Carstairs and John Wing. For many years, Christine Vaughan and Julian Leff, a psychologist and a psychiatrist, have published together. A more recent example is the work of Melvin Karno, a psychiatrist, and Janis Jenkins, an anthropologist. The financial and organizational requirements of team research are often so great that it can only be sustained if supported by large-scale research institutes such as the National Institute of Mental Health or the World Health Organization.

In Chapter 4 I identified a number of core processes—integration, encompassment, and exclusion—that organized relationships among members of a clinical team. It is possible that these processes may also pertain to the organization of research teams, though I have no direct ethnographic evidence to support this proposition. What is clear, however, is that integration, encompassment, and exclusion are all features of the knowledge about schizophrenia generated by such teams.

In the bio-psycho-social model, integration of a diversity of perspectives is achieved by the multifactorial approach. Biological or psychosocial aspects are rendered into causal fac-

tors, or variables, and then arranged into an additive or inter-
active sequence as if they belong in a mathematical equation
that results in schizophrenia. The puzzle of schizophrenia to
be solved by psychiatric science is how these factors might
interact.[16] According to the systems theory, on which the bio-
psycho-social model is based, factors are hierarchically organized. Each factor is a subsystem in open communication with
other subsystems and is encompassed by the whole. Pathology
within any single subsystem reverberates throughout the entire
system. Thus schizophrenia is not just a neurochemical abnormality but a disorder of the encompassing whole. The
whole patient is pervaded by disorder. The puzzle of schizophrenia is how to comprehend the nature of this systemic
disorder.

The idea of imbalance, derived originally from humoral
medicine, is one way of thinking about such a disordered system. In health, homeostatic feedback mechanisms maintain
an equilibrium. In schizophrenia, the whole bio-psycho-social
system teeters on the edge of imbalance because it is exqui-
sitely sensitive to the environment and because normal feedback mechanisms do not work. The patient is vulnerable to
both understimulation and overstimulation. 'On the one
hand, too much social stimulation, experienced by the patient
as social intrusiveness, may lead to an acute relapse. On the
other hand, too little stimulation will exacerbate any tendency
already present toward social withdrawal' (Wing 1978a). These
ideas of schizophrenia as the essence of disequilibrium are the
scientific correlates of common-sense images of the psychotic
patient as unbalanced ('tipping up', 'tipping over' 'off his
rocker'), as explored in Chapter 6.

At the same time that they encompass a range of perspectives, bio-psycho-social theories maintain medical dominance
by giving precedence to biological knowledge,[17] in keeping
with the underlying emphasis and tenor of the institutions
where such theories are developed. In England much of the

---

[16] See Rosenthal and Kety (1968) for an early representative collection of studies
into the interaction of genetic and experiential factors in schizophrenia.
[17] See Goodman (1991) on the dualism that underlies the bio-psycho-social theory
and its failure to adequately account for a causal relationship between mind
and brain.

influential bio-psycho-social research has emanated from the Medical Research Council Social Psychiatry Unit (Wing 1980) based at the Institute of Psychiatry, the home of biological research. The term bio-psycho-social itself suggests that biological factors are regarded as more fundamental and prior.[18] When the model is represented diagrammatically as a set of concentric circles or squares (see Fig. 4.2), biology occupies the innermost core, with successively peripheral zones designated psychological, interpersonal, social, and cultural. In another common representation, factors are arranged hierarchically in an ascending order, combining spatial images (from microscopic to macroscopic) and societal images (from individuals to nation states). Engel's (1980) version ascends from subatomic particles, to atoms, to molecules, to organelles, cells, tissues, organs or organ systems, the nervous system, the person, the family, community, culture, society, nation, and finally the biosphere. The ideas that inform these representations are reflected in the language of bio-psycho-social psychiatry. The adjective 'biological' is usually associated with nouns such as 'roots', 'basis', 'substrate' or 'core', whereas 'cultural' usually refers to 'overlay'.

The bio-psycho-social model is commonly reduced to a linear sequence representing a causal chain, drawing on the analogy of the mathematical equation. Biological factors appear on the left side of the equation, where they operate as primary causes. Psychosocial factors are located toward the right side. If they are attributed any influence at all, it is the weak influence of a secondary factor that does not cause the illness but modifies its subsequent course and outcome. Lower social class, migration, and social isolation had formerly been attributed a causal role in schizophrenia; but with the introduction of the bio-psycho-social model, these factors underwent a shift to the right to become secondary aspects of the illness or merely factors affecting its prognosis. This linear sequence translates easily into the life history of an individual, where biological factors mainly come into play at or before birth (a genetic endowment, intra-uterine insults, or perinatal

---

[18] Carpenter (1987:21) is an exception in that he rejects conventional assumptions of biological priority: 'When multiple levels simultaneously subserve an observed dysfunction, it is not *a priori* evident which is primary.'

trauma); and the psychological and social factors come into play much later when they trigger the illness (Birley and Brown 1970) or influence the recovery process. The distinctive genre of bio-psycho-social psychiatry is the multi-author volume, where the priority of biology is evident in the chapter sequence. First come the biological topics, such as genetics and neuropathology, followed by discussions of psychological and family factors, and finally topics dealing with cultural issues, economics, and community care (for examples, see Brenner and Böker 1989; Powchik and Schulz 1993).

The bio-psycho-social approach does not exhaust Western thought on schizophrenia, as there are alternative theories and metaphors that this form of psychiatry seeks to exclude as illegitimate or to keep on the margins of accredited knowledge. For example, the radical biological stance of the orthomolecular movement asserts that schizophrenia is a disorder of vitamin balance. Proponents of this view adopt a position first promoted by the chemist Linus Pauling (Hawkings and Pauling 1973). Their popular constituency lies mainly among adherents of the 'healthy living' movement, with a small but active following among some patients and their families. Bio-psycho-social psychiatry discredits the orthomolecular model as lacking scientific validity (Wing 1978b:45; Briggs 1981). Likewise, supernatural or religious interpretations are discredited as irrelevant to a modern secular definition of schizophrenia. Such interpretations are likened to occult, magical, or spirit possession beliefs of tribal peoples or of mediaeval Europe (Wing 1978b:14–20), and are thereby relegated to history or primitivism. It is often patients themselves who hold these extreme somatic or religious views. They may explain their symptoms as a result of poisoning. They may interpret their situation in terms of good and evil forces, possession by God or the Devil, or external control over their body and mind. Thus an important effect of the bio-psycho-social model is to exclude some of those ideas about schizophrenia advanced by the patients.

Bio-psycho-social science has also excluded the earlier family theories of schizophrenia from the arena of legitimate knowledge. A carefully controlled experiment was set up to test Singer and Wynne's theories of communication deviance.

It demonstrated no detectable difference between families of people with schizophrenia and families of people who do not have this illness (Hirsch and Leff 1975). Experiments to test the double bind hypothesis also found that it is neither specific to, nor selective for, schizophrenia. Antipsychiatry retreated in the face of bio-psycho-social psychiatry. In the preface to the second edition of *Being Mentally Ill*, Scheff (1984) offered a major retraction of labelling theory, confessing that it is 'ambiguous, ideologically biased, . . . [and] not literally true'. He acknowledged the possible role of neurotransmitters and stated that psychiatric treatment is not necessarily a labelling reaction.

Thus psychiatric science has dominated family therapy and antipsychiatry by domesticating them, incorporating them into an overarching bio-psycho-social model that reasserts the priority of biology. It is under the umbrella of the bio-psycho-social approach that biological reasoning has again assumed a dominant position in psychiatric thought. Psychoanalysis, the family approach, and antipsychiatry have endeavoured to develop an empathic understanding of the patient, but as each of these interpretive perspectives has been subsumed by bio-psycho-social science, it has become operationalized and rendered into a causal factor. These changes entail a shift from an interpretive to an empirical paradigm, from understanding schizophrenia to explaining it.

Deinstitutionalization and the EE family

It has often been commented that the bio-psycho-social version of schizophrenia exonerates family members. McLean (1990) has shown how, in the United States, this practice has been largely due to the influence of organizations that represent families of people with mental illness. She traces the rise of the National Alliance for the Mentally Ill (NAMI) from a small group of 284 people in 1979 into an organization of more than 80,000 in 1989. It gained a reputation as a powerful, effective lobbying force in Congress. NAMI actively sought to modify the professional discourse and scientific theories of mental illness, and it played an influential role in shaping policy within the National Institute of Mental Health (NIMH), fostering the development of biological rather than psycho-social research. NAMI's most persuasive advocate in this re-gard was Shervert Frazier, previously the director of the NIMH. 'Clearly the redefinition of schizophrenia as a disease of the brain, with emphasis on organic processes, was largely an effort by families to once and for all exculpate themselves from generations of blame and indignity imposed by mental health professionals espousing family aetiology theories of mental illness' (McLean 1990:977). In England the relation-ship with family organizations has been less confrontational. Psychiatry has cultivated a constituency among families by en-dorsing the Schizophrenia Fellowship and by articulating a sustained critique of Laing and others who appeared to be blaming family members. In response, these organizations have come to function as major outlets for the distribution of the bio-psycho-social model to the general public. In Australia the Schizophrenia Fellowship distributes films and video re-cordings, educational pamphlets, and books that espouse this model.

The new alliance between psychiatry and the family is a direct consequence of deinstitutionalization and the increas-ing responsibility it has placed on family members to care for their mentally ill relatives. At the beginning of the asylum movement, urban life and the family were regarded as noxious and excitatory influences. A cure could be effected only by removing the patient to the calm of an asylum located in a natural rural setting and by discouraging family visits. Now, at the end of the asylum movement, these values are reversed. A cure can be effected only by removing the patient from the noxious influence of the institution to his or her natural set-ting, the community, and the family. Thus the family is no longer regarded as a primary causal factor in the evolution of the illness. Instead, it becomes a weaker, secondary factor that either interferes with or facilitates recovery. The family has been shifted from the left side of the schizophrenia equation to the right side, from a strong influence to a weak influence, from a causal factor to a recovery factor.

From the structural terrain of deinstitutionalization and the conceptual terrain of bio-psycho-social thought, a new body of knowledge has emerged to do with expressed emotion (EE) in families. Building on the idea of emotional overstimulation, it began with a series of studies that demonstrated patients run a high risk of relapse if they return to live with relatives who are emotionally expressive (Brown *et al.* 1962; Brown, Birley, and Wing 1972; Vaughn and Leff 1976). Three types of emotion directed toward the patient, all negative, were found to be relevant: critical comments, hostility, and overinvolvement. Standardized interviews were developed to rate the expression of these emotions. Critical comments were the easiest to quantify because it was possible to count their number during a specified period of time. The intensity of emotional expression varied from low, through mid-range, to high. However, the statistical design of this research dictated that families be apportioned to two groups so that EE could be treated as a dichotomous variable whose association with relapse could be determined by statistical means, such as the chi-square test (Brown, Birley & Wing 1972). The number of critical comments was the main criterion: seven critical comments or more meant that a family was designated 'high EE'; fewer than seven meant 'low EE'. It is preferable when using the chi-square test to have two groups of approximately equal size.[19] In this 1972 study a cut-off point was chosen, which meant that 45 of 101 families were designated high EE and 56 low EE. In a later replication of this study, the cut-off point was lowered to six critical comments because this number gave a more distinct separation of relapse rates. 'In view of the arbitrary nature of the original cutoff point, we felt justified in making an adjustment in the level of criticism required for allocation to the high EE subgroup' (Vaughn and Leff 1976).

Expressed emotion has been celebrated as the most important recent advance in our knowledge of the psychosocial dimensions of schizophrenia. A large-scale international research enterprise has developed that explores the many facets of EE (Kavanagh 1992), including its cross-cultural significance (Karno and Jenkins 1993). A new style of family intervention has been developed to help families lower their EE level (Koenigsberg and Handley 1986).

---

[19] This is to ensure that the number of cases in any one cell of a four-cell design does not fall below the minimum required for a legitimate comparison of data.

The EE approach flows logically from the bio-psycho-social model in its linear form. When schizophrenia is regarded as an equation, the family, if it is not to be attributed a causal role, must become a secondary factor that influences the course of illness. To render the family a factor, psychiatric science measures some aspect of it and treats it as a variable. EE researchers have elected to make this variable dichotomous, thereby creating new entities: the high EE family and the low EE family.

Apart from this logical connection, there is a substantive link between EE research and the bio-psycho-social model. EE is a parameter for categorizing families according to whether they support current definitions of schizophrenia. Drawing on data collected in their 1976 study, Vaughn and Leff (1981) provided stereotypes of high and low EE families. They characterized high EE family members as intrusive. They are intolerant of disturbed behaviour and doubt that their relative is genuinely ill. 'Frequently the patient is blamed or held responsible for his condition'. By contrast, low EE family members are concerned but cool and controlled. They respect the patient's need for distance and tolerate disturbed behaviour. They acknowledge that their relative has a legitimate illness and do not hold him or her responsible for its symptoms. These stereotypes have a currency despite the arbitrary nature of the cut-off point by which they were created.

Thus psychiatry has absolved the family of the blame for the schizophrenia. In exchange, it asks that the family support its bio-psycho-social definition of illness and charges the family with the responsibility of behaving in a manner that facilitates the patient's recovery. To those families who do not, it offers therapy. It is in this substantive sense that the bio-psycho-social model and EE research are mutually supportive.

I have demonstrated that the dichotomous (high/low) nature of the EE construct flows from the overstimulation/understimulation model of schizophrenia and, more importantly, is dictated by the statistical methodology of the original research. It has become widely accepted in psychiatric practice because clinicians, following the example of Vaughn and Leff (1981), can easily render it into stereotypes that are used to characterize families thought to be helpful or difficult. A family who accepts and tolerates the illness might be described as providing 'the perfect low EE environment', but an argumentative, emotional, blaming family is today described as 'a typical high EE family'. Although the organizations representing families have found EE research more acceptable than the previous generation of family studies, there is growing concern that it serves to 'conceal subjective judgements of families behind the objective veneer of a complex scientific methodology' (Kanter, Lamb, and Loeper 1987) and that the EE construct can be used by mental health professionals as a pseudoscientific means of negatively stereotyping some families (Hatfield 1987). The future direction taken by this research will largely be determined by the interplay of power between national family organizations, state psychiatric services, and national research organizations.

Where does the patient sit amid all these organizations and definitions? The institutions of psychiatry and the family, with their concepts of schizophrenia as a bio-psycho-social entity in an EE environment, tend to construct the patient as a 'victim', a 'sufferer,' or a 'burden' (Thompson and Doll 1982; Fadden, Bebbington, and Kuipers 1987). Less stigmatizing characterizations must await the development of the fledgling organizations that represent patients (for example, the Hearing Voices Network in the United Kingdom) to the point where they too can exert some influence in the medico-political arena within which schizophrenia is defined.

Institutions, schizophrenia, and the person

In this chapter I have developed the argument that aetiological theories of schizophrenia reflect the institutional background of the people who develop them as much as they reflect the patients who have this condition. That is, it is possible to 'read' the latest theories for what they tell us about the organizations that produce them. Schizophrenia is a pastiche of concepts, which attests to the number and diversity of institutions that have a say in its definition, beginning in the nineteenth century with the asylum and the university research institute and expanding during the twentieth century to include philanthropic trusts such as the Rockefeller Foundation, national research funds such as the NIMH and the MRC, the pharmaceutical industry, psychoanalysis, various reform movements such as family therapy and antipsychiatry, and the many scientific disciplines that surround psychiatry, such as genetics, biochemistry, virology, sociology, and anthropology. These various institutions, with their paradigms, policies, and sectional interests, can be seen in the different models of schizophrenia, either as a background context or manifested explicitly. The influence of such institutions is most clearly evident in the different languages used to talk about a patient with schizophrenia: the 'proband' of the geneticist, the 'schizophrenic brain' of the biochemist, the 'regressed ego' of the psychoanalyst, the 'divided self' of the antipsychiatrist.

As institutions evolve, so does the definition of schizophrenia. The most remarkable change during the twentieth century has been the move away from the asylum. It has entailed a geographic shift from the rural idyll to the urban centre. Psychiatric practice is moving toward general hospitals; the production of psychiatric theories is moving to research institutes; and many patients are moving back to live with their families. The model of schizophrenia as a bio-psycho-social entity located in an EE environment is a knowledge correlate of these new institutional patterns. It legitimates the collaborative structure of the research institute and at the same time serves as a blueprint for the treatment of patients by the multi-disciplinary team. As a consequence, the patient is captured in a new language derived from team ideology, and his or her family is evaluated in the new language of EE generated by the grammar of statistics.

In the scientific literature it is recognized that theories of schizophrenia are historically contingent. They are often referred to as 'current theories'. Wing (1978a) calls them 'concepts of schizophrenia in vogue at present'. Paykel (1980) describes various biochemical hypotheses as 'topical' or 'fashionable'. In *fin de siècle* Europe, when literary and art movements revealed a general preoccupation with sexuality, medicine also began to claim sexuality as its province. Accordingly, when the new disease category of dementia praecox was formulated, its cause was attributed to an abnormality of the sexual organs. As medicine's infatuation with sexuality passed, it lost interest in these theories. During the late twentieth century, medicine's focus has become ultra-microscopic. In an era of molecular biology and gene mapping, the cause of schizophrenia is sought at the level of specific neurotransmitters and their receptor sites, or abnormalities in amino acid sequences at specific loci on individual chromosomes.

The history of art, as Samuel Butler said, is the history of revivals. The history of schizophrenia may be seen in the same light. The nineteenth century theme of the split person resurfaced at the beginning of the twentieth century in a psychoanalytic form as 'ego splitting' and again at mid-century in an existential form as the 'divided self'. The idea of evolutionary degeneration was reformulated by psychoanalysis as regression to a primitive level of functioning and by neurobiology as a dysfunction of the primordial parts of the brain leading to a disintegration of higher, more complex cerebral functions. Although they might appear to be disparate disciplines, psychoanalysis and neurobiology have much in common. Both have breathed new life into the early Jacksonian 'dissolution' concept of pathology as an escape of primitive functions from higher control. Underlying the most modern of all models of schizophrenia are the ancient humoral theories of imbalance and excess. The sophistication and creativity with which old themes are refashioned, as well as the diversity of languages in which they are expressed, gives the area of schizophrenia studies a special cultural richness and depth and makes it a fertile field for anthropological analysis. This richness and diversity comes from a productive tension between science and madness when they confront each other. Science explains certain aspects of schizophrenia, but it also defines it, in large measure, as beyond explanation—just about to be grasped by the latest technological advance. Thus for science schizophrenia is elusive, mysterious, and enigmatic.

At the beginning of Chapter 7 I identified interpretation—by which I meant the ability to interpret the actions of others and to be interpreted by others as engaging in meaningful action—as the most fundamental criterion for defining what we mean by a person. The various approaches to schizophrenia discussed in this chapter pertain to the issue of interpretation. The *biological approach* states that people with schizophrenia are categorically different from other people. They do not have the capacity for accurate interpretation, nor can their actions be interpreted as meaningful. Their symptomatic behaviour must be explained in terms of a genetic or cerebral mechanism, though this explanation is not yet available to science. *Psychosocial approaches* state that people with schizophrenia are essentially the same as other people. They have the capacity to interpret others accurately, and their own speech and behaviour can be empathically understood, but not as one might interpret the speech and behaviour of a full person, only that of a primitive, a child, or a split person. The bio-psycho-social model encompasses both approaches, though it more closely resembles the biological approach.

Elements of all three approaches are found in day-to-day hospital practice. At Ridgehaven the staff were well versed in the theories outlined in this chapter, and it was common to find them drawing on each in turn as the situation demanded, oscillating between a biological explanation and a psychoanalytic understanding, between an antipsychiatry perspective and a bio-psycho-social synthesis. When different approaches were pieced together in this way, they produced a composite definition of the person with schizophrenia as partly the same as others, partly different; partly intelligible, partly unintelligible; partly endowed with the capacity for interpretation, partly lacking it; partly a person, partly a nonperson. In this setting of ambiguity, the patient with schizophrenia became an anomalous category of person, both endowed with and lacking the core attributes of personhood.

9

Schizophrenia for practical purposes

Irrespective of the status of current theories and whether there is sufficient evidence to prove them, schizophrenia finds its principal use in psychiatry as a working concept that is good enough, more or less, for practical purposes. This chapter looks at schizophrenia as a pragmatic category by studying how the patients and staff of Ridgehaven Hospital talked about the illness in their day-to-day interactions with each other. It forms an ethnographic coda to the previous chapters, examining how people drew on myriad sources—theoretical perspectives, lay understandings, underlying cultural metaphors—to negotiate with each other what schizophrenia meant. The analysis is based on data I recorded during the course of an education programme in which the staff taught patients about schizophrenia. Although not the only opportunity for patients and staff to discuss psychiatric illness, it was a setting in which a team of professionals worked together with patients and in which differing definitions of schizophrenia were aired. The staff oscillated between the biological and the psychosocial approaches within an encompassing bio-psycho-social framework. Biologically speaking, schizophrenia was seen as an entity located in the patient's body but separate from his or her self. It was also portrayed as a set of ideas and actions for which the patient was not held responsible. Psychosocially speaking, schizophrenia was reintegrated with the person and relocated within the patient's sphere of responsibility. Patients contributed actively, partly embracing and partly rejecting the representations of schizophrenia put forward by the staff.

Education programme: structure of the course, its curriculum, and teaching styles

The education programme was developed at a time when the scope of the Schizophrenia Team was expanding to offer a more comprehensive range of services. At the suggestion of the Team Leader, a psychiatrist whom I have called Dr Guthrie set up a multidisciplinary education team, inviting interested clinicians from each profession to participate. The most enthusiastic response to this invitation came from a group of psychiatric nurses who worked in the subacute ward, Forest House, which I have previously described as a setting in which team principles and psychiatric hegemony gave way to ward principles and nursing dominance. Independently of the psychiatrists and social workers on the Team, nurses in Forest House already ran a rehabilitation programme for chronic patients that had a psychotherapeutic orientation, chiefly comprising group therapy techniques that involved role-playing, assertiveness training, and specific exercises to build self-esteem. Though not opposed to a biological model of schizophrenia, their approach was a partial critique of this model with its focus on psychopathology, its tendency to perceive patients as passive and controlled by their illness, and its propensity to make patients dependent on the hospital. The Forest House nurses sought to revalue chronic patients, emphasizing health rather than illness. They aimed to reinvest patients with a sense of responsibility and self-control. To do it, they drew on a range of theoretical approaches, such as traditional psychoanalytic concepts, gestalt therapy, and Maslow's concept of self-actualization, reflected in a nursing policy statement:

> Each individual's essential value and uniqueness is emphasized. Whilst much of the group discussion centres around the clinical features of schizophrenia, a concept of wellness and of normality is constantly reinforced. Participants are encouraged to take responsibility for their thoughts, feelings and behaviour in an effort to live more autonomous lives.

In this setting of therapeutic enthusiasm and nursing activism, three nurses wrote a series of booklets—*So They Say You're Crazy, Delusions: Is This For Real, Man? You and Your Voices,* and

Life is for Living—which formed the curriculum for the education programme. They wrote in a distinctive literary style that attempted to capture 'the language of the patient', although, as it turned out, what the patients actually said was often more sophisticated than the booklets suggested. Symptoms were described in bold, simple statements. The layout was uncluttered, with one or two major points on each page. There was frequent use of upper-case lettering, underlining, asterisks, and exclamation marks to draw the reader's attention to key ideas. Sometimes there was a light-hearted tone, with rhyming jingles:

> When you're setting out to impress,
> Don't leave yourself open to STRESS.
> If you want to stay whole,
> Polish up on CONTROL,
> And you'll find you're a roaring success!

Other sections contained crisp instructions, 'STORE IT, IGNORE IT', or 'ZIP IT!!'. Cartoons were used to illustrate the main ideas. For example, a kangaroo illustrated how thoughts and conversation could jump from one subject to another; a railway train that was stopped by a brick wall illustrated the blocking of a train of thought. Taken as a whole, the style of the booklets was reminiscent of children's books. Indeed, people with schizophrenia were often depicted as an infant with three or four strands of hair, as a teenager, or as a little person dressed in pyjamas.

A number of problems arose in the hospital in relation to the ownership of these booklets, ultimately solved by a compromise in which copyright was invested in the authors, and the hospital, as a corporate body, acted as publishers and received the proceeds of sale. Once these problems were ironed out, the booklets were ceremonially launched by the state Minister for Health. In no time there was a demand for them from psychiatric professionals and hospitals both within Australia and from overseas, an indication of the extent to which they reflected contemporary practice in relation to schizophrenia.

Thus at the core of the education programme were a group of nurses who were actively involved in developing their own distinctive style, who were being enveloped by the tolerant psychiatric hegemony of the team, while at the same time encountering the administrative authority of the hospital.

Each course comprised eight two-hour sessions run over four weeks. Patients were referred to the course coordinator by members of their Treatment Team. Most of them were young adults, ranging in age from 18 to 30 years. All had a well established diagnosis of schizophrenia or schizo-affective disorder, and all had been receiving treatment for more than two years; patients who were actively psychotic were not accepted into the course. The high ratio of men to women probably reflected the preponderance of young male patients with a poor prognosis treated by the Schizophrenia Team. As many as eight patients at a time participated in each course.

The psychiatrist, Dr Guthrie, delivered the first two sessions during which schizophrenia was defined. For the middle section of the course two psychiatric nurses, Phillipa and Patrick, took a leading role on alternate sessions. Brenda, a social worker, led the final session on community resources, and Frank, a community psychiatric nurse, played an active role throughout. The course was conducted in a large room in Forest House, used at other times for recreation.

I observed two contrasting pedagogic styles: workshop and therapeutic. Dr Guthrie's sessions had a workshop atmosphere, with patients and staff seated around a large square table, handouts placed in front of them, and an overhead projector on the table. From time to time, Dr Guthrie stood in front of the class and wrote on a blackboard. The second style was employed by Patrick more than any other team member. During his sessions the table was removed, and patients sat in a circle facing each other as might be expected in a group therapy session. Corresponding to these different styles, two ways of defining illness were used in the education course. In one, schizophrenia was defined as separate from the patient; in the other, it was reintegrated with the patient. The first style was used mainly at the beginning of the course and the second during subsequent sessions.

Separating schizophrenia from the person

The overarching definition of schizophrenia was presented by the psychiatrist during the first two sessions. Dr Guthrie taught a bio-psycho-social view of the illness: patients were born with an inherited predisposition to schizophrenia, and emotional stress that occurred during adolescence or adult life could precipitate an episode of illness. He taught that schizophrenia occurs the world over at similar rates, irrespective of race or culture.[1] Thus he accorded psychological factors (stress) and social factors (culture) a minor precipitating or modifying role compared to the biological origins of the illness. To underscore this biological basis, Dr Guthrie compared schizophrenia to diabetes. This analogy is commonly used for schizophrenia education. Symptoms of diabetes can be linked to a measurable abnormality in blood glucose; and although medical science cannot provide a full account of its aetiology, many of the causal mechanisms are known and can be explained to patients. (By way of contrast, schizophrenia is not used as a model of disease for diabetes education.) The analogy serves to convey the idea of an incurable but controllable illness and the need for long-term medication to achieve this control, the idea of insulin being more acceptable than major tranquillizers.

The important pedagogic techniques of Dr Guthrie's workshops were reading and writing. He either read from the booklets, demonstrated the main points by means of an overhead projector, or wrote up patients' accounts of their experiences on the blackboard under psychiatric headings. I have shown in my analysis of case records how clinical interactions that involve reading and writing produce a segmented account of the patient because the interview dialogue must be truncated and transformed to fit the subdivisions of the document. The end result is a rendition of the patient as divided into segments. Hand in hand with this process of division is the transformation of private experiences into the public domain of written discourse and their translation into a technical idiom that serves to distance them from the patient. Similar effects occurred in the education course when Dr Guthrie wrote three headings across the top of the blackboard, *Behaviour,* *Thinking,* and *Feeling.* Beginning with a definition of schizophrenia as an abnormality in each of these segments of the

---

[1] See Leff (1981), Murphy (1982), and Prince (1983) for contrasting opinions on the incidence and prevalence of schizophrenia in different cultures.

person, he invited patients to discuss their own abnormal experiences under each heading.

Tim, the first patient to talk, offered an account of how he had once jumped onto the back of a staff member during a football match. Dr Guthrie did not accept this behaviour as abnormal, as it could be interpreted within the common-sense understanding of a football tackle. Tim replied that it was not part of the match: the football was at the other end of the field when he did it. Only then was 'jumping onto a staff member's back' written under the heading of abnormal behaviour. Norman, another patient, stated that he once threw a pair of shoes away. Again, the psychiatrist declined to accept this action as an example until Norman added that the shoes were brand new and that he threw them away because his voices told him to do so. Now that this act was defined as unintelligible within a common-sense framework of understanding, his contribution was entered without further modification onto the list of abnormal behaviours. As the other patients observed these negotiations, they learned how to phrase an acceptable description. By the time the third patient, Craig, spoke up, he was able to provide a fully furnished account of abnormal behaviour without any need for negotiation. He once threw his clock and his long playing records into a fire. It was a stupid thing to do, he admitted, but he did it because his voices told him to.

Under the next heading, *Thinking,* Tony said that he had a delusion that he was a communist spy. In a long monologue, he described how he thought he had taken photographs of secret plans and defected to another country, and that other communist spies wanted to kill him. This account was delivered in the confident style of a raconteur, prompting Dr Guthrie to ask Tony in a quizzical tone whether or not he really believed this happened. Tony replied that it was 'sort of real and sort of make-believe'. For it to be a delusion, Dr Guthrie stated, Tony would have to be fully convinced that it was real. During the final interchange, Tony said he *was* fully convinced at the time, and Dr Guthrie wrote it on the blackboard as a delusion.

Sometimes the negotiation led to a patient's account being excluded from the definition of schizophrenia. When Tony said he had experienced 'thought blocking' (defined as a sudden stopping of thoughts, leaving a blank mind), Dr Guthrie asked whether his thoughts disappeared from his mind entirely so that he could not recall them. Tony could remember what he had been thinking before his mind went blank. As a result, this experience, said Dr Guthrie, was not part of his schizophrenia. No entry was made on the blackboard.

The patients exercised less control over the negotiative process than did Dr Guthrie. They were seated around the table in a public forum, offering accounts of their private mental experiences, many of which did not neatly fit the categories of normal or abnormal. Standing by the blackboard, chalk in hand, Dr Guthrie exercised control by shaping these amorphous accounts so they clearly fitted into one or other of these categories. As the discussion moved from *Behaviour,* to *Thinking,* to *Feeling,* examples of bizarre behaviour, unintelligible thinking, and strange feelings began to flow easily from the patients, keeping the psychiatrist writing quickly.

The schizophrenia education booklets were used for the same purpose as writing on the blackboard. In a way that was reminiscent of a school classroom, one patient at a time was asked to read from a booklet, pausing after the description of each symptom so the other patients could provide examples from their own experience.

Norman:	[reading from *So They Say You're Crazy*]: You may hold beliefs which others do not share, e.g., you may believe that other people are 'out to get you'. You may believe that you are a powerful, perfect person. You may believe that your body is being 'changed' in some way. You may believe that other people can read your thoughts or that you can tell what other people are thinking.
Dr Guthrie:	Have any of you experienced any of these?
Ron:	I had thoughts I was Jesus Christ.
Norman:	I thought I was the Devil.

Although the initial process of elicitation and writing was based on a division of the person into three areas (behaviour, thinking, and feeling), as the session progressed a more basic division emerged between person and schizophrenia. In-

cluded under the rubric of the person were normal, understandable thoughts and perceptions that were located inside
the head and that were owned and controlled by the patient.
Under the rubric of schizophrenia fell abnormal thoughts and
perceptions, those that were not amenable to common-sense
interpretation, that were externally located, and that were not
owned or controlled by the patient.

Once this potentially blurred distinction had been clarified,
the education programme focused on how these two entities,
the person and the schizophrenia, should properly relate to
each other. There was an expectation that the person should
suffer from the schizophrenia, as illustrated by the oft repeated
dictum: 'You are not a schizophrenic, you are a person who
suffers from schizophrenia'. With an onset during adolescence
or early adulthood, this suffering had a tragic dimension. Patients were seen as having been struck down in their prime.

Descriptions of suffering were elicited from patients and
then amplified by the education programme. When asked to
describe their feelings, they volunteered 'fear', 'anger' and
'helplessness'. Throughout the course, the staff directed their
empathy toward such expressions of suffering and thereby encouraged and reinforced them. When discussing the symptom
of 'thought broadcast' ('You may believe that other people can
read your thoughts') Dr Guthrie said, 'It must make you feel
exposed!' When the class was asked to catalogue their emotions, one patient revealed how he had thought he was going
to die. Dr Guthrie spontaneously offered, 'Could I add
"panic" and "terror" to our list; wouldn't most people panic
if they thought they were going to die?' Asked how they felt
when they first discovered they suffered from schizophrenia,
Tim replied, 'Shock!', and this was written on the blackboard.
Craig said he had found out from other patients and it did
not worry him much. This off-hand response was ignored.
Similarly, positive emotions were excluded from the definition
of schizophrenia. When discussing grandiose delusions ('You
may believe that you are a powerful, perfect person'), many
of the patients began to smile. Craig said that his delusions
made him feel 'good' and 'powerful' but these adjectives were
neither acknowledged nor recorded. During the discussion of
'thought broadcast', Tim asked if it meant that people could

work out what is going on in your head by observing your body language. Dr Guthrie replied, 'No, it is specific to the illness and it is *frightening*'. Suffering emerged as a key criterion by which symptoms were judged a legitimate part of schizophrenia.

The theme of suffering was continued in subsequent sessions of the course that dealt with hallucinations and delusions. These sessions were run by Phillipa, the psychiatric nurse. She stated that hallucinations resulted from suffering, and that they created even more suffering. In the booklet *You and Your Voices*, this view was conveyed by a pictorial representation of a patient in a state of anguish as a result of hallucinations. Asked how they might feel, the patients offered, 'frightened' and 'insecure'. Phillipa also reinterpreted pleasant hallucinations in terms of suffering. Although they might appear on the surface to be enjoyable, they were held to represent an escape from the problems of loneliness and isolation. Delusions too, even if enjoyable, were defined as an unconscious defence against 'feeling bad about you and your life', a way of 'escaping from harsh reality'.

The only way to deal with suffering, it was argued, was to exert control over the schizophrenia. A combat metaphor, widely used in medicine to talk about treatment, was also used in this setting to exhort patients to fight their illness, battle its symptoms, and thereby overcome the suffering. Courage and determination were the requisite qualities.

The patients, however, did not fully accept that they 'suffered' from schizophrenia. The stance adopted by Ron is illustrative. During the third session of the course, when Phillipa was explaining how delusions stemmed from life problems, Ron related how bad his life had been as a result of unemployment and arguments within his family. He compared his delusion of being Jesus to a ball that neatly filled a hole in his life. Eventually the ball became too big for the hole so it no longer fitted. It was a fantasy, said Ron, that had grown too large and had begun to take over his life. This testimony was greeted with admiration and respect from the staff. However, Ron added that his delusion was not all bad, and that some good things had come from it. Phillipa acknowledged Ron's point, agreeing that there were many positive aspects associated with delusions. During this interchange Ron adopted a stance characteristic of many patients, partly accepting the role of sufferer and partly rejecting it. Given the persuasive force of Ron's personal account, Phillipa altered the main thrust of her argument for that session by acknowledging that schizophrenia could have some positive as well as negative aspects.

Similarly, when Phillipa talked about the relationship between hallucinations and suffering, patients agreed that the figure depicted in the cartoon was suffering; but a different picture emerged when they recounted their own experiences. Norman asserted: 'I wasn't frightened of my voices. They were telling me who I was. Sometimes they told me I was good, and sometimes they told me I was bad.' In reply, Phillipa suggested that there might have been things in Norman's life that were going wrong prior to the onset of the voices, but Norman disagreed: 'Life was good, I felt really important.' This conflict of interpretations led to an impasse that could not be resolved.

Some members of the team appeared perplexed or sceptical when patients reported they did not suffer from their symptoms. When Brenda, the social worker, asked Walter about his voices, he replied:

Walter:	They were thought forms. They came from Lucifer's mistress on Saturn. They understood me . . . understood what I was getting at. They would just chat with me.
Brenda:	How did you feel?
Walter:	[smiling bashfully]: In love.
Brenda:	Not frightened?
Walter:	[pausing to consider his reply]: Not really.
Brenda:	[quizzically]: Not really? . . . Mmmm.

When they wished to make their resistance more pointed, patients would redefine the experience of schizophrenia as humorous and its treatment as pleasurable, as discussed in Chapter 6. Thus when asked about delusions, Craig built up a series of fantastic portraits of himself as Flash Gordon, Sitting Bull, Bruce Lee, and a werewolf, which had the other patients in fits of laughter, but not the staff, who remained stony silent. At a later session concerned with how patients could change their lifestyle to gain control over their illness, Tony suggested going for a holiday, smoking marijuana, and having a warm shower; or, as he said, 'having a shower just a little on the hot side of warm'. The staff tended to pass over such comments, return to the booklet, and move on to the next section, thereby reasserting the structure of the course and the formal definition of schizophrenia and suffering.

Thus far I have described a number of disparate domains that came together into a coherent constellation when staff interacted with patients. There was the domain of psychiatric knowledge comprising the bio-psycho-social model of schizophrenia with its special emphasis on biological abnormality. This knowledge domain was linked to the domain of inter-professional relationships. As the person who presented the bio-psycho-social model, it was the psychiatrist who laid out an encompassing framework for the team as a whole. As I have previously demonstrated, this model could serve as a blueprint for team integration while at the same time facilitating psychiatric hegemony. Thirdly, there was the domain of staff–patient interaction. I have described a reading and writing educational technique that had the effect of portraying patients as divided into segments, the most important division being that between person and schizophrenia—between what was understandable and what was 'ununderstandable'. This division went hand in hand with the idea of biological schizophrenia as a repository or an explanatory framework for thoughts, feelings, or actions deemed not amenable to common-sense understanding. The staff expected that patients should suffer from their schizophrenia because suffering established a proper channel for empathy. Whereas it was inappropriate for the staff to empathize with feelings of love toward Lucifer's mistress and they could not relate to the predicament of a spy who had defected, they *could* direct their empathy onto the suffering patient. Finally, there was the domain of resistance. Patients partly rejected the idea of suffering, not when the psychiatrist was laying out the definition of schizophrenia and setting the framework for the team but later, during the discussions with the psychiatric nurse and the social worker.

Although these domains were disparate, what brought them together was the nexus between the language of bio-psycho-social psychiatry, the public medium of reading and writing, the power to deploy a team, and the power to define a patient as split in two. Patients lacked the power to organize the team. They lacked the power to define themselves and their schizophrenia, to adjudicate in matters of what was a hallucination and what was not. Their power lay in the arena of private emotions, where they controlled the definition of what was suffering and what was pleasure. This power endowed them with the capacity to reject empathy—to resist at the point where the staff really put their hearts into it.

Reintegrating schizophrenia with the person

Starting from the overarching definition that was set up by the psychiatrist, the nurses moved toward a psychosocial definition of schizophrenia that sought to reintegrate it with the person. Phillipa drew on psychoanalytic constructs, explaining how people are divided into an unconscious and a conscious part and how symptoms of schizophrenia could be understood as a communication between the two. Hallucinations, she said, were messages from the unconscious mind that tell you about the good and bad feelings you have toward yourself, an idea expressed in *You and Your Voices*:

> For instance, guilt, fear and anger—especially towards loved ones—are hard to accept consciously. But these thoughts have to be expressed in some form or another. Your unconscious mind produces voices to express the thoughts for you.

Delusions too, in Phillipa's view, originated in attempts by the unconscious to protect the conscious self, as was well expressed in *Delusions: Is This For Real, Man?*:

> Your delusions show how your unconscious self thinks and feels about you and your surroundings. Feeling bad about yourself and your life is very hard to accept. (We tend to believe that we must feel good and cope well all the time. This is not so.) When you feel bad your unconscious mind protects you. One way in which it protects you is to create a fantasy world.

In contrast to what Dr Guthrie taught about the unintelligible nature of schizophrenic symptoms, Phillipa stressed that they could be understood. They were not separate from the person, they arose from within, albeit from within a person divided into two parts.

This reincorporation of schizophrenic symptoms into the person was enacted at the fourth session conducted by Patrick. Patrick began in the reading and writing mode used by Dr Guthrie. He drew a vertical chalk line on the blackboard and wrote *True* on one side and *Delusional* on the other. The main point he conveyed was that the patients could learn to detect, by watching the reactions of others, when they were talking in a delusional way and when they were telling the truth. Following this exercise there was an abrupt transition in presentational style. Leaving the blackboard, Patrick sat down with the group, telling everyone to place their booklets to one side. The table used for previous sessions had already been removed so the staff and patients could be seated in a circle, facing each other as in a group therapy session. Patrick offered patients a choice. Either they could rid themselves of their delusions entirely, or they could control their delusions by storing them away in the back of their minds. Some patients expressed uncertainty about this offer. Ron said that in some ways he wanted to remove his delusions, but in other ways he did not. Patrick reassured everyone that if they chose to store their delusions away, these delusions would still be there at any time in the future if they were needed. He then asked all participants to close their eyes. Some simply lowered them. Talking in a soothing tone of voice, he encouraged everyone to conjure up their delusions ('all those ideas that people have said you were crazy for'), to bring them to the front of their minds, examine them, then push them into 'some dark corner'. 'Say goodbye to these ideas,' he said (in the words of the booklet, 'Store it, ignore it'). Finally, Patrick gave the instruction to open their eyes and replace the delusions they had stored away with good ideas about themselves.

In keeping with the tendency to partially accept and partially reject what the staff were teaching, Ron said that this session made him feel 'pressured' and that the group had been 'too close' for him. This statement had the effect of undermining Patrick's psychosocial approach and his attempt to reintegrate delusions in some meaningful way with the person. His response to this threat was to return to a more standard illness model of schizophrenia, as initially outlined by the psychiatrist.

> *Patrick*: This is only education. If you come down with an ill-ness then . . . . .
>
> *Tim*: Like a broken leg!
>
> *Patrick*: Yes!

The return to a biological analogy was accompanied by a re-turn to the reading and writing mode. Patrick asked everyone to get out their booklets, and they recommenced the written curriculum.

In the same way that some patients were unwilling to accept the idea of suffering, they also regarded the internalization of schizophrenia as a contentious issue. Craig exemplified this attitude better than any other patient. Although he accepted his diagnosis of schizophrenia, he nevertheless did not accept that hallucinations and delusions came from within him: 'It doesn't matter what you say, I still think it was God. It is not your own thoughts. The voices mean you *are* possessed by the Devil.'

Taking apart and putting back together again

During the overall sequence of this education course, delu-sions, hallucinations, and other symptoms of schizophrenia were first separated from the person and then were packed back into the person again. This sequence was depicted in the booklets with simplistic clarity by means of cartoon figures rep-resenting patients. Symptoms were represented by agencies located outside the head. Small demons, perched near the patient's ear, inserted and withdrew thoughts through a hole in the skull. A malevolent figure emerging from a cloud con-trolled the patient like a puppet on strings. Delusions were represented by a 'thought bubble' above the patient's head. Sometimes the skull itself was depicted as disintegrating—

either cracking like a jigsaw puzzle coming to pieces or opening up like an orange being peeled. These were graphic images of a person coming apart. Not only did the symptoms spill out into the surrounding environment, but the person, thus opened up, was vulnerable to external control.

Other images showed the skull beginning to repair, the boundary between inside and outside represented by a zigzag line, a motif commonly employed in the iconography surrounding schizophrenia. Some cartoons in *You and Your Voices* showed the skull closed over again. They illustrated the fully formed schizophrenic identity. In one, the cranial cavity was depicted as divided into two halves. Inside the left half were representations of goodness, light, and youth. There were soft, curved shapes resembling clouds. The right side contained evil, darkness, old age, and sharp straight lines resembling cobwebs. In other examples the cranium was drawn as if viewed from the side, the light compartment located at the front, the dark compartment at the back. Demons that had previously been represented outside the person were now inside, cringing in the darkness. It was here at the back of the head, in a dingy space like a cellar, that delusions were to be locked away in an old trunk, allowing the patient to present a youthful, healthy self to the outside world. Thus schizophrenia was relocated inside the person, and in the process there was a transformation into a split schizophrenic identity.

The sequence from biological to psychosocial, from taking apart to putting back together again, was evident in the overall structure of this course and in the design of its illustrated material. In addition, I observed that the staff oscillated from one aspect of this sequence to the other. This oscillation was possible within a single session or even within the space of a brief interchange with a patient. It occurred particularly when staff found it difficult to defend what they were teaching, as when Patrick returned to a biological analogy in order to re-establish control of the situation. An important aspect of this oscillation was that in a biological idiom symptoms such as hallucinations were defined as nonsensical, whereas in a psychosocial idiom they made sense. The overall impression imparted to patients was that their schizophrenia was both unintelligible and understandable.

The staff also moved back and forth between a bio-psycho-social definition of schizophrenia and ideas of 'madness' and 'craziness'. In an earlier chapter I made the point that these 'lay' notions of mental illness were an important strategic resource used by the staff in their day-to-day talk about patients. The schizophrenia education course began with a focus on 'craziness', legitimated by the aspiration to write in the language of patients. The import of the first booklet, *So They Say You're Crazy*, was to assure patients that they were not in fact crazy, were not dangerous lunatics, and did not have a split personality. As the course proceeded, the focus of attention and the language of instruction changed from 'lay' to professional, from craziness to schizophrenia. Patients were now encouraged to bring their symptoms out, to speak freely about their hallucinations and delusions. Private experiences were opened up to a public forum. Toward the end of the course the focus shifted back from schizophrenia to craziness in order to convey the message that patients should not act on their delusions or hallucinations and especially should not speak about them to anyone else apart from their treating psychiatrist or nurse. Hearing voices does not mean you are crazy, it was argued, but if you tell people about your voices they will regard you as crazy. To have delusions does not make you crazy, providing you do not act on them. Symptoms should not be made public, they should be kept private. The prospect of being regarded as 'crazies' was used to encourage patients to internalize their hallucinations and delusions, best captured in the injunction to '*Zip it*'. Translated into a more professional discourse, patients were encouraged to 'encapsulate' their delusions and hallucinations by speaking about these experiences to no one except their psychiatrists, nurses, or social workers.

Finally, there was an oscillation between difference and sameness. In Chapter 8 I suggested that a biological model of schizophrenia posited a difference between the patient and other people, whereas psychosocial models emphasized continuity. This suggestion was borne out in practice. When patients complained that they were being treated as different, staff reminded them that they were just the same as other people. Conversely, when patients argued that they were the same as others, staff returned to the essential difference implied by schizophrenia.

Clive: For me there is little difference between sane and insane. When I am crazy my thoughts might get a bit mixed up, but the two states are basically the same.

Patrick: We are all a little bit crazy, but the difference is that we don't talk about our crazy ideas.

Well-rounded formulations of schizophrenia would combine sameness and difference into a single statement:

Phillipa: We all need fantasies, but we don't all have delusions.

The bio-psycho-social model of schizophrenia was especially suited to the production of statements that simultaneously affirmed sameness and difference.

Patrick: We all go through stress, but not all of us come down with schizophrenia as a result of this stress.

One effect of this was to suspend patients in a structure of ambiguity. The 'schizophrenic' identity negotiated by staff and patients was always composed of two parts: one the same as other people, the other different.

This chapter has explored ethnographically the movement between four polarities: between the 'ununderstandable' and the understandable, between biological and psychosocial aspects of the bio-psycho-social model, between professional and 'lay' language, and, finally, between attributes of similarity and difference. It has demonstrated how these four polarities all come to bear on the definition of schizophrenia when it is negotiated by staff and patients. The underlying metaphor organizing each of these movements is one in which the patient is opened up and shut down, taken apart and put back together again—a fundamental process of therapeutic work in a psychiatric hospital.

10

The person, the case, and schizophrenia

This book is about the social definition of schizophrenia. It has examined how this illness is constituted and endowed with meaning within the institutional and cultural context of modern society. I have explored this relationship between illness and context by studying the Schizophrenia Team at Ridgehaven Hospital, where there was a concentration of people who experienced this disorder and where the daily work of clinical staff was to diagnose schizophrenia, think about it, talk about it, write about it, and treat it. I have used an ethnographic research strategy in order to ground schizophrenia, as a category of practical knowledge, in the collective intellectual work and the day-to-day interactions of these patients, psychiatrists, nurses, and social workers. I have also linked illness to social context by turning back to the earliest formulations of schizophrenia, dementia praecox, and their precursors to see how they were first conceived within the European asylums and universities of the nineteenth century. I am interested in the way these formulations reflected the intellectual climate of that era and, in particular, how they were predicated on theories of personhood that were current at that time.

As a synchronic analysis of Ridgehaven Hospital in the 1980s and as a diachronic analysis spanning two centuries of psychiatric thought, the purpose of this book has been to examine psychiatric institutions, their ideas and practices, and how they define what it is to be a person, what it is to be a case of psychiatric illness, and what it is to have schizophrenia.

From hospital organization to case

The problems I addressed in this book were initially formulated from within a theoretical framework of social phenomenology, as this movement in philosophy has been received and employed within anthropology and sociology over the past three decades. I began with the study of two phenomenal categories—time and space—asking how they might be invested with meaning within a psychiatric hospital. At Ridgehaven time was signified chiefly in terms of progress, a theme that not only linked the hospital to a wider progressivist society but also unified the hospital internally by pervading its many disparate domains: its logo, style of leadership, oral and written histories, future goals, concept of science, and, most importantly, the professional identity of the people who worked there. The intersection of time and space was evident in the 'hospitalscape' of Ridgehaven, with its new, modern, open wards at the front, closest to the nearby suburbs, and the old decrepit back wards hidden away at the rear, near the empty paddocks. There was a moral dimension to this spatio-temporal continuum, for modernity was valued over backwardness, 'the community' was valued over 'the institution'. The best features of the hospital were proudly displayed at the front and the bad features tucked away at the back; positive images of the hospital were projected into its future, whereas the negative images were relegated to its dark past. Located along this moral continuum were the staff and patients. The most prestigious clinical work took place in the wards at the front of the hospital and in the wider community, where the most promising patients were located. The staff who worked in the old wards at the back were more vulnerable to demoralization, as it was here that the more dangerous patients and those unlikely to improve were locked away.

Autonomy was highly valued by the psychiatrists, nurses, and social workers of Ridgehaven, who defined their respective professional identities in terms of the unique perspectives they could bring to the understanding and treatment of psychiatric illness. The pursuit of autonomy and the assertion of distinctiveness were played out in the way the staff organized their time (the daily and weekly rhythms of their clinical interactions as well as their long-term career patterns) and their space (the various rooms and areas inside and outside the hospital in which they practised). Work time and work space had important implications for the way in which staff formulated cases. A case was more than just an individual instance of a general category of psychiatric disorder. It was a distinctive representation of the person attributed with temporal and spatial dimensions—case time and case space.

Psychiatrists, who belonged to the most powerful and autonomous of the three professions, maintained a temporal and spatial distance from patients. This distance was combined with a focus on private, intimate information to produce a depth perspective on the case, viewing it as if it had a hidden interior core. Whether they used a biological or a psychodynamic orientation, psychiatrists always claimed these deeper aspects of the case as their privileged domain of knowledge and practice. The notion of inner depth has influenced medical and psychiatric thought since the late eighteenth century. It was borrowed initially from the Romantic movement, with its idea of a self-reflecting 'inner man' as a deep wellspring of feelings, and from the moral therapy movement, where the ideal product of treatment was a person who could achieve internal self-restraint.

Although psychiatric nursing was less powerful and autonomous as a professional body, nurses nevertheless derived an advantage from the proximity of their work to patients and their capacity collectively to maintain a continuous form of observation on them. It conferred an authority to define what was 'real', 'true' or 'actual' about a case, as exemplified by the nurses' ability to detect whether the person was presenting a façade or was genuine.

Social workers had mobility. Their daily routine took them into the suburbs as they negotiated between the hospital, the family, the proprietors of hostels and boarding houses, and the various instrumentalities of state welfare. They gave breadth to the case, for their distinctive contribution was a knowledge of the wider context in which people lived.

Thus the case was implicitly a three-dimensional spatial entity with a deep domain that was the preserve of psychiatry, a surface zone that was the preserve of psychiatric nursing, and a broader context, the preserve of social work.

The dimension of time was also fundamental to the way a case was constituted. Time first became a focus of attention in the early nineteenth century asylums, when the biographical method was introduced to clinical psychiatry and when scientific attention began to focus on the curability and the long-term outcome of insanity. At Ridgehaven, a psychiatric case would have been difficult to imagine if it did not have a deeply retrospective biographical component and a prospective sense of evolution and progress. Temporal and spatial dimensions of a case condensed into a single set of mutually defining images. The feelings, thoughts, and drives that lay deep within the inner core were said to have arisen from deep within the patient's past. In keeping with their depth perspective, psychiatrists placed great store on eliciting an extended developmental history, whereas nurses, with their surface orientation, emphasized the 'here and now'.

The case, with its implicit spatio-temporal dimensions, was a distinctive construction of the person. It was the focus and product of psychiatric work. It was the very basis on which psychiatric work was possible.

Case, whole person, anyone: categories of person

Initial assessment: deconstructing a person to form a segmented case

When a person was admitted to hospital, the assessment process resulted in a case format that was divided into segments. Segmentation was integral to the creation of a written case history with its many divisions and subdivisions. Interview questions, as well as the interpretive procedures for documenting the answers, were oriented to eliciting, shaping, and rearranging the person's account of self and illness so it fitted into these subdivisions. For example, questions that sought to specify the duration of the illness and its various symptoms led to a case history divided into the time segments called Presenting Complaint, Past Psychiatric History, Premorbid Personality, and Developmental History.

The most salient division to emerge was that which separated the psychiatric illness from the person. The patient was encouraged to discriminate between experiences that arose internally and belonged to the self and experiences that seemed to arise externally and did not belong to the self. The latter were singled out and rendered into an increasingly technical language, from 'voices' to 'hallucinations' to 'schizophrenia'. It was often a problem for clinicians and patients alike to discriminate between illness and person, but through the process of documentation the two were separated and rendered distinct. Ultimately, in the *DSM-III* diagnostic formulation, they were formed into separate 'axes', an illness axis and a personality axis.

The hospital was a schismatic organization within which each profession promoted autonomy and distinctiveness. The segmented case, with its matrix of cross-cutting divisions, reflected this division of professional labour. The case was a multifaceted worksite within which each profession could establish an exclusive niche.

Rendering the case an object

Segmentation was accompanied by objectification, as clinical assessment aimed to produce an objective analysis of the factors, variables, and influences that caused psychiatric illness. There was a deliberate effort on the part of clinicians to keep their own subjective feelings and biases out of the case record or at least to keep a check on them. During the interview they adopted a stance of empathic understanding in order to elicit the patient's subjective experiences, yet these experiences were often documented in distancing idioms such as: 'thinks he can ... ', 'believes he is ... ', 'only admits to ... ', or 'claims that. ... '. When patients tried to build up conversational themes that might convey how they made sense of their world, they were frequently interrupted by an incisive style of interviewing that aimed to pinpoint symptoms and specify their duration. Thus the techniques of the interview and the conventions and idioms of its documentation left little room to describe the patient as a subjective person who could mean-ingfully interpret his or her situation. As persons endowed with subjectivity, both patient and clinician actively contrib-uted to the construction of meaning. Together they built up intersubjective understandings by processes of negotiation that drew on shared common-sense assumptions, particularly about the nature of mental illness. These nuances and nego-tiations were edited out of the record. Instead, it read as a compilation of the objective facts of the case. The case record and the case itself became an object—a deterministic con-struct stripped of subjective intentionality. Symptoms and be-haviour were explained in the language of mechanistic cause and effect as the result of interactions between the various segments of the case—between genetic predisposition, devel-opmental influences, family dynamics, recent stressors, and so on.

With the division of the case into an illness segment and a patient segment, the illness was vested with principles of power and control, whereas the patient was portrayed as a passive object whose actions, thoughts, and feelings were controlled. There was a parallel contrast between clinician and patient. The ideal case record portrayed the clinician as an active, ra-tional decision-maker. The patient was depicted as an irra-tional object who could be legitimately controlled by the cli-nician's decisions. Portrayed as controlled by the psychiatric illness and the management decisions of the treating staff, there was no space in the record to describe a person's be-haviour in terms of conscious intent.

The fully worked-up case: reconstructing a 'whole person'

When psychiatrists, nurses, and social workers combined into a team they put together a comprehensive assessment known as the 'fully worked-up case', bringing the various segments into relation with each other to reconstruct what was called a 'whole person'. The earliest expression of this holistic ap-proach within psychiatry was associated with the German an-thropological movement of the late eighteenth and early nine-teenth centuries, which extolled the psycho-physical unity of mankind. It has received new impetus during the second half of this century in the bio-psycho-social model.

In Chapter 4 I identified encompassment, integration, and exclusion as three of the processes that mediated interprofessional relationships within a multidisciplinary team. All three had important implications for the way teams defined cases. Psychiatrists established hegemony within the team by encompassing it, successfully identifying themselves and their psychiatric principles with the team as a whole, its goals, values, and its very *raison d'être*. In the same way that psychiatrists encompassed their nursing and social work colleagues, the multidisciplinary team as a whole encompassed the case by means of a totalizing approach, as epitomized in the slogan 'total patient care'. They carried out a comprehensive form of assessment that explored and documented its every facet and dimension, culminating in a 'fully worked-up case'. Another way of encompassing a case was to encapsulate it, and thus a hallmark of good clinical writing was the ability to summarize succinctly the relevant clinical information about a patient. Likewise, a hallmark of accomplished clinical oratory was an ability to put a case 'in a nutshell'. At case conferences team members communicated with each other using abbreviated case summaries, which I have called epigrammatic appraisals, thereby reducing the case to a few telling phrases, an illustrative story, or a brief thumbnail sketch.

Just as the multidisciplinary team, in its ideal form, worked as an integrated unit, so it produced an integrated formulation of the case in which the separate segments were shown to be related to each other. Thus the patient's personality was shown to influence the psychiatric illness or vice versa. Such a formulation could show how biological factors interacted with psychological factors, and how both were affected by family factors; or it could demonstrate the relation between genetic predisposition, developmental influences, and psychosocial stressors that acted to precipitate the illness.

The fully worked-up case thus differed from the segmented case in that it was synthesized into a cohesive whole. It was totally explored, encapsulated, and integrated. Yet it remained an objectified account. It sought to explain the psychiatric illness and the patient as elements within a causal equation.

Even the 'whole person', though laudable in its scope and promise, was an object. It was a product of team ideology rather than someone with whom one could sit and talk and thereby enter into an intersubjective understanding.

Management and progress: reinvesting the person with subjectivity

When the initial assessment and the 'full work-up' had been completed, team members began to rely less on the case record and more on clinical discussion as they concentrated on management and monitoring progress. In the transition from writing to talking about patients, there was a change in the way they were conceptualized. The staff endowed them with a cluster of qualities, among which subjectivity was paramount. Staff interacted with individual patients as if each were a person endowed with subjectivity–as if they had the capacity to interpret their situation accurately, to create intersubjective understandings with others, and thereby to engage in meaningful social interaction. Closely related to subjectivity, though not synonymous with it, was volition. The staff approached a patient as if he or she were a person who had the capacity for rational, purposive action. Moreover, such a person was perceived as unified rather than segmented, insofar as he or she was regarded as a single source of conscious motivation. Increasingly, the thumbnail sketches, illustrative stories, and telling phrases addressed questions of patients' cooperation in the therapeutic task: What were these people trying to gain by being in hospital? Were they just biding their time until they could be discharged? Instead of treating them as powerless patients whose behaviour was controlled by the psychiatric illness and by the decisions of the treating team, they were treated as people who could exert self-control, control over their illness, and control over other people, in particular the team members themselves. Instead of regarding behaviour as determined by unconscious psychodynamic or biological factors, it was understood in terms of the person's conscious motivation. Instead of seeing someone's actions as determined by past influences, they were understood in terms of the future outcome which the person was intentionally trying to bring about.

Patients were now treated as moral beings who were responsible for their actions and capable of distinguishing right from wrong. Holding them to account meant evaluating them as good or bad. At Ridgehaven, such judgements were predicated on whether patients appeared to be suffering from their illness, working on getting better, and showing progress, or whether they were enjoying the symptoms, playing at being ill, slipping backward, or stagnating. The staff were critical of themselves for making these judgemental evaluations, regarding them as unprofessional, subjective, and biased. Evaluative statements appeared in clinical talk rather than in case records because the staff did not wish to be held legally accountable for them. The tendency for hospital staff to talk about patients in this way has been regretted or decried as unprofessional in the psychiatric and sociological literature. Here I have demonstrated that this evaluative work is central to the therapeutic process of transforming a case into a morally competent person. Effecting this transformation and monitoring its progress of necessity involves assigning motive, responsibility, and value.

The final product of hospital work was a person endowed with subjectivity, volition, unity of consciousness, and moral value. It is difficult to find a succinct designation for this category of person because the hospital staff themselves had no name for it. Such a person was neither a case, a patient, a client, nor even a 'whole person'. This lack of designation suggests that, for the staff, it was a concept of the person that lay within the realm of common-sense thinking. The terms 'any person' or 'anyone' best convey this idea and have been adopted for the purpose of this ethnographic description. The overall goal of hospital treatment was thus to return a patient to the mundane world of everyday social interaction within which personhood itself could be taken for granted—where he or she could be treated just like 'anyone' else.

Tensions: part versus whole, subjectivity versus object

In the first part of this book I have drawn a map of the spatio-temporal dimensions of the psychiatric case as an ethnographically specific representation of the person. I have used this map to explore a tension between part and whole that is inherent in the way the person is constituted in Western thought and that is accentuated within the case. On the one hand, there are widely available common-sense notions of the person as an entity that is divisible into halves (for example, mental versus physical, thoughts versus feelings, nature versus nurture) or into competing roles. The psychiatric hospital adds its own imprint, deepening these divisions to produce a segmented case. At the same time there is a widely promulgated ideology of individualism in Western culture that posits a concept of the person as an autonomous indivisible whole. The 'whole person' of hospital psychiatry is an amplified version of this concept. Whereas the segmented case is a product of the division of professional labour, the whole person is the product of the integration of labour into a multidisciplinary team.

I have also explored a tension between subjectivity and objectification that is inherent in the constitution of the person. The subjective aspect of the person is commonly identified with the flow of conscious thoughts. Such a subjectivity is attributed the ability to endow his or her environment with meaning, to engage in intersubjective understandings with other subjectivities and thereby interact within the social world. At the same time, there is a process of objectification, which is essential to the idea of the person as a reflexive self. Other people establish distance from you and regard you as an object, but you can also do the same. You can direct your conscious thinking back onto your own thoughts, establishing the same degree of distance that others do and thereby relate to yourself as an object. The capacity for self-reflection is regarded as so fundamental it is sometimes claimed as a distinguishing feature of humans, separating them from lower creatures.

The tension between the subjective person and the person as an object is taken up and elaborated in psychiatric models of the person. The segmented case removes subjectivity to portray a patient as a passive object whose behaviour is determined by forces that lie beyond conscious control. On the other hand, the idea of 'any person' or 'anyone' implies the opposite: that he or she is a being invested with subjectivity, a unified centre of consciousness, volition, and moral responsibility.

These tensions, whether they pertain to the person in general or to its more specific psychiatric representations, can be teased apart and clarified by means of a plane diagram in which part versus whole stands on the vertical axis, and object versus subjectivity lies on a horizontal axis (Figure 10.1). This presentation contains four possibilities, designated A, B, C, and D, which help to visualize several representations of the person. They have a static appearance because they have been drawn in boxes. To counteract this impression it is necessary to remember that they refer to the emergent properties of social processes: they are models of the person that emerge from the interactions of staff and patients within the hospital. A, B, C, and D should thus be regarded as fluid rather than static: any one of them can be merged with or change into any of the others.

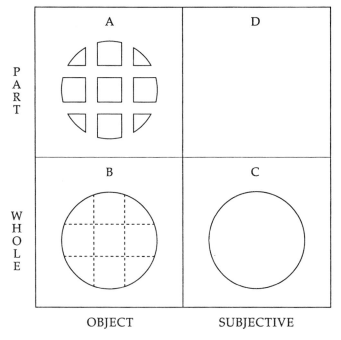

Fig. 10.1.   Model of the subjective person and the person as an object; in relation to the part person and the whole person. See text for discussion.

The segmented case is represented by A. It is based on the concept of the divisible person. It lacks a full circular boundary, indicating that the parts have precedence over the whole. B is a representation of the 'fully worked-up case' or the 'whole person'. It is based on the concept of the individual. The segments have been joined to form a cohesive whole with the result that the internal divisions appear less prominent: wholeness and unity prevail over division. A and B are both objects of clinical work, the former a product of individual work by psychiatry, nursing, and social work, the latter a product of integrated teamwork. Both differ from the person as a unified, conscious subjectivity (C), which I have represented by means of a circle.

The transitions between A, B, and C represent some of the major transformations in a person effected by psychiatric hospital treatment. The first transformation involves creation of a segmented object (A). This occurs at the initial assessment, during which the person is divested of subjectivity. The second transformation is brought about by the 'full work-up'. It is represented by a movement from A to B. The separate parts are integrated and subordinated to a whole. The hospital staff were aware of the processes described so far, as they were the consciously articulated goals of hospital assessment—to carry out an objective analysis of the case culminating in a synthesized case formulation. By contrast, the third transformation, represented by the shift from B to C, was not a goal that was articulated by the staff. However, on the basis of the ethnographic evidence presented in this book, I contend that it is an essential dynamic of psychiatric treatment. An object is transformed into a person endowed with subjectivity, a person who can again be regarded as just 'anyone'.

The sequence of psychiatric assessment and treatment bears resemblance to cultural processes of transformation that have been described elsewhere in the anthropological literature. It is a triphasic process that first divests a person of subjectivity, deconstructs and reconstructs the resultant object, and finally reinvests this new object with subjectivity to create a different person. Whatever else is accomplished or not accomplished, this is the most basic thing that happens to a person when admitted to, treated in, and discharged from a psychiatric hospital.

Multiple definitions of the person and schizophrenia

Physiological and ontological versions of schizophrenia

The representations of the person that I have delineated, with their inherent tensions and their potential to be transformed from one state to another, were germane to most people with a psychiatric disorder treated in the hospital, irrespective of their diagnosis. In the second half of the book, I have explored their relevance to schizophrenia. When the segmented case is reintegrated into a 'whole person', what happens to the schizophrenia? If schizophrenia does not go away, what becomes of it when there is a shift to a more volitional concept of the person?

To answer these questions it is necessary to recall that people think about schizophrenia using the same metaphors and images with which they think about a person. This is not surprising because, as I have argued in the body of the book, the category itself emerged historically from a framework of Western concepts of the person. In the same way that there is a subjectivity–object tension within the person, this tension can be found in the concept of schizophrenia, though it takes a somewhat different form.

In Chapter 8 I distinguished between two versions of schizophrenia. One was based on a so-called physiological or functional view of disease as a reaction of the individual organism to its environment. Expressed in pure form in some of the psychosocial theories, this version of schizophrenia is represented as a severe reaction of the person to major physical or psychological influences, especially those that affect his or her development. Because it posits that schizophrenia is a *state of the person*, this version incorporates ideas of subjectivity and volition. Schizophrenia itself may be personified, attributed qualities that we usually associate with a person.

The second version does not take subjectivity into account but construes the illness as an object. It is based on a so-called ontological view of disease: the assumption, usually tacit, that it is a real object or thing, rather than a logical type, and that it has an existence independent of its particular expression in an individual case. This version can be found in some forms of biological theorizing about the cause of schizophrenia, where the schizophrenic 'thing' is thought to be a genetic abnormality or a faulty neurotransmitter.

In the everyday practical reasoning of clinical work there was a slippage between these two versions. This conclusion is not to accuse the staff of being sloppy or logically inconsistent but to reveal how, in moving between them, they were able to effect transformations in the people they treated. These transformations can be examined with the assistance of Figure 10.2, which I have drawn by adding schizophrenia to Figure 10.1. I have used dots to represent schizophrenia so that it can be depicted as a discrete entity or a diffuse influence.

Acute psychosis as absence: the person 'away with the fairies'

Acute schizophrenia was portrayed as an absence of the person, conceived of as a conscious subjectivity and centre of volition. As I have demonstrated, the process of clinical documentation ensured that subjectivity was excluded from the case records. To discover its fate, it is necessary to look to clinical discussions about patients with florid psychosis, as talk was the medium of communication in which the staff grappled with subjectivity. They spoke about patients in images that located them as persons in external metaphoric space: outside their own self and away from the mundane world of social interaction. The person was 'out of it', 'out of his tree', 'away with the birds', 'away with the fairies', 'in cloud cuckoo land', 'off in her own little world,' 'off the air' or 'off the planet'. The ubiquitous term 'off' succinctly expressed the sense that the person was spatially away. (If I were to represent this idea in relation to Figure 10.2, I would have to draw a circle somewhere off the page or outside this book, or append a small helium-filled balloon to the book.) What was left behind, be it body, mind, or behaviour, was likened to a physical object or a member of a lower species of animal—entities that lay outside the realm of humankind. These graphic terms were used in conjunction with idioms that conveyed a sense of extreme madness, craziness, imbalance, and explosiveness. Thus

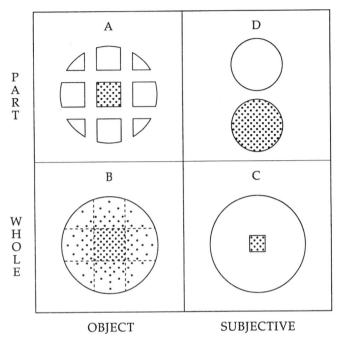

Fig. 10.2.   Model of the person in relation to schizophrenia. See text for discussion.

there was a counterpoint between external subjectivity and the person as an automaton. People with psychosis themselves used the same imagery, especially when they reported voices coming from the external environment and when they talked about their thinking, actions, or bodily movements being controlled by an external conscious agency. Similar images could be found in the educational booklets I described in Chapter 9, which contained cartoon illustrations of external agencies located outside the head. They included little demons inserting and withdrawing thoughts through the skull or a nasty figure in a cloud controlling a puppet by pulling its strings. Whether I read the case records or the educational booklets, whether I listened to the staff members speaking at a case conference or asked the patients directly, acute schizophrenic psychosis was conceived of as a particular state of the person, one in which subjectivity, consciousness, and volition were altogether absent.

Segmenting: the case of schizophrenia

When the clinical assessment procedures rendered the disordered person into a segmented case (Fig. 10.2A), one of the segments became the schizophrenia itself. The assessment interview encouraged a sharp distinction between schizophrenia and other segments. The intense focus on the time and mode of onset of the illness established a temporal demarcation between the illness and the person's premorbid state. Dichotomous choice questions posited two mutually exclusive entities, person and schizophrenia, and allocated experiences to one or the other. Those experiences with which the staff could empathize were allocated to the person; those that seemed bizarre or beyond empathic understanding were attributed to schizophrenia. The case record contained the clearest representations of this demarcation, and it was by attending to the questions that were repeatedly put to them from their record that patients further learned to distinguish between themselves and their illness and to see themselves as *a case of schizophrenia.*

Objectifying and internalizing: chemical abnormality within the brain

Constructing a case entailed an important shift from a physiological version of schizophrenia to an ontological version. From viewing it as a state of the person, characterized by the absence and external location of subjectivity and volition, it was transformed into an object in the brain, usually explained as a faulty chemical causing hallucinations and delusions. In other words, a great deal of effort was put into convincing people to see that experiences they thought were coming from an agency located outside them in fact arose from a *chemical abnormality within their brain.*

It was a double transformation—from outside to inside and from subjectivity to object. It was so central to the therapeutic process that when patients resisted treatment they would characteristically make a stand on this issue, maintaining that the voices or controlling forces *did* come from some person-like being located outside them, from God or the Devil perhaps, and *did not* arise from their own disordered brain.

Integrating and totalizing: the whole person as a 'schizophrenic'

The 'full work-up' located schizophrenia at the core of the case, which I have depicted in Figure 10.2B, by a concentration of dots at the centre of the circle. A thorough family history sought to identify schizophrenia or other psychopathology in family members and thereby associated schizophrenia with the patient's genetic code. It was postulated that this genetic disorder led to a neurotransmitter abnormality situated somewhere deep within the central integrating connections of the brain, in the mesolimbic or mesocortical pathways. A detailed developmental history, beginning with the gestation and birth of the patient, sought to trace the source of the illness to the beginning of case time and, in particular, to perinatal insults to the brain. The developmental history often served to show that attenuated forms of schizophrenia, schizoid or paranoid traits, had been evolving and growing within the patient's personality structure for many years. Schizophrenia was thus identified with the core of the case in both space and time.

To speak about the core of an object, its inner kernel and its earliest origins, is to speak about its essential nature. The essence of the case thus became defined in terms of schizophrenia. Furthermore, to speak of the essence of something is to speak of its totality. Schizophrenia came to permeate every aspect of the fully worked-up case. In Figure 10.2 I have depicted this concept by a diffusion of dots spreading across to the edge of the circle.

Through their meticulous, round-the-clock observations, psychiatric nurses were able to demonstrate how schizophrenia could pervade the patient's everyday behaviour. Through their assessment of the patient's context, social workers were able to show how it influenced and was influenced by the family environment. Integrated into a comprehensive team assessment, these perspectives led to a totalizing bio-psycho-social definition of schizophrenia. Systems theory, on which the bio-psycho-social approach is based, posits a model of the person as a hierarchy of subsystems, each in open communication with other subsystems, all of them encompassed by the whole system. Thus the neurotransmitter abnormality of schizophrenia, though it was only a disorder of one subsystem, ramified throughout other subsystems. Schizophrenia thus became a disorder of the encompassing whole.

Within the conceptual frame of the 'full work-up', the bio-psycho-social approach, and systems theory, schizophrenia could become an all-pervasive construct that was coextensive with the boundaries of the 'whole person'. This construction created the possibility of treating someone as a schizophrenia object—a '*schizophrenic*'.

Reinvesting subjectivity: the person in control of schizophrenia

According to the spatial metaphors described above, recovery was depicted as a trajectory from 'off' to 'settled', which meant a return journey back into the self, back to the everyday world, back to the here and now. Someone who had traversed this path might be described as 'much more settled within himself', 'with it', 'back to reality', or 'facing reality issues'. The person as a subjective and volitional being had come back, though not to displace the illness altogether, because even when it was inactive schizophrenia was thought to have an enduring presence and an ongoing potential to become active again in the future. For the time being, however, it was in a state of remission.

In this ideal state of remission the person and his or her schizophrenia stood opposed. In terms of the whole–part tension, the person was associated with integration and wholeness, whereas the schizophrenia came to be seen as a small part of the overall picture. The part was subsumed within and subordinated to the whole. In terms of the subjectivity–object tension, subjectivity was attributed to the person, whereas the schizophrenia remained a mere inactive object. Apportioning volition to the person placed him or her in control of the schizophrenia. In Figure 10.2, this might be represented by a composite image that takes a model of schizophrenia from A and subordinates it to a model of the person depicted in C.

This ideal end product was the *person with schizophrenia*. Such persons were bounded and inner-focused: they could distinguish clearly between the self and the external environment and could see that thoughts, perceptions, and actions stemmed from within. Internally, they were integrated, subjective, self-controlled persons who could separate their schizophrenia as a small part inside them and treat it as an object that could be contained and controlled. They had *insight* into their schizophrenia. The hallmark of such persons was the capacity to engage in meaningful social interaction to the extent that their personhood no longer remained a focus of attention. It could be taken for granted. They could be treated as anyone. Given the enduring potential for relapse attributed to schizophrenia, this state was the closest possible approximation to complete recovery.

Emphasizing volition: 'putting on' schizophrenia

A variant of this ideal, though one that was negatively rather than positively valued, gave special emphasis to the volitional aspect of the person. Here the person became a rational, calculating, self-interested strategist. This way of thinking about schizophrenia has been exemplified in the writings of Thomas Szasz. At Ridgehaven it emerged among the staff when they were in a mood of sceptical mistrust, particularly when they had to perform the gate-keeping role of admitting genuine patients to hospital while excluding those who were undeserving. In this setting, schizophrenia was transformed from a fundamental and central part of the person into a superficial veneer or cloak, something the person 'put on' to manipulate others into giving them things they did not deserve. Instead of illustrating this state by drawing schizophrenia near the centre of the person, it might be depicted as a thin dotted band running around the edge of the circle, thus being portrayed as a superficial presentation, or façade, that could be used as an instrument for personal gain.

Personifying the illness: you and your schizophrenia

There was another possible way of thinking, represented in Figure 10.2D, in which neither the person nor the schizophrenia were subsumed within a whole. Each was thought of as a separate entity and, in the transition from the left side of Figure 10.2 to the right, both entities were invested with subjectivity and volition. In other words, not only could the patient be approached as a person, so could the illness. Schizophrenia could be personified. It could be conceptualized as if it were an autonomous being with the capacity to think, feel, perceive, and engage in social interaction. It could be attributed volition and the power to control, victimize, and inflict suffering. It could be endowed with moral qualities, usually negative ones.

This model of schizophrenia was widely prevalent. At Ridgehaven I found it to be one of the most common ways of thinking and talking about schizophrenia. When a staff member said to someone, 'That is your illness talking, not you', they were employing the metaphor of schizophrenia as a person. It was also implicit in legal reasoning, where it underpinned the concept of diminished responsibility or the verdict of 'not guilty by virtue of insanity'. The patient's responsibility was diminished insofar as the schizophrenia was attributed a capacity to form intent and to bring about actions in fulfilment of this intent. Like any other person in society, schizophrenia could be tried at law and shouldered with responsibility for a crime.

There were several ways of imagining the relationship between someone and their personified schizophrenia. During the early stages of illness, the treating staff were keen to establish that schizophrenia caused the person to suffer. A major effort was made to convince people that they were victims who *suffer from schizophrenia*. It was expected that they would fight and struggle against their schizophrenia, working hard to recognize it, contain it, and control it. Whereas most needed little convincing that they were suffering, some vigorously resisted this idea. They interpreted their voices or ideas as intriguing, enjoyable, or helpful and appeared to show little inclination to work on or struggle against their illness.

In the longer term, it was a matter of *learning to live with the schizophrenia*, like two old foes who must learn to get on with each other. Gradually the schizophrenia became more a nuisance than a danger, and professional advice consisted mainly of practical tips for getting around it or putting up with it.

The education programme, because it was a setting in which staff and patients built and worked with practical definitions of schizophrenia, largely employed personified images of illness. In Chapter 9 I described a sequence of cartoons that depicted the process of internalization as a transition from a skull that was cracked or peeled apart, the inside communicating freely with the external world, to one that was completely closed. In the process of closing over, the agencies and demons that had previously perched outside now crouched within the head. During the formation of a segmented case (Fig. 10.2A), internalization meant rendering schizophrenia into an object. Here (Fig. 10.2D), however, internalization led to the formation of schizophrenia as a little person inside the skull. This image was reinforced by graphic representations of a skull divided into two equal but opposite halves, one containing a youthful, outgoing healthy person and the other a decrepit old demon, causing trouble by noisily blasting 'voices' through a megaphone, cowering in a dark corner, or completely locked up in a chest covered with cobwebs. Given a psychoanalytic accent, the schizophrenic half was identified with the unconscious mind and the healthy person with conscious thoughts. From its unconscious site, schizophrenia could communicate with the conscious self. It seemed to take on a helpful and caring complexion rather than a victimizing role, as if trying to protect that self. Thus hallucinations were messages from the unconscious that could help individuals understand feelings about themselves, particularly those that were difficult to accept, and delusions helped protect them from feeling bad about their lives.

Schizophrenia as a disintegrated person or a split person

Because the state depicted in Figure 10.2D combines the principles of division and personification, it provides a framework for thinking of *schizophrenia as a split person* (where there are two halves) or *schizophrenia as a disintegrated person* (where there are many parts), ideas that harken back to the very origin of the concept itself. I have argued that the opposition between wholeness as health and splitting or disintegration as pathology is deeply rooted within European thought. Its penetration of medical thought can be traced to late eighteenth century Romanticism (with its concern for integration of the inner self through the reconciliation of contradictory forces) and Kantian idealism (with its related concern for a unity that transcends man's division into two selves that live in two separate worlds). The link between splitting and pathology permeated European literature, hypnotism, psychoanalysis, neuropathology, and psychopathology. Kraepelin was influenced by this tradition to the extent that he identified a loss of inner unity as the single defining feature of dementia praecox, as was Bleuler when he renamed it schizophrenia and elevated the idea of splitting into the name of the disease. During the twentieth century the theme of splitting can be found in several important causal theories of schizophrenia that have been formulated by psychoanalysts, antipsychiatrists, and those who would find its origins in the emotionally contradictory schizophrenogenic mother or a double-binding, schismatic family.

Schizophrenia continues to convey the idea of a split person: for the uneducated, who regularly think of it as a split personality; and for those involved in educating them, who repeatedly assert that schizophrenia is *not* a split personality. In doing so, mental health educators bring these two cognate ideas into close conjunction within the same phrase, paragraph, or public health slogan, ironically reproducing the fundamental connection between them. If schizophrenia did not, at some deeper level, have to do with splitting, it would not be necessary to labour the point so. To always evoke that image, even if only to deny it, keeps it before the public.

With the exception of 'loosening of associations', images of splitting or disintegration no longer feature prominently as formal diagnostic criteria in the manuals published by the American Psychiatric Association or the World Health Organization. However, I found that the theme of disintegration surfaced when the hospital staff talked informally about their patients 'going to pieces', 'cracking up', 'falling apart' or undergoing 'psychotic disintegration'. A person with incipient psychosis was sometimes described as 'fragile' or 'a bit loose at the edges'; and a first episode of frank schizophrenia was occasionally referred to as a 'first break'. The word 'crazy' is itself an expression of this theme, as it is derived from roots that primarily mean cracked or liable to fall to pieces (*OED*). A disintegration motif could also be found on the dust jackets of books on schizophrenia and in the imagery of advertisements for antipsychotic drugs. Typical images included split faces, disarticulated torsos and limbs, and a characteristic fractured typescript.

Schizophrenia as reversal: upsurge of the primitive

A major proposition advanced in this book is that schizophrenia, as a conceptual category, is grounded in Western concepts of the person as an encapsulated whole that encompasses, orders, and integrates its component parts such that there is a more or less harmonious and balanced interaction among them. The essence of schizophrenia becomes disintegration, where the whole can no longer exert order and control; and as a consequence the parts begin to act separately and in opposition to one another. This situation leads to a reversal of normal hierarchical relationships so individual parts can come to dominate and control the whole person. Thus biological research postulates a disorder of the integrative functions of the brain that, according to the Jacksonian idea of dissolution, enables the lower functions to escape from higher control. Schizophrenia becomes a reversal of an internal hierarchy— an upside-down person. Primordial parts of the brain dominate the complex parts. Primitive forces within a person, represented by a surge of neurotransmitters, rise up to dominate and control the person as a whole. Although differing in many ways from these biological propositions, psychoanalytic formulations are based on the same ideas of disintegration and the reversal of hierarchy. For the psychoanalyst, psychosis involves an upsurge of instinctual drives that are normally repressed, as unconscious material erupts into consciousness, primary process thinking overwhelms secondary process thinking, and magical thinking comes to dominate rational thought. For analyst and biologist, schizophrenia is an uprising of the primitive within the civilized person.

Four modes of connecting schizophrenia to the person

The four modes of relating schizophrenia to the person elucidated in Figure 10.2 account for the multiple ways in which people speak about, write about, and socially define this disorder. Only in the hands of extremists are A, B, C, or D expressed in pure form. For the most part, they form the intellectual building blocks people use to construct complex definitions of schizophrenia as a multiple reality. The underlying changes from part to whole and from object to subjectivity that necessarily occur during the transitions between A, B, C, and D are integral to the transformations effected in a person's identity as he or she undergoes treatment for schizophrenia in a psychiatric hospital. The path from A to C, for example, represents the recovery trajectory, and the ideal state of remission incorporates elements from both A and C. Figure 10.2 helps to elucidate the compound rhetorical statements frequently made to convince people about the 'true' nature of schizophrenia. The statement that schizophrenia is a treatable illness, not a split personality, invokes D to explain that it is not D but in fact A. This analysis goes some way to explaining why ideas about incurable disintegration and split personality, which invoke images of marginality, danger, and stigma, persist in the face of community awareness programmes. They continue to surface because they are inevitable outcomes of the cultural logic of schizophrenia, as it has been historically constituted in relation to the person. Finally, Figure 10.2 encompasses some of the contradictions within the discourse on schizophrenia. In a progressive hospital patients are taught: 'You are not a schizophrenic, you are a person with a schizophrenic illness'. That is, you are not B, you are C. Yet in other domains of discourse, for example the *British Journal of Psychiatry*, they are often referred to as 'schizophrenics'.

As a category of knowledge, schizophrenia has long been regarded as multifaceted. It is often said that, like the elephant to the blind men, it cannot be grasped in its entirety from any single perspective. The image of a fragmented body of knowledge in itself reproduces the underlying idea of disintegration, the historical root of the category schizophrenia. This analysis has laid bare the cultural logic by which the multiple versions of schizophrenia are generated.

Figure 10.2 is not an exhaustive map of all possibilities, but it does provide a guide to the ideational terrain across which you constantly travel, back and forth, up and down, when you become involved with schizophrenia, either treating it or experiencing it yourself.

Temporal images of schizophrenia: deterioration and stasis

Figure 10.2 is a two-dimensional spatial representation that, although concerned with change and transformation, does not fully capture the temporal images with which people think about schizophrenia and its treatment. An ideology of progress characterizes the modern capitalist state, with its economy predicated on growth and expansion. It is within this ideological framework that the person is constituted as continually evolving, developing, maturing, and ascending: from young to old, from dependent to productive, from unsocialized to socialized, from primitive to sophisticated, from rudimentary to complex. I have shown how this ideology penetrated every corner of the psychiatric hospital, influencing the way people within it defined themselves. At Ridgehaven the professional person exemplified the ideal, as power, self-esteem, and personal satisfaction were associated with careers that progressed steadily upward through the hospital ranks to positions of authority or outward into the private sphere where autonomy of practice was greatest. The recovering patient was another example of this ideal, as recovery was progress (evidence of it was recorded in the Progress sheets of the case record).

From its inception, schizophrenia has been formulated as the obverse of progress. Degeneration theory, borrowed from eighteenth century natural history by Morel, formed the conceptual basis for *démence précoce* as a rapid, incurable mental and physiological decline to a state of dementia. This theory was widely influential during the late nineteenth century, and it structured Kraepelin's ideas about dementia praecox. So fundamental is the principle of degeneration to the way schizophrenia has been constituted historically that this illness is still equated with incurable deterioration by the lay population and by many mental health professionals, despite evidence to the contrary from long-term follow-up studies.

Because time and space are so interwoven and mutually defining, temporal images of degeneration are inseparable from spatial images of disintegration and splitting. Whereas the ideal person (and therefore the aim of all therapeutic intervention) is defined in terms of a progressive evolution toward higher levels of integration and wholeness, a powerful spatiotemporal image of schizophrenia is one of decline and devolution, culminating in disintegration and splitting.

Time is particularly germane to the definition of 'chronic schizophrenia', though the term 'chronic' means more than long-term. It is a state in which the process of schizophrenic deterioration and decline has come to a standstill or has 'burned out'. Therapeutic efforts to achieve improvement and recovery are no longer making headway. Progress has halted, and the patient has 'plateaued' or is going around in circles in a 'revolving door'. Neither descending nor ascending, neither deteriorating nor progressing, the chronic patient has come to a standstill. The idea of a trajectory is no longer applicable. The passage of time no longer marks change. Chronic schizophrenia is a state of being suspended outside time, as time is endowed with meaning and value within the world of the hospital. Often the patient is merely referred to as a 'chronic', a term that has come to mean static, severe, and not very interesting, rather than long-term in a more strictly chronological sense.

Acute schizophrenia is primarily depicted in spatial metaphors: a state of being in which subjectivity and volition are located outside the self and outside social space; somewhere away from the hospital (for example, in 'cloud cuckoo land'). Chronic schizophrenia is depicted primarily in temporal metaphors: a state of being outside the time frame of development and maturation that is normally attributed to persons and outside the socially defined time of the hospital where illness is equated with regression and recovery with progress. Acute and chronic schizophrenia are defined outside space and time— outside the fundamental phenomenological dimensions of the social world.

Schizophrenia as an anomalous category of person

There is a theme of schizophrenia as an anomalous category running throughout this book. That is, schizophrenia is socially defined as an interstitial state located between conventional cultural categories, as a marginal state on the edge of these categories, or as outside them altogether. The setting in which people were diagnosed and treated, Ridgehaven Hospital, was itself situated in a marginal zone between city and country, amid a group of institutions that dealt with other marginal social categories (the intellectually retarded, the blind, the criminal, and the slaughtered beast).

When I examined causal theories of schizophrenia, I noted that within the biological approach the patient was categorized as different from others: someone whose actions could not be interpreted as meaningful and who lacked the capacity to interpret the world. From a psychosocial perspective, the person was seen as essentially the same as others: someone who could be empathically understood and who could make sense of the world in which he or she lived. In the world of psychiatric theory, these alternative approaches were dovetailed into the bio-psycho-social model of schizophrenia. However in day-to-day practice the staff oscillated between these approaches, such that people with schizophrenia were constituted as interstitial beings: partly the same as others, partly different; partly intelligible, partly unintelligible; partly attributed interpretive ability, partly not. People with schizophrenia were partly endowed with, and partly lacking, the core attributes of personhood.

When I examined the various trajectories of recovery, I also noted that schizophrenia was situated in-between a number of social categories. I showed how recovery entailed a transition from being an object whose actions were determined to being a person invested with subjectivity who was capable of exercising self-control. The positively valued trajectory toward recovery was associated with suffering and hard work and the negatively valued one with enjoyment and play. The category of chronic schizophrenia lay in the interstices between these states, between the trajectories that connected them, and between the moral values they carried. Clinical descriptions were thus interspersed with a curious mixture of voluntaristic and deterministic metaphors. The person was depicted as both active and passive, controlling and controlled, able to use an illness and its symptoms to manipulate the staff while, at the same time, suffering from this illness. Such persons were attributed neither the positive value that comes from suffering and working nor the negative value associated with enjoyment of an illness and taking pleasure in its treatment. Instead, they were invested with values that are commonly attributed to anomalous cultural categories. They were seen as uninteresting, described in metaphors of pollution, and treated as a socially dangerous category of person capable of levels of violence and disruption which they rarely manifested.

People with schizophrenia are defined as external to the fundamental categories of the social world. Not only are they located outside the phenomenal categories of time and space but also beyond the possibility of knowledge itself. Schizophrenia is defined as an *ununderstandable* state, an alien mode of experiencing the world that cannot be empathically understood by ordinary people. Thus terms such as 'bizarre' become central to its definition. Science reproduces these ideas in its own idioms. The biological literature on schizophrenia abounds with adjectives such as obscure, perplexing, puzzling, complex, enigmatic, elusive, baffling, mysterious, murky, and clouded. Science takes up madness as an ununderstandable state and transforms it into schizophrenia as an inexplicable disease. As science marches forward, conquering new domains of knowledge, it continually reconstitutes schizophrenia as a category that lies just beyond its capacity for explanation, always enticingly just over the horizon. Whether in terms of empathic understanding or scientific explanation, schizophrenia is constituted as lying beyond the realm of the knowable.

Directions

Theoretical directions: power that is taken for granted

This book has been concerned with power and its relation to knowledge, stimulated mainly by the ideas of Foucault, who contends that power is exercised within the modern state in a diffuse and decentralized manner. For Foucault, power is not repressive, it is a productive force that generates categories of knowledge and practice. This approach has generated penetrating analyses of the history of ideas, yet it has limited application to everyday social interaction. This is because Foucault does not incorporate the participating subject into his account of power. Indeed he silences it, as he is interested only in the way that the conscious subject is historically constituted as such. For this reason, the works of Foucault and those inspired by him often lack specificity. They have a tendency to become trapped within the metaphor of 'the gaze' without extending their own gaze. They have tended to reproduce again and again what has now achieved the status of an adage, that power is everywhere and nowhere.

Here I have sought to extend Foucault's approach by holding it in tension with social phenomenology, particularly with the work of Alfred Schutz and those who have subsequently applied his ideas to sociological research. Consequently, this book has focused attention on the everyday world of the psychiatric hospital and the tacit assumptions that people routinely make in their day-to-day work. It has examined psychiatry's stock of knowledge, both theoretical and practical, and taken special interest in the words and metaphors of common-sense reasoning within the hospital. This approach attends to the voices of meaning-giving subjects (here the clinicians and the people they treat) and asks how it is possible for them to create intersubjective understanding. By this strategy I have been able to give ethnographic specificity to Foucault's concept of power. Power is more or less everywhere, it is true; but it is not nowhere. It is exercised within the domain of taken-for-granted knowledge and practice.

At Ridgehaven, power was enacted through the definition of cases and their deployment across the hospital. The taken-for-granted dimensions of these cases—their depth, surface, and context—were the most important resources through which members of the different professions exercised their power of definition. Another aspect of power was the capacity to shape the way by which the team as a whole defined cases and to control the deployment of team members. This was effected by means of hegemonic domination, which secured leadership by enlisting consent rather than by the exercise of bureaucratic authority. Psychiatrists did not issue orders; they developed an organizational structure of teams that were aligned with psychiatric principles rather than with nursing or social work principles. My analysis of writing emphasized the power of the mundane cycle of interviewing and documenting, with its capacity to shape patients' understanding and renditions of their illnesses. At the case conference, I was intrigued by the curious mixture of technical and 'lay' language that gave a unique quality to the clinical discussions. It was through this distinctive language, its tone, and its key that power was exercised over the team as a whole and the way by which it defined cases.

By focusing on what is taken for granted, this book has revealed underlying tensions between whole and part and between object and subjectivity in the constitution of the person. It thereby serves to correct the undue concentration on individualism, wholeness, and unity of consciousness that has dominated recent analyses of the Western person within sociology and anthropology. The psychiatric hospital is a principal site, among modern institutions, in which distinctive form is given to the abstract category of the person. This study has clarified the particular varieties of person that psychiatric hospitals generate: the 'case', the 'whole person', the 'patient', the 'client', the 'professional patient', or 'anyone' as the taken-for-granted person. It has identified the particular ways by which such persons are endowed with or divested of subjectivity and has thereby given specificity to a Foucauldian analysis of power in a way that is possible only via the ethnographic method. People who work in psychiatric hospitals exercise power to transform persons by effecting subtle shifts in the way they are defined as parts or wholes, objects or subjectivities.

Furthermore, the book has examined the power of psychiatric institutions to generate a disease category, schizophrenia, as a pathological variant of the category of the person. The phenomenological approach has clarified the different guises taken on by a person when viewed through this category: the 'case of schizophrenia', the 'schizophrenic', the 'sufferer', the person 'from another planet', the carrier of an inherited bio-chemical abnormality, the 'schizophrenic brain', the 'chronic', the 'person with insight', the 'regressed infant', the 'primi-tive', the 'split person', the 'schizo'.

Reflexivity and field-work

This study has implications for the conduct of anthropological inquiry, and they chiefly turn on the reflexive nature of the enterprise. A major theme of my work has revolved around the tension between object and subjectivity. The theoretical underpinnings of the study contain this tension, as I have em-ployed one perspective that addresses the historical and insti-tutional conditions within which people are constituted as ob-jects; however, I held this perspective in counterpoint with a phenomenological perspective that takes account of the way these same people subjectively endow their world with mean-ing. Carrying out the field-work and subsequently writing the analysis involved the same tension. As a practicing psychiatrist at Ridgehaven I would become immersed in the everyday world of the hospital, paying scant attention to the words and phrases I automatically used or the tacit interpretive processes I employed to make sense of my daily work. On the other hand, I was an ethnographer who struggled to distance him-self from these processes in order to write about what I and my colleagues normally took for granted. Finally, the object–subjectivity tension emerged as central to this analysis of the person and its complex relationship to schizophrenia. Thus the theoretical basis of this study, its research method, its field of study, its substantive findings, and my own personal expe-rience in carrying it out were all expressions of a fundamental object–subject duality. It is no wonder that a problem of re-flexivity arises when one seeks to understand the dualistic na-ture of persons and their illnesses; but all one has to bring to bear on this question is one's own dualistic self and a long tradition of Western dualistic thought. This problem arises when *homo duplex* studies *homo duplex* and *schizo-phrenia.*

Another side to the recursive nature of ethnographic work is that it inevitably becomes part of the object it holds up for examination. Institutions such as Ridgehaven are sites in which people with psychiatric illness are studied and treated, but they are also sites for the production of knowledge about psychiatric illness. This book is another example. It is an anthropological study of schizophrenia that enters the very discourse that constitutes schizophrenia. It is not only a study of a psychiatric institution; it is also a product of a psychiatric institution. Such institutions have a long history of generating their own critique. Thus I fit a familiar organizational stereotype—the sceptical insider—who has been stalking around since the very inception of the asylum. Like many before me, my task has been to produce a critical examination of the institution in which I work.

Research directions

An ethnography of this nature demands the comparative study of similar problems in different cultural settings. I am currently undertaking a study of *gila* (madness) among the Iban people of Sarawak. It also demands further ethnographic research, which leaves the psychiatric institution behind in order to ground the problem of schizophrenia in the perspectives of those who experience the disorder and in the perspectives of their family members. Hannan's (1990) ethnographic study of people with chronic mental illness in an Australian community contains many points of correspondence with this study. She found that people commonly perceived their failure as an essential inner attribute and came to regard themselves as persons who were inherently different from others. They sometimes depicted themselves as aliens from outer space, and they reported a sense of time standing still or a feeling of being caught in a 'time warp'. They too regarded themselves as outside space and time; yet Hannan's ethnographic material shows the extent to which they nevertheless build a rich and intricate world of social interaction.

The implications of this study may extend beyond schizophrenia. It has delineated a relationship between illness and personhood that may pertain to other psychiatric and medical conditions. Chronic pain, alcohol abuse, and borderline personality disorder are some of the ambiguous long-term conditions that might fruitfully be compared with schizophrenia.

It may also be useful to examine illnesses such as rheumatoid arthritis or epilepsy in the light of this ethnography. I suspect that disorders of mood, such as bipolar affective disorder, may not be fraught with the same conceptual tensions, first because they refer to abnormalities in emotional life, with which it is easier to empathize, and second because they are understood within cultural metaphors of ups and downs, cycles and roller coasters, rather than deterioration or disintegration. Hence it is less likely for a patient with manic depressive disorder to be designated chronic, even when the condition has been present for decades.

It is also conceivable that many of the social processes I have studied are found in other modern institutions where there are professionals who deal primarily with people. The interpretive work of interviewing people and then writing about them, treating them as objects, deconstructing them, reconstructing them, and reinvesting them with subjectivity may be common to a number of modern people-processing institutions such as those concerned with medicine and the law. It may also pertain to several of the people-researching disciplines such as psychology and sociology. The staff members of a psychiatic hospital treat individuals with psychiatric illness, whereas social anthropologists study individuals as they relate to groups. Yet these tasks both entail talking, note-taking, and 'writing-up'; and they employ remarkably similar interpretive strategies.

This study also has implications for psychiatric research. I have demonstrated that it is difficult to disentangle culture from biology. Because geneticists and neurochemists are people, they have a tendency to think and write about their investigations using concepts and metaphors that are culturally based. The research literature is replete with these metaphors. A literary analysis of primary reports and review articles on schizophrenia reveals that they are pervaded by themes of schizophrenia as a mystery, as disintegration, as a primitive condition, as something central, or as a state of excess, imbalance, or reversal. These cultural images set the agenda for research, directing attention, for example, to certain central neural pathways that are difficult to study because they are so complex, minuscule, and inaccessible.

When we gather together a group of people with schizophrenia in order to study this illness, it must be recognized that we are categorizing them on the basis of cultural principles that first began to form in eighteenth century Europe, crystallized during the nineteenth century, and have become consolidated and transformed in the twentieth century. It would be astonishing indeed were we to identify a singular biochemical process or gene to account for such a dynamic cultural category. For the purpose of conducting research, psychiatry may find it useful to suspend belief in schizophrenia temporarily and to focus biological investigations on groups of people categorized in other ways that are less steeped in our cultural history, for example people who experience hallucinations or who manifest thought disorder.

Clinical directions: therapeutic implications of social processes

For my clinical colleagues, I anticipate that this study will shed some light on their ordinary day-to-day practice, as it has for me. I hope that it will illuminate the words, phrases, and metaphors they use and the powerful interactional processes of mundane clinical work that normally go unnoticed. I hope that it will also lead to a better understanding of the basic cultural work—internalization, objectification, segmentation, integration, resubjectification—carried out on a person who is admitted to a hospital, treated as a case, put together as a 'whole person', and then, on recovery, becomes just anyone again. Thinking as a clinician, these transformations could be regarded as fundamental processes of therapy and, as with any form of therapy, it may be useful to consider their efficacy and unwanted side effects.

For example, if the objectification and segmentation that occur during the writing of a case history do indeed help patients create distance from their symptoms and separate themselves from their illness, it may be possible to explore ways of enhancing these effects. Some patients may find it useful to be actively involved in writing their case record rather than being excluded from it. Usually patients' writings arc included only if they illustrate psychopathology, but it may be equally important for patients to contribute written accounts of principal symptoms and current problems as well as written plans to deal with these problems. Similarly, if disintegration and breakdown are deeply rooted ways of thinking about psychiatric illness and if reintegration is one of the important metaphors of recovery, it may be beneficial to devise techniques that harness such powerful metaphors. Patients may find it useful to be aware that reintegration is an underlying agenda of treatment so they can actively participate in this process of putting themselves 'together' again. Others may find it useful to meet with the entire team in conjunction with friends or family members in order to make explicit that there is a degree of social integration around them.

This study has looked at various ways the hospital staff morally evaluate their patients and has proposed that the evaluative process itself is crucial in transforming a person from a case to a moral being invested with volition and responsibility. Presently, these practices are regarded as an embarrassment. Evaluative terminology is restricted to the medium of talk and relegated to the tea room because it is thought to be too unprofessional for the record. Yet it does not go away. Once there is recognition that moral evaluation is integral to therapy, not epiphenomenal or evidence of bad practice, it may be possible to devise procedures for making it explicit, so team members can become aware of the moral judgements they apply to patients and how these might influence clinical decision making. It would involve developing a new clinical language with which to describe a person in terms of their willpower, their strategic ability, the level of enjoyment they obtain from treatment, their proclivity to influence the staff, their ability to exert control over mental health resources, and their capacity for negotiation.

It is also important to recognize that these processes may have harmful side-effects. Objectification can easily lead a person to assume the identity of a 'schizophrenic'. Premature insistence that suffering is the only way a person can relate to their schizophrenia can cut off the treating staff from the varieties of experience that patients may wish to communicate to them. Trying too hard to force people into an ideal of the autonomous, self-contained, self-possessed person who can act and relate independently in the world may have more to do with the reproduction of a Western cultural stereotype than with providing assistance.

For patients I am hopeful that this study will facilitate their more active contribution to the understanding and treatment of this disorder. What I have learned from the staff and patients of Ridgehaven Hospital can be used as a map of the various ways of thinking about the illness, a guide for other patients to explore and understand their own relationship with schizophrenia. Some patients may find the concept of schizophrenia useful because it helps make sense of their experiences. Others may find that it needs to be jettisoned because it carries too many deeply rooted cultural associations with danger and split personality. It is difficult enough to deal with voices and disrupted thoughts without, in addition, having to regard oneself as fundamentally bizarre and different from others, an anomaly in this world.

References

Abrahamson, D. (1993) Institutionalisation and the long-term course of schizophrenia. *British Journal of Psychiatry*, **162**, 533–8.

Abrams, R. & Taylor, M. A. (1983) The genetics of schizophrenia: a reassessment using modern criteria. *American Journal of Psychiatry*, **140** (2), 171–5.

Ackerknecht, E. H. (1982) *A Short History of Medicine*. Baltimore: Johns Hopkins University Press.

Akhtar, S. & Byrne, J. (1983) The concept of splitting and its clinical relevance. *American Journal of Psychiatry*, **140** (8), 1013–16.

Al-Issa, I. (1982) *Culture and Psychopathology*. Baltimore: University Park Press.

Allderidge, P. (1991) The foundation of the Maudsley Hospital. In *150 Years of British Psychiatry 1841–1991*, ed. G. E. Berrios & H. Freeman, pp. 79–88. London: Gaskell.

Allen, D. F. & Postel, J. (1992) Introduction to P. Pinel: 'On periodic or intermittent mania.' *History of Psychiatry*, **3** (3), 351–6.

Alpert, M. & Friedhoff, A. (1980) An un-dopamine hypothesis of schizophrenia. *Schizophrenia Bulletin*, **6** (3), 387–90.

American Psychiatric Association. (1980) *Diagnostic and Statistical Manual III*. Washington, DC: American Psychiatric Association.

Andreasen, N. C. (1990) Positive and negative symptoms: historical and conceptual aspects. In *Schizophrenia: Positive and Negative Symptoms and Syndromes*, ed. N. C. Andreasen, pp. 1–42. Basel: Karger.

Arieti, S. (1955) *Interpretation of Schizophrenia*. New York: Robert Brunner.

Armstrong, D. (1984) The patient's view. *Social Science and Medicine*, **18** (9), 737–44.

Arney, W. R. & Bergen, B. J. (1983) The anomaly, the chronic patient and the play of medical power. *Sociology of Health and Illness*, **5** (1), 1–24.

Arney, W. R. & Bergen, B. J. (1984) *Medicine and the Management of Living: Taming the Last Great Beast*. Chicago: University of Chicago Press.

Atkinson, P., Reid, M. & Sheldrake, P. (1977) Medical mystique. *Sociology of Work and Occupations*, **4** (3), 243–80.

Barham, P. (1984) *Schizophrenia and Human Value: Chronic Schizophrenia, Science and Society*. Oxford: Basil Blackwell.

Baron, M., Gruen, R., Rainer, J., Kane, J., Asnis, L. & Lord, S. (1985) A family study of schizophrenic and normal control probands: implications for the spectrum concept of schizophrenia. *American Journal of Psychiatry*, **142** (4), 447–55.

Bateson, G. (1958) *Naven: A Survey of the Problems Suggested by a Composite Picture of the Culture of a New Guinea Tribe Drawn from Three Points of View*. Stanford, CA: Stanford University Press.

Bateson, G. (1973) *Steps to an Ecology of Mind*. Frogmore, St. Albans: Granada.

Bateson, G., Jackson, D., Haley, J. & Weakland, J. (1956) Toward a theory of schizophrenia. *Behavioral Science*, **1**, 251–64.

Beer, D., trans. (1992) The manifestations of insanity, by E. Kraepelin. *History of Psychiatry*, **3** (4), 504–29.

Belknap, I. (1956) *The Human Problems of a State Mental Hospital*. New York: McGraw-Hill.

Benda, C. E. (1966) What is existential psychiatry? *American Journal of Psychiatry*, **123** (3), 288–96.

Ben-Sira, Z. & Szyf, M. (1992) Status inequality in the social worker-nurse collaboration in hospitals. *Social Science and Medicine*, **34** (4), 365–74.

Berger, P. L. & Luckman, T. (1967) *The Social Construction of Reality: A Treatise in the Sociology of Knowledge*. London: Allen Lane.

Berrios, G. E. (1991) Positive and negative signals: a conceptual history. In *Negative Versus Positive Schizophrenia*, ed. A. Marneros, N. C. Andreasen & M. T. Tsuang, pp. 8–27. Berlin: Springer-Verlag.

Berrios, G. E. & Hauser, R. (1988) The early development of Kraepelin's ideas on classification: a conceptual history. *Psychological Medicine*, **18**, 813–21.

Berze, J. (1987) Primary insufficiency of mental activity [1914]. In *The Clinical Roots of the Schizophrenia Concept: Translations of Seminal European Contributions on Schizophrenia*, ed. J. Cutting & M. Shepherd, pp. 51–58. Cambridge: Cambridge University Press.

Birley, J. L. T. & Brown, G. W. (1970) Crises and life changes preceding the onset or relapse of acute schizophrenia: clinical aspects. *British Journal of Psychiatry*, **116**, 327–33.

Bittner, E. (1974) The concept of organization. In *Ethnomethodology: Selected Readings*, ed. R. Turner, pp. 69–81. Harmondsworth: Penguin Books.

Bleuler, E. (1950) *Dementia Praecox or The Group of Schizophrenias*. New York: International Universities Press.

Bleuler, E. (1987) The prognosis of dementia praecox: the group of schizophrenias [1908]. In *The Clinical Roots of the Schizophrenia Concept: Translations of Seminal European Contributions on Schizophrenia*, ed. J. Cutting, M. Shepherd, pp. 59–74. Cambridge: Cambridge University Press.

Bleuler, M. (1974) The long-term course of the schizophrenic psychoses. *Psychological Medicine*, **4**, 244–54.

Bleuler, M. (1984) What is schizophrenia? *Schizophrenia Bulletin*, **10** (1), 8–10.

Blumer, H. (1971) Society as symbolic interaction. In *Human Behaviour and Social Processes: An Interactionist Approach*, ed. A. M. Rose, pp. 189–92. London: Routledge and Kegan Paul.

Boon, J. A. (1985) Anthropology and degeneration: birds, words and orangutans. In *Degeneration: The Dark Side of Progress*, ed. J. E. Chamberlin & S. L. Gilman, pp. 24–48. New York: Columbia University Press.

Borges, J. L. (1970) Borges and I. In *Labyrinths*, pp. 282–3. Harmondsworth: Penguin Books.

Bowen, W. T., Maler, D. C. & Androes, L. (1965) The psychiatric team: myth and mystique. *American Journal of Psychiatry*, **122**, 687–90.

Bowers, M. B. (1980) Biochemical processes in schizophrenia: an update. *Schizophrenia Bulletin*, **6** (3), 393–403.

Bowler, P. J. (1984) *Evolution: The History of an Idea*. Berkeley: University of California Press.

Braginsky, B. M., Braginsky, D. D. & Ring, K. (1969) *Methods of Madness: The Mental Hospital as a Last Resort*. New York: Holt, Rinehart and Winston.

Brenner, H. D. & Böker, W., eds. (1989) *Schizophrenia as a Systems Disorder*. London: Royal College of Psychiatrists (*British Journal of Psychiatry*, **155**, Suppl. 5).

Briggs, M. (1981) *Vitamins in Human Biology and Medicine*. Boca Raton, FL: CRC Press.

Brightwell, R. (1982) *Human Brain – Madness* [film]. London: British Broadcasting Corporation.

Brody, E. B. (1956) Interprofessional relations, or psychologists and psychiatrists are human too, only more so. *American Psychologist*, **11**, 105–11.

Brown, G. W., Birley, J. L. T. & Wing, J. K. (1972) Influence of family life on the course of schizophrenic disorders: a replication. *British Journal of Psychiatry*, **121**, 241–58.

Brown, G. W., Monck, E. M., Carstairs, G. M.& Wing, J. K. (1962) Influence of family life on the course of schizophrenic illness. *British Journal of Preventative and Social Medicine*, **16**, 55–68.

Bucher, R. & Strauss, A. (1961) Professions in process. *American Journal of Sociology*, **66** (4), 325–34.

Buchsbaum, M. S. & Haler, R. J. (1987) Functional and anatomical brain imaging: impact on schizophrenia research. *Schizophrenia Bulletin*, **13** (1), 129–46.

Burke, K. (1969a) *A Rhetoric of Motives*. Berkeley: University of California Press.

Burke, K. (1969b) *A Grammar of Motives*. Berkeley: University of California Press.

Bynum, W. F. (1984) Alcoholism and degeneration in 19th century European medicine and psychiatry. *British Journal of Addiction*, **79**, 59–70.

Bynum, W. F. (1991) Tuke's *Dictionary* and psychiatry at the turn of the century. In *150 Years of British Psychiatry, 1841–1991*, ed. G. E. Berrios & H. Freeman, pp. 163–79. London: Gaskell.

Cadet, J. L. (1984) Disorders of the isodendritic core of the brainstem. *Schizophrenia Bulletin*, **10** (1), 1–3.

Carlson, E. T. (1985) Medicine and degeneration: theory and praxis. In *Degeneration: The Dark Side of Progress*, ed. J. E. Chamberlin & S. L. Gilman, pp. 121–44. New York: Columbia University Press.

Carlsson, A. (1977) Does dopamine play a role in schizophrenia? *Psychological Medicine*, **7**, 583–97.

Carlsson, A. (1978) Does dopamine have a role in schizophrenia? *Biological Psychiatry*, **13** (1), 3–21.

Carlsson, A. & Lindqvist, M. (1963) Effect of chlorpromazine or haloperidol on formation of 3-methoxytyramine and normetanephrine in mouse brain. *Acta Pharmacologica et Toxicologica*, **20**, 140–4.

Carpenter, W. T. (1983) What is schizophrenia? *Schizophrenia Bulletin*, **9** (1), 9–10.

Carpenter, W. T. (1987) Approaches to knowledge and understanding of schizophrenia. In *Special Report: Schizophrenia*, ed. D. Shore, pp. 17–24. Rockville MD: National Institute of Mental Health.

Carpenter, W. T., McGlashan, T. H. & Strauss, J. J. (1977) The treatment of acute schizophrenia without drugs: an investigation of some current assumptions. *American Journal of Psychiatry*, **134** (1), 14–20.

Carrigan, D. R. & Waltrip, R. W. (1990) Viral theories of schizophrenia. *Current Opinion in Psychiatry*, **3**, 14–18.

Castel, R., Castel, F. & Lovell, A. (1982) *The Psychiatric Society*. New York: Columbia University Press.

Caudill, W. (1958) *The Psychiatric Hospital as a Small Society*. Cambridge, MA: Harvard University Press.

Cauwenbergh, L. S. (1991) J. Chr. A. Heinroth (1773–1843): a psychiatrist of the German romantic era. *History of Psychiatry*, **2** (4), 365–83.

Chapman, J. (1966) The early symptoms of schizophrenia. *British Journal of Psychiatry,* **112,** 225–51.

Cicourel, A. V. (1968) *The Social Organization of Juvenile Justice.* New York: Wiley.

Cicourel, A. V. (1974) Interviewing and memory. In *Pragmatic Aspects of Human Communication,* ed. C. Cherry, pp. 51–82. Dordrecht: Reidel.

Clay, B. J. (1986) *Mandak Realities: Person and Power in Central New Ireland.* New Brunswick, NJ: Rutgers University Press.

Cohen, J. D. & Servan-Schreiber, D. (1993) A theory of dopamine function and its role in cognitive deficits in schizophrenia. *Schizophrenia Bulletin,* **19** (1): 85–104.

Collins, R. (1980) Erving Goffman and the development of modern social theory. In *The View from Goffman,* ed. J. Ditton, pp. 170–209. London: Macmillan.

Collins, S. (1985) Categories, concepts or predicaments? Remarks on Mauss's use of philosophical terminology. In *The Category of the Person: Anthropology, Philosophy, History,* ed. M. Carrithers, S. Collins & S. Lukes, pp. 46–82. Cambridge: Cambridge University Press.

Comaroff, J. & Maguire, P. (1981) Ambiguity and the search for meaning: childhood leukaemia in the modern clinical context. *Social Science and Medicine,* **15B,** 115–23.

Conrad, J. (1960) The secret sharer [1912]. In *Three Tales from Conrad,* ed. D. Brown, pp. 127–74. London: Hutchinson Educational.

Coser, R. L. (1979) *Training in Ambiguity: Learning Through Doing in a Mental Hospital.* New York: Free Press.

Coulter, J. (1973) *Approaches to Insanity.* London: Martin Robertson.

Crayton, J. W. (1990) The dopamine hypothesis of schizophrenia. *Current Opinion in Psychiatry,* **3,** 19–22.

Creese, I., Burt, D. R. & Snyder, S. H. (1976) Dopamine receptor binding predicts clinical and pharmacological potencies of antischizophrenic drugs. *Science,* **192** (4238), 481–3.

Crighton, J. L. (1990) Introduction to C. F. Nasse, 'Zeitschrift für psychische Ärzte' [preface to the first issue; 1818]. *History of Psychiatry,* **1** (2), 233–5.

Crow, T. J. (1980) Molecular pathology of schizophrenia: more than one disease process? *British Medical Journal,* **280** (6206), 66–68.

Crow, T. J. (1984) A re-evaluation of the viral hypothesis: is psychosis the result of retroviral integration at a site close to the cerebral dominance gene? *British Journal of Psychiatry,* **145,** 243–53.

Crow, T. J. (1989) A current view of the type II syndrome: age of onset, intellectual impairment, and the meaning of structural changes in the brain. *British Journal of Psychiatry,* **155** (suppl. 7), 15–20.

Daniels, A. K. (1975) Professionalism in formal organizations. In *Processing People: Cases in Organizational Behaviour,* ed. J. B. Mc-Kinley, pp. 303–38. London: Holt, Rinehart and Winston.

Darwin, C. (1965) *The Expression of the Emotions in Man and Animals.* Chicago: University of Chicago Press.

Davidson, K. W. (1990) Role blurring and the hospital social worker's search for a clear domain. *Health and Social Work,* **15** (3), 228–34.

Day, R. (1977) A review of the current state of negotiated order theory: an appreciation and a critique. *Sociological Quarterly,* **18**, 126–42.

Dingwall, R. & Murray, T. (1983) Categorization in accident departments: 'good' patients, 'bad' patients and 'children'. *Sociology of Health and Illness,* **5** (2), 127–48.

Ditton, J., ed. (1980) *The View from Goffman.* London: Macmillan.

Doerner, K. (1981) *Madmen and the Bourgeoisie: A Social History of Insanity and Psychiatry.* Oxford: Basil Blackwell.

Donnelly, M. (1983) *Managing the Mind: A Study of Medical Psychology in Early Nineteenth-Century Britain.* London: Tavistock.

Dostoevsky, F. (1916) *A Raw Youth.* London: Heinemann.

Douglas, M. (1966) *Purity and Danger: An Analysis of the Concepts of Pollution and Taboo.* London: Routledge and Kegan Paul.

Dowbiggin, I. (1985) Degeneration and hereditarianism in French mental medicine 1840–90: psychiatric theory as ideological adaptation. In *The Anatomy of Madness: Essays in the History of Psychiatry, Vol. I: People and Ideas,* ed. W. F. Bynum, R. Porter & M. Shepherd, pp. 188–232. London: Tavistock.

Dreyfus, H. L. & Rabinow, P. (1982) *Michel Foucault: Beyond Structuralism and Hermeneutics.* Brighton, Sussex: Harvester Press.

Duff, R. S. & Hollingshead, A. B. (1968) *Sickness and Society.* New York: Harper and Row.

Dumont, L. (1980) *Homo Hierarchicus: The Caste System and Its Implications,* rev. ed. Chicago: University of Chicago Press.

Dumont, L. (1986) *Essays on Individualism: Modern Ideology in Anthropological Perspective.* Chicago: University of Chicago Press.

Durkheim, E. (1965) *The Elementary Forms of the Religious Life: A Study in Religious Sociology.* New York: Free Press.

Eagles, J. M. (1992) Are polioviruses a cause of schizophrenia? *British Journal of Psychiatry,* **160**, 598–600.

Ehrmann, J. (1968) *Game, Play and Literature.* Boston: Beacon Press.

Ellenberger, H. F. (1970) *The Discovery of the Unconscious: The History and Evolution of Dynamic Psychiatry.* London: Allen Lane/Penguin.

Engel, G. L (1977) The need for a new medical model: a challenge for biomedicine. *Science,* **196**, 129–36.

Engel, G. L. (1980) The clinical application of the biopsychosocial model. *American Journal of Psychiatry*, **137** (5), 535–44.

Engel, G. V. & Hall, R. H. (1971) The growing industrialization of the professions. In *The Professions and Their Prospects*, ed. E. Freidson, pp. 75–88. Beverly Hills, CA: Sage Publications.

Engelhardt, H. T. (1975) The concepts of health and disease. In *Evaluation and Explanation in Biomedical Science*, ed. H. T. Engelhardt & S. F. Spiker, pp. 125–41. Dordrecht: Reidel.

Engstrom, E. J. (1991) Emil Kraepelin: psychiatry and public affairs in Wilhelmine Germany. *History of Psychiatry*, **2** (2), 111–32.

Engstrom, E. J. (1992) Introduction to E. Kraepelin 'Psychiatric observations on contemporary issues'. *History of Psychiatry*, **3** (2), 253–6.

Erikson, K. T. (1957) Patient role and social uncertainty: a dilemma of the mentally ill. *Psychiatry*, **20**, 263–72.

Erikson, K. T. & Gilbertson, D. E. (1969) Case records in the mental hospital. In *On Record: Files and Dossiers in American Life* ed. S. Wheeler, pp. 389–412. New York: Russel Sage Foundation.

Erksteins, M. (1985) History and degeneration: of birds and cages. In *Degeneration: The Dark Side of Progress*, ed. J. E. Chamberlin & S. L. Gilman, pp. 1–23. New York: Columbia University Press.

Estroff, S. E. (1981) *Making it Crazy: An Ethnography of Psychiatric Clients in an American Community*. Berkeley: University of California Press.

Etzioni, A. (1960) Interpersonal and structural factors in the study of mental hospitals. *Psychiatry*, **23**, 13–22.

Evans-Pritchard, E. E. (1973) Some reminiscences and reflections on field work. *Journal of the Anthropological Society of Oxford*, **4** (1), 1–12.

Ewing, K. P. (1990) The illusion of wholeness: culture, self, and the experience of inconsistency. *Ethos*, **18** (3), 251–78.

Fabrega, H., Jr. (1982) Culture and psychiatric illness: biomedical and ethnomedical aspects. In *Cultural Conceptions of Mental Health and Therapy*, ed. A. J. Marsella & G. M. White, pp. 39–68. Dordrecht: Reidel.

Fadden, G., Bebbington, P. & Kuipers, L. (1987) The burden of care: the impact of functional psychiatric illness on the patient's family. *British Journal of Psychiatry*, **150**, 285–92.

Farde, L., Wiesel, F-A., Hall, H., Halldin, C., Stone-Elander, S. & Sedvall, G. (1987) No D_2 receptor increase in PET study of schizophrenia. *Archives of General Psychiatry*, **44**, 671–2.

Farde, L., Wiesel, F-A., Stone-Elander, S., Halldin, C., Nordström, A-L., Hall, H. & Sedvall, G. (1990) D_2 dopamine receptors in neuroleptic-naive schizophrenic patients: a positron emission tomography study with [^{11}C] raclopride. *Archives of General Psychiatry*, **47**, 213–19.

Federn, P. (1952) *Ego Psychology and the Psychoses.* New York: Basic Books.

Forchuk, C. (1989) Establishing a nurse-client relationship. *Journal of Psychosocial Nursing,* **27** (2), 30–34.

Forster, M. (1993) Hegel's dialectical method. In *The Cambridge Companion to Hegel,* ed. F. C. Beiser, pp. 130–70. Cambridge: Cambridge University Press.

Fortes, M. (1981) On the concept of the person among the Tallensi. In *La Notion de Personne in Afrique Noire,* pp. 283–319. Paris: Éditions du Centre National de la Récherche Scientifique.

Foucault, M. (1967) *Madness and Civilization: A History of Insanity in the Age of Reason.* London: Tavistock.

Foucault, M. (1972) *The Archeology of Knowledge.* London: Tavistock.

Foucault, M. (1977) *Discipline and Punish: The Birth of the Prison.* Harmondsworth: Penguin Books.

Foucault, M. (1978) The eye of power [interview]. *Semiotexte,* **3** (2), 6–20.

Foucault, M. (1980) *Power/ Knowledge: Selected Interviews and Other Writings, 1972–1977,* ed. C. Gordon. Brighton, Sussex: Harvester Press.

Fox, R. C. & Willis, D. P. (1983) Personhood, medicine, and American society. *Milbank Quarterly,* **61** (1), 127–47.

Frank, G. (1979) Finding the common denominator: a phenomenological critique of the life history method. *Ethos,* **7**, 68–94.

Frankenberg, R. (1988) Gramsci, culture, and medical anthropology: Kundry and Parsifal? or rat's tail to sea serpent. *Medical Anthropology Quarterly,* **2** (4), 324–37.

Freidson, E. (1970) *Profession of Medicine: A Study in the Sociology of Applied Knowledge.* New York: Harper and Row.

Freidson, E., ed. (1971) *The Professions and Their Prospects.* Beverly Hills, CA: Sage Publications.

Freidson, E. (1986) *Professional Powers: A Study of the Institutionalization of Formal Knowledge.* Chicago: University of Chicago Press.

Freidson, E. & Rhea, B. (1972) Processes of control in a company of equals. In *Medical Men and Their Work,* ed. E. Freidson & J. Lorber, pp. 185–99. New York: Aldine.

Freud, S. (1950) The project for a scientific psychology (1895). In *The Standard Edition of the Complete Psychological Works of Sigmund Freud. Vol. I,* ed. J. Strachey & A. Freud, pp. 283–98. London: Hogarth Press and Institute of Psychoanalysis.

Freud, S. (1957a) Five lectures on psycho-analysis: first lecture (1910). In *The Standard Edition of the Complete Psychological Works of Sigmund Freud. Vol. XI,* ed. J. Strachey & A. Freud, pp. 9–22. London: Hogarth Press and Institute of Psychoanalysis.

Freud, S. (1957b) On the history of the psycho-analytic movement (1914). In *The Standard Edition of the Complete Psychological*

Works of Sigmund Freud. Vol. XIV, ed. J. Strachey & A. Freud, pp. 7–66. London: Hogarth Press and Institute of Psychoanalysis.

Fromm-Reichmann, F. (1948) Notes on the development of treatment of schizophrenics by psychoanalytic psychotherapy. *Psychiatry*, **11**, 263–73.

Gaines, A. D. (1992) Ethnopsychiatry: the cultural construction of psychiatries. In *Ethnopsychiatry: The Cultural Construction of Professional and Folk Psychiatries*, ed. A. D. Gaines, pp. 3–49. Albany, NY: State University of New York Press.

Garfinkel, H. (1974) 'Good' organizational reasons for 'bad' clinic records. In *Ethnomethodology: Selected Readings*, ed. R. Turner, pp. 109–27. Harmondsworth: Penguin Books.

Geertz, C. (1983) *Local Knowledge: Further Essays in Interpretive Anthropology*. New York: Basic Books.

Gellner, E. (1964) *Thought and Change*. Chicago: University of Chicago Press.

George, V. & Dundes, A. (1978) The Gomer: a figure of American hospital folk speech. *Journal of American Folklore*, **91**, 568–80.

Glaser, B. & Strauss, A. L. (1964) The social loss of dying patients. *American Journal of Nursing*, **64**, 119–21.

Glaser, B. & Strauss, A. L. (1965) *Awareness of Dying*. Chicago: Aldine.

Glaser, B. & Strauss, A. L. (1967) *The Discovery of Grounded Theory: Strategies for Qualitative Research*. Chicago: Aldine.

Glaser, B. & Strauss, A. L. (1968) *Time for Dying*. Chicago: Aldine.

Glowinski, J., Tassin, J. P. & Thierry, A. M. (1984) The mesocortico-prefrontal dopaminergic neurons. *Trends in Neuroscience*, **7**, 415–18.

Goethe, J. W. (1987) *Faust: Part One*, trans. D. Luke. Oxford: Oxford University Press.

Goffman, E. (1959) *The Presentation of Self in Everyday Life*. Garden City, NY: Doubleday, Anchor Books.

Goffman, E. (1968) *Asylums: Essays on the Social Situation of Mental Patients and Other Inmates*. Harmondsworth: Penguin Books.

Goffman, E. (1970) *Strategic Interaction*. Oxford: Basil Blackwell.

Goffman, E. (1972) Role distance. In *Encounters: Two Studies in the Sociology of Interaction*, pp. 73–134. Harmondsworth: Penguin Books.

Goldstein, J. (1987) *Console and Classify: The French Psychiatric Profession in the Nineteenth Century*. Cambridge: Cambridge University Press.

Goodman, A. (1991) Organic unity theory: the mind-body problem revisited. *American Journal of Psychiatry*, **148**, 553–63.

Goody, J. (1980) Thought and writing. In *Soviet and Western Anthropology*, ed. E. Gellner, pp. 119–34. London: Duckworth.

Goody, J. (1982) Alternative paths to knowledge in oral and literate cultures. In *Spoken and Written Language: Exploring Orality and Literacy*, ed. D. Tannen, pp. 201–15. Norwood, NJ: Ablex.

Gottesman, I. I. & Shields, J. (1982) *Schizophrenia: The Epigenetic Puzzle*. Cambridge: Cambridge University Press.

Gramsci, A. (1971) *Selections from the Prison Notebooks of Antonio Gramsci*, ed. Q. Hoare & G. N. Smith. London: Lawrence and Wishart.

Gray, A. (1983) *Unlikely Stories Mostly*. Edinburgh: Canongate.

Gray, D. E. (1986) Community and institutional roles: evaluations by Australian psychiatric nurses. *Community Mental Health Journal*, **22** (2), 147–59.

Gruzelier, J. & Manchanda, R. (1982) The syndrome of schizophrenia: relations between electrodermal response, lateral asymmetries and clinical ratings. *British Journal of Psychiatry*, **141**, 488–95.

Hall, B. A. (1988) Specialty knowledge in psychiatric nursing: where are we now? *Archives of Psychiatric Nursing*, **2** (4), 191–9.

Hall, P. M. (1973) A symbolic interactionist analysis of politics. *Sociological Inquiry*, **42** (3), 35–75.

Halliwell, L. (1977) *Halliwell's Film Guide*. London: Granada.

Hallmayer, J., Kennedy, J. L., Wetterberg, L., Sjogren, B., Kidd, K. K. & Cavalli-Sforza, L. L. (1992) Exclusion of linkage between the serotonin 2 receptor and schizophrenia in a large Swedish kindred. *Archives of General Psychiatry*, **49**, 216–19.

Handelman, D. (1978) Bureaucratic interpretation: the perception of child abuse in urban Newfoundland. In *Bureaucracy and World View: Studies in the Logic of Official Interpretation*, ed. D. Handelman & E. Leyton, pp. 15–68. Social and Economic Studies No. 22. Institute of Social and Economic Research. Memorial University of Newfoundland. Toronto: University of Toronto Press.

Hannan, L. (1990) *Stigma, Felt Identity and the Chronically Mentally Ill: An Ethnographic Study of the Chronically Mentally Ill in an Australian Community*. Ph.D. thesis, University of Sydney.

Haracz, J. (1982) The dopamine hypothesis: an overview of studies with schizophrenic patients. *Schizophrenia Bulletin*, **8** (3), 438–69.

Hardie, R. J. (1991) Principles of management of neurological disability. In *Neurology in Clinical Practice: Principles of Diagnosis and Management*, ed. W. G. Bradley, R. B. Daroff, G. M. Fenichel & C. D. Marsden, pp. 749–87. Boston: Butterworth-Heinemann.

Harding, C. M., Zubin, J. & Strauss, J. S. (1992) Chronicity in schizophrenia: revisited. *British Journal of Psychiatry*, **161** (suppl. 18), 27–37.

Harris, G. G. (1989) Concepts of individual, self, and person in description and analysis. *American Anthropologist,* **91** (3), 599–612.

Haslam, J. (1988) *Illustrations of Madness* [1810], ed. R. Porter. London: Routledge.

Hatfield, A. B. (1987) The expressed emotion theory: why families object. *Hospital and Community Psychiatry,* **38** (4), 341.

Hawkins, D. & Pauling, L. (1973) *Orthomolecular Psychiatry: Treatment of Schizophrenia.* San Fransisco: W. H. Freeman.

Hawthorn, G. (1990) The impossible sociology of post-modern persons. *Australian Journal of Anthropology,* **1** (2–3), 168–79.

Hawthorn, J. (1983) *Multiple Personality and the Disintegration of Literary Character: From Oliver Goldsmith to Sylvia Plath.* London: Edward Arnold.

Hay, G. G. (1983) Feigned psychosis: a review of the simulation of mental illness. *British Journal of Psychiatry,* **143**, 8–10.

Heaslip, B. (1971) *Saints and Strait Jackets: An Intimate View of Life in an Australian Psychiatric Hospital.* [Australian City]: The Author.

Heath, S. B. (1982) Protean shapes in literacy events: ever-shifting oral and literate traditions. In *Spoken and Written Language: Exploring Orality and Literacy,* ed. D. Tannen, pp. 91–118. Norwood, NJ: Ablex.

Heston, L. L. (1966) Psychiatric disorders in foster home reared children of schizophrenic mothers. *British Journal of Psychiatry,* **112**, 819–25.

Heston, L. L. (1970) The genetics of schizophrenic and schizoid disease. *Science,* **167** (3916), 249–55.

Hirsch, S. R. & Leff, J. P. (1975) *Abnormalities in Parents of Schizophrenics: A Review of the Literature and an Investigation of Communication Defects and Deviances.* London: Oxford University Press.

Hirst, P. & Woolley, P. (1982) *Social Relations and Human Attributes.* London: Tavistock.

Hoenig, J. (1991) Jaspers's view on schizophrenia. In *The Concept of Schizophrenia: Historical Perspectives,* ed. J. G. Howells, pp. 75–92. Washington, DC: American Psychiatric Press.

Holt, A. (1979) [*Ridgehaven Hospital*]: *The First Fifty Years.* [Australian City: Ridgehaven Hospital].

Holzberg, J. D. (1960) The historical traditions of the state hospital as a force of resistance to the team. *American Journal of Orthopsychiatry,* **30**, 87–94.

Howells, J. G. (1991) Introduction. In *The Concept of Schizophrenia: Historical Perspectives,* ed. J. G. Howells, pp. ix–xxiv. Washington, DC: American Psychiatric Press.

Huertas, R. (1992) Madness and degeneration. I. From 'fallen angel' to mentally ill. *History of Psychiatry,* **3** (4), 391–411.

Huertas, R. (1993a) Madness and degeneration. II. Alcoholism and degeneration. *History of Psychiatry*, **4** (1), 1–21.

Huertas, R. (1993b) Madness and degeneration. III. Degeneration and criminality. *History of Psychiatry*, **4** (2), 141–58.

Husserl, E. (1960) *Cartesian Meditations: An Introduction to Phenomenology*. The Hague: Martinus Nijhoff.

Hymes, D. (1972) Models of the interaction of language and social life. In *Directions in Social Linguistics: The Ethnography of Communication*, ed. J. J. Gumperz & D. Hymes, pp. 35–71. New York: Holt, Rinehart and Winston.

Institute of Psychiatry, The Bethlem Royal and Maudsley Hospital (1991) *Annual Report 1990*. London: Institute of Psychiatry.

Jackson, D. D. (1960) A critique of the literature on the genetics of schizophrenia. In *The Etiology of Schizophrenia*, ed. D. D. Jackson, pp. 37–87. New York: Basic Books.

James, H. (1957) The jolly corner [1908]. In *Selected Short Stories*, ed. Q. Anderson, pp. 321–57. New York: Holt, Rinehart and Winston.

Jamous, H. & Peloille, B. (1970) Professions or self-perpetuating systems? Changes in the French university-hospital system. In *Professions and Professionalization*, ed. J. A. Jackson, pp. 109–52. London: Cambridge University Press.

Janson, H. W. (1986) *History of Art*. Englewood Cliffs, NJ: Prentice-Hall.

Janzarik, W. (1992) 100 years of Heidelberg psychiatry. *History of Psychiatry*, **3** (1), 5–27.

Jaspers, K. (1963) *General Psychopathology*. Manchester: Manchester University Press.

Jaspers, K. (1974) Causal and 'meaningful' connexions between life history and psychosis. In *Themes and Variations in European Psychiatry*, ed. S. Hirsch, M. Shepherd & L. Kalinowsky, pp. 81–93. Charlottesville, VA: University Press of Virginia.

Jeffrey, R. (1979) 'Normal rubbish': deviant patients in casualty departments. *Sociology of Health and Illness*, **1** (1), 90–107.

Jehenson, R. (1973) A phenomenological approach to the study of formal organization. In *Phenomenological Sociology: Issues and Applications*, ed. G. Psathas, pp. 219–47. New York: Wiley.

Jimenez, M. A. (1988) Chronicity in mental disorders: evolution of a concept. *Social Casework*, **69**, 627–33.

Johnson, T. (1977) The professions in the class structure. In *Industrial Society: Class, Cleavage and Control*, ed. R. Scase, pp. 93–110. London: George Allen and Unwin.

Johnston, T. B., Davies, D. V. & Davies, F. (1958) *Gray's Anatomy: Descriptive and Applied*. London: Longmans.

Jones, P. & Murray, R. M. (1991) The genetics of schizophrenia is the genetics of neurodevelopment. *British Journal of Psychiatry*, **158**, 615–23.

Jung, C. G. (1982a) The psychology of dementia praecox [1907]. In *The Collected Works of C. G. Jung*, Vol. 3, ed. H. Read, M. Fordham & G. Adler, pp. 3–151. Princeton, NJ: Princeton University Press.

Jung, C. G. (1982b) The content of the psychoses [1908]. In *The Collected Works of C. G. Jung*, Vol. 3, ed. H. Read, M. Fordham & G. Adler, pp. 154–78. Princeton, NJ: Princeton University Press.

Kadushin, C. (1962) Social distance between client and professional. *American Journal of Sociology*, **67**, 517–31.

Kahn, R. S. & Davidson, M. (1993) Serotonin, dopamine and their interactions in schizophrenia. *Psychopharmacology*, **112**, S1–S4.

Kallman, F. J. (1946) The genetic theory of schizophrenia: an analysis of 691 schizophrenic twin index families. *American Journal of Psychiatry*, **103**, 309–22.

Kant, I. (1974) *Anthropology from a Pragmatic Point of View* [1798]. The Hague: Martinus Nijhoff.

Kanter, J. (1989) Clinical case management: definition, principles, components. *Hospital and Community Psychiatry*, **40** (4), 361–8.

Kanter, J., Lamb, R. H. & Loeper, C. (1987) Expressed emotion in families: a critical review. *Hospital and Community Psychiatry*, **38** (4), 374–80.

Kapferer, B. (1988) *Legends of People, Myths of State: Violence, Intolerance, and Political Culture in Sri Lanka and Australia*. Washington, DC: Smithsonian Institution Press.

Karlsson, J. L. (1968) Genealogic studies of schizophrenia. In *The Transmission of Schizophrenia*, ed. D. Rosenthal & S. Kety, pp. 85–94. Oxford: Pergamon Press.

Karno, M. & Jenkins J. H. (1993) Cross-cultural issues in the course and treatment of schizophrenia. *Psychiatric Clinics of North America*, **16** (2), 339–50.

Karno, M. & Norquist, G. (1989) Schizophrenia: epidemiology. In *Comprehensive Textbook of Psychiatry*, ed. H. I. Kaplan & B. J. Sadock, pp. 699–705. Baltimore: Williams and Wilkins.

Karp, D. A. (1992) Illness ambiguity and the search for meaning: a case study of a self-help group for affective disorders. *Journal of Contemporary Ethnography*, **21** (2), 139–70.

Kavanagh, D. (1992) Recent developments in expressed emotion and schizophrenia. *British Journal of Psychiatry*, **160**, 601–20.

Kendler, K. S. (1983a) Overview: a current perspective on twin studies of schizophrenia. *American Journal of Psychiatry*, **140** (11), 1413–25.

Kendler, K. S. (1983b) Heritability of schizophrenia [letter to the editor]. *American Journal of Psychiatry*, **140** (1), 131–2.

Kendler, K. S. & Diehl, S. R. (1993) The genetics of schizophrenia: a current genetic-epidemiological perspective. *Schizophrenia Bulletin*, **19** (2), 261–85.

Kendler, K. S. & Robinette, C. D. (1983) Schizophrenia in the National Academy of Sciences–National Research Council twin registry: a 16-year update. *American Journal of Psychiatry*, **140** (12), 1551–63.

Kennedy, J., Giuffra, L., Moises, H., Cavalli-Sforza, L., Pakstis, A., Kidd, J., Castiglione, C., Sjogren, B., Wetterberg, L. & Kidd, K. (1988) Evidence against linkage of schizophrenia to markers on chromosome 5 in a northern Swedish pedigree. *Nature*, **336**, 167–9.

Kety, S. S., Rosenthal, D., Wender, P. H. & Schulsinger, F. (1971) The types and prevalence of mental illness in the biological and adoptive families of adopted schizophrenics. In *The Transmission of Schizophrenia*, ed. D. Rosenthal & S. Kety, pp. 345–62. Oxford: Pergamon Press.

Kitcher, P. (1984) Kant's real self. In *Self and Nature in Kant's Philosophy*, ed. A. W. Wood, pp. 113–47. Ithaca: Cornell University Press.

Koehler, H. (1979) First rank symptoms of schizophrenia: questions concerning clinical boundaries. *British Journal of Psychiatry*, **137**, 234–48.

Koenigsberg, H. W. & Handley, R. (1986) Expressed emotion: from predictive index to clinical construct. *American Journal of Psychiatry*, **143** (11), 1361–73.

Kolakowski, L. (1978) *Main Currents of Marxism: Its Origins, Growth and Dissolution. I. The Founders*. Oxford: Oxford University Press.

Kraepelin, E. (1919) *Dementia Praecox and Paraphrenia*, trans. R. M. Barclay. Edinburgh: Livingstone.

Kraepelin, E. (1987) Dementia praecox [1896]. In *The Clinical Roots of the Schizophrenia Concept: Translations of Seminal European Contributions on Schizophrenia*, ed. J. Cutting & M. Shepherd, pp. 13–24. Cambridge: Cambridge University Press.

Kraepelin, E. (1992a) Die Erscheinungsformen des Irreseins [The manifestations of insanity (trans. D. Beer)]. *History of Psychiatry*, **3** (4), 509–29.

Kraepelin, E. (1992b) Psychiatrische Randbemerkungen zur Zeitgeschichte [Psychiatric observations on contemporary issues: (trans. E. J. Engstrom)]. *History of Psychiatry*, **3** (2), 256–69.

Kuhn, T. (1962) *The Structure of Scientific Revolutions*. Chicago: University of Chicago Press.

Labov, W. & Fanshel, D. (1977) *Therapeutic Discourse: Psychotherapy as Conversation*. Orlando, FL: Academic Press.

La Fontaine, J. S. (1985) Person and individual: some anthropological reflections. In *The Category of the Person: Anthropology, Philosophy, History*, ed. M. Carrithers, S. Collins & S. Lukes, pp. 123–40. Cambridge: Cambridge University Press.

Laing, R. D. (1965) *The Divided Self: An Existential Study in Sanity and Madness*. Harmondsworth: Penguin Books.

Laing, R. D. (1967) *The Politics of Experience and The Bird of Paradise.* Harmondsworth: Penguin Books.

Lanzic, M. (1992) Karl Ludwig Kahlbaum (1828–1899) and the emergence of psychopathological and nosological research in German psychiatry. *History of Psychiatry,* **3** (1), 53–58.

Leff, J. (1981) *Psychiatry Around the Globe: A Transcultural View.* New York: Marcel Dekker.

Leigh, H. (1987) Multidisciplinary teams in consultation-liaison psychiatry: the Yale model. *Psychotherapy and Psychosomatics,* **48**, 83–89.

Lewis, A. (1967) *The State of Psychiatry: Essays and Addresses.* London: Routledge and Kegan Paul.

Lewis, A. (1979a) Paranoia and paranoid: a historical perspective. In *The Later Papers of Sir Aubrey Lewis,* pp. 153–63. Oxford: Oxford University Press.

Lewis, A. (1979b) Edward Mapother and the making of the Maudsley Hospital. In *The Later Papers of Sir Aubrey Lewis,* pp. 1135–52. Oxford: Oxford University Press.

Lidz, T., Fleck, S. & Cornelison, A. R. (1965) *Schizophrenia and the Family.* New York: International Universities Press.

Lieberman, J. A. (1993) Understanding the mechanism of action of atypical antipsychotic drugs: a review of compounds in use and development. *British Journal of Psychiatry,* **163** (suppl. 22), 7–18.

Liederman, D. B. & Grisso, J-A. (1985) The Gomer phenomenon. *Journal of Health and Social Behavior,* **26**, 222–32.

Liégeois, A. (1991) Hidden philosophy and theology in Morel's theory of degeneration and nosology. *History of Psychiatry,* **2** (4), 419–27.

Liptzin, S. (1973) *Historical Survey of German Literature.* New York: Cooper Square Publishers.

List, S. J. & Cleghorn, J. M. (1993) Implications of positron emission tomography research for the investigation of the actions of antipsychotic drugs. *British Journal of Psychiatry,* **163** (suppl. 22), 25–30.

Littlewood, R. (1986) Russian dolls and Chinese boxes: an anthropological approach to the implicit models of comparative psychiatry. In *Transcultural Psychiatry,* ed. J. Cox, pp. 37–58. London: Croom Helm.

Locke, J. (1976) *An Essay Concerning Human Understanding.* London: Dent and Sons.

London, N. J. (1973) An essay on psychoanalytic theory: two theories of schizophrenia. Part I. Review and critical assessment of the development of the two theories. *International Journal of Psychoanalysis,* **54**, 169–78.

Lorber, J. (1975) Good patients and problem patients: conformity and deviance in a general hospital. *Journal of Health and Social Behavior,* **16** (2), 213–25.

Ludwig, A. M. (1983) What is schizophrenia? *Schizophrenia Bulletin,* **9** (3), 334–5.

Ludwig, A. M. & Farrelly, F. (1967) The weapons of insanity. *American Journal of Psychotherapy,* **21** (4), 737–49.

Lukes, S. (1973) *Individualism.* Oxford: Basil Blackwell.

Macfarlane, A. (1978) *The Origins of English Individualism: The Family, Property and Social Transition.* Oxford: Basil Blackwell.

Magan, S. J. & Mrozek, R. (1990) Nursing theory applications: a practice model. *Issues in Mental Health Nursing,* **11,** 297–312.

Malek-Ahmadi, P. & Fried, F. (1976) Biochemical correlates of schizophrenia. *Comprehensive Psychiatry,* **17** (4), 499–509.

Malone, J. (1991) The DSM-III-R versus nursing diagnosis: a dilemma in interdisciplinary practice. *Issues in Mental Health Nursing,* **12** (3), 219–28.

Mark, B. (1980) From 'lunatic' to 'client': 300 years of psychiatric patienthood. *Journal of Psychiatric Nursing and Mental Health Services,* March, 32–36.

Marriott, M. (1976) Hindu transactions: diversity without dualism. In *Transaction and Meaning: Directions in the Anthropology of Exchange and Symbolic Behavior,* ed. B. Kapferer, pp. 109–42. Philadelphia: Institute for the Study of Human Issues.

Martinot, J-L., Peron-Magnan, P., Huret, J-D., Mazoyer, B., Baron, J-C., Boulenger, J-P., Loc'h, C., Maziere, B., Caillard, V., Loo, H. & Syrota, A. (1990) Striatal D_2 dopaminergic receptors assessed with positron emission tomography and [^{76}Br] bromspiperone in untreated schizophrenic patients. *American Journal of Psychiatry,* **147** (1), 44–50.

Marx, K. & Engels, F. (1975) The Holy Family, or critique of critical criticism. In *Collected Works,* Vol. 4, pp. 5–211. London: Lawrence and Wishart.

Marx, O. M. (1990) German romantic psychiatry. Part 1. *History of Psychiatry,* **1** (4), 351–81.

Marx, O. M. (1991) German romantic psychiatry. Part 2. *History of Psychiatry,* **2** (1), 1–25.

Maslow, A. H. (1970) *Motivation and Personality.* New York: Harper and Row.

Matthews, W. M. (1960) Psychotherapy in an orthopsychiatric setting: background and principles. *American Journal of Orthopsychiatry,* **30,** 49–52.

Mauss, M. (1985) A category of the human mind: the notion of person; the notion of self. In *The Category of the Person: Anthropology, Philosophy, History,* ed. M. Carrithers, S. Collins & S. Lukes, pp. 1–25. Cambridge: Cambridge University Press.

McGue, M. & Gottesman, I. I. (1989) Genetic linkage in schizophrenia: perspectives from genetic epidemiology. *Schizophrenia Bulletin,* **15** (3), 453–64.

McGuffin, P., Farmer, A. E., Gottesman, I. I., Murray, R. M. & Reveley, A. M. (1984) Twin concordance for operationally defined schizophrenia: confirmation of familiality and heritability. *Archives of General Psychiatry*, **41**, 541–5.

McHenry, L. C. (1969) *Garrison's History of Neurology*. Springfield, IL: Charles C. Thomas.

McHugh, P. (1968) *Defining the Situation: The Social Organization of Meaning in Social Interaction*. New York: Bobbs-Merrill.

McHugh, P. (1970) A common-sense conception of deviance. In *Deviance and Respectability: The Social Construction of Moral Meanings*, ed. J. Douglas, pp. 61–68. New York: Basic Books.

McKinlay, J. B., ed. (1975) *Processing People: Cases in Organizational Behaviour*. London: Holt, Rinehart and Winston.

McLean, A. (1990) Contradictions in the social production of clinical knowledge: the case of schizophrenia. *Social Science and Medicine*, **30** (9), 969–85.

Mead, G. H. (1934) *Mind, Self and Society: From the Standpoint of a Social Behaviorist*. Chicago: University of Chicago Press.

Meltzer, H. Y. (1982) What is schizophrenia? *Schizophrenia Bulletin*, **8** (3), 433–4.

Menhennet, A. (1981) *The Romantic Movement*. London: Croom Helm.

Menninger, K. (1963) *The Vital Balance: The Life Process in Mental Health and Illness*. New York: Viking Press.

Merquior, J. G. (1985) *Foucault*. London: Fontana Press.

Merton, R. K. (1957) The role set: problems in sociological theory. *British Journal of Sociology*, **8**, 106–20.

Miller, K. (1985) *Doubles: Studies in Literary History*. Oxford: Oxford University Press.

Miller, P. (1980) The territory of the psychiatrist. *Ideology and Consciousness*, **7**, 63–103.

Mishler, E. G. (1984) *The Discourse of Medicine: Dialectics of Medical Interviews*. Norwood, NJ: Ablex.

Mizrahi, T. (1985) Getting rid of patients: contradictions in the socialization of internists to the doctor-patient relationship. *Sociology of Health and Illness*, **7** (2), 214–35.

Moffic, S., Patterson, G. K., Laval, R. & Adams, G. L. (1984) Paraprofessionals and psychiatric teams: an updated review. *Hospital and Community Psychiatry*, **35** (1), 61–67.

Movahedi, S. (1975) Loading the dice in favour of madness. *Journal of Health and Social Behavior*, **16** (2), 192–7.

Munn, N. (1992) The cultural anthropology of time: a critical essay. *Annual Review of Anthropology*, **21**, 93–123.

Murphy, H.B.M. (1982) *Comparative Psychiatry: The International and Intercultural Distribution of Mental Illness*. Berlin: Springer-Verlag.

Myer, A. (1973) Frederic Mott, founder of the Maudsley Laboratories. *British Journal of Psychiatry*, **122**, 497–516.

Nason, F. (1981) Team tension as a vital sign. *General Hospital Psychiatry*, **3** (1), 32–36.

Nason, F. (1984) Diagnosing the hospital team. *Social Work in Health Care*, **9** (2), 25–45.

Neale, J. M. & Oltmanns, T. F. (1980) *Schizophrenia*. New York: Wiley.

Nehls, N., Blahnik, L., Nestler, K. & Richardson, D. (1992) A collaborative nurse-physician practice model for helping persons with serious mental illness. *Hospital and Community Psychiatry*, **43** (8), 842–3.

Noll, R. (1985) Review of D. G. Benner & C. S. Evans, 'Unity and multiplicity in hypnosis, commissurotomy, and multiple personality disorder'. *Transcultural Psychiatric Research Review*, **22** (4), 237–40.

Nye, R. A. (1985) Sociology and degeneration: the irony of progress. In *Degeneration: The Dark Side of Progress*, ed. J. E. Chamberlin & S. L. Gilman, pp. 40–71. New York: Columbia University Press.

O'Toole, A. W. (1981) When the practical becomes theoretical. *Journal of Psychiatric Nursing and Mental Health Services*, **19** (2), 11–19.

Owen, M. (1992) Will schizophrenia become a graveyard for molecular geneticists? *Psychological Medicine*, **22**, 289–93.

Owen, M., Craufurd, D. & St Clair, D. (1990) Localization of a susceptibility locus for schizophrenia on chromosome 5. *British Journal of Psychiatry*, **157**, 123–7.

Papper, S. (1970) The undesirable patient. *Journal of Chronic Disease*, **22**, 777–9.

Parsons, T. (1952) *The Social System*. London: Tavistock.

Pashukanis, E. G. (1978) *Law and Marxism: A General Theory*. London: Ink Links.

Pato, C. N., Lander, E. S. & Schulz, S. C. (1989) Prospects for the genetic analysis of schizophrenia. *Schizophrenia Bulletin*, **15** (3), 365–72.

Paykel, E. S. (1980) Psychopharmacological and social aspects of schizophrenia: recent developments. *Australian and New Zealand Journal of Psychiatry*, **14**, 241–7.

Peters, U. H. (1991) The German classical concept of schizophrenia. In *The Concept of Schizophrenia: Historical Pesrpectives*, ed. J. G. Howells, pp. 59–73. Washington, DC: American Psychiatric Press.

Pichot, P. (1983) *A Century of Psychiatry*. Paris: Edition Rojer da Costa.

Pincus, H. A. & Fine, T. (1992) The 'anatomy' of research funding of mental illness and addictive disorders. *Archives of General Psychiatry*, **49**, 573–9.

Polanyi, M. (1958) *Personal Knowledge: Towards a Post-Critical Philosophy*. Chicago: University of Chicago Press.

Pollock, D. (1985) *Personhood and Illness Among the Culina of Western Brazil.* Ph.D. dissertation, University of Rochester.

Pollock, D. (1992) Structured ambiguity and the definition of psychiatric illness: adjustment disorder among medical inpatients. *Social Science and Medicine,* **35** (1), 25–35.

Poe, E. A. (1872) *The Works of Edgar Allan Poe.* London: John Camden Hotten.

Pope, H. G., Jonas, J. M., Cohen, B. M. & Lipinski, J. F. (1982) Failure to find evidence of schizophrenia in first-degree relatives of schizophrenic probands. *American Journal of Psychiatry,* **139** (6), 826–8.

Pope, H. G., Jonas, J. M., Cohen, B. M. & Lipinski, J. F. (1983) Dr. Pope and associates reply [letter to the editor]. *American Journal of Psychiatry,* **140** (1), 132–3.

Powchik, P. & Schulz, S. C., eds. (1993) *Schizophrenia.* Psychiatric Clinics of North America, 16 (2).

Prince, R. (1983) Review of 'Comparative psychiatry' by H. B. M. Murphy. *Transcultural Psychiatric Research Review,* **20** (3), 114–18.

Radcliffe-Brown, A. R. (1952) *Structure and Function in Primitive Society: Essays and Addresses.* London: Cohen and West.

Raffel, S. (1979) *Matters of Fact: A Sociological Inquiry.* London: Routledge and Kegan Paul.

Rattner, J. (1983) *Alfred Adler.* New York: Frederick Ungar.

Reed, P. G. (1987) Constructing a conceptual framework for psychosocial nursing. *Journal of Psychosocial Nursing,* **25** (2), 24–28.

Renvoise, E. (1991) The Association of Medical Officers of Asylums and Hospitals for the Insane, the Medico-Psychological Association, and their presidents. In *150 Years of British Psychiatry, 1841–1991,* ed. G. E. Berrios & H. Freeman, pp. 29–78. London: Gaskell.

Rhodes, L. A. (1991) *Emptying Beds: The Work of an Emergency Psychiatric Unit.* Berkeley: University of California Press.

Rhodes, L. A. (1992) The subject of power in medical/psychiatric anthropology. In *Ethnopsychiatry: The Cultural Construction of Professional and Folk Psychiatries,* ed. A. D. Gaines, pp. 51–66. Albany, NY: State University of New York Press.

Ricoeur, P. (1967) *Husserl: An Analysis of His Phenomenology.* Evanston, IL: Northwestern University Press.

Ricoeur, P. (1976) *Interpretation Theory: Discourse and the Surplus of Meaning.* Fort Worth, TX: Christian University Press.

Ricoeur, P. (1979) The model of the text: meaningful action considered as a text. In *Interpretive Social Science: A Reader,* ed. P. Rabinow & W. M. Sullivan, pp. 73–101. Berkeley: University of California Press.

Ricoeur, P. (1981) *Hermeneutics and the Human Sciences: Essays on Language, Action and Interpretation.* Cambridge: Cambridge University Press.

Roach Anleu, S. L. (1992) The professionalisation of social work? A case study of three organisational settings. *Sociology*, **26** (1), 23–43.

Roberts, G. W. (1991) Schizophrenia: a neuropathological perspective. *British Journal of Psychiatry*, **158**, 8–17.

Roccatagliata, G. (1991) Classical concepts of schizophrenia. In *The Concept of Schizophrenia: Historical Perspectives*, ed. J. G. Howells, pp. 1–27. Washington, DC: American Psychiatric Press.

Rogler, L. H. & Hollingshead, A. B. (1965) *Trapped: Families and Schizophrenia.* New York: Wiley.

Rose, A. M. (1971) A systematic summary of symbolic interaction theory. In *Human Behavior and Social Processes: An Interactionist Approach*, ed. A. M. Rose, pp. 3–19. London: Routledge and Kegan Paul.

Rosenhan, D. L. (1973) On being sane in insane places. *Science*, **179**, 250–8.

Rosenhan, D. L. (1981) The contextual nature of psychiatric diagnosis. In *The Sociology of Mental Illness: Basic Studies*, ed. O. Grusky & M. Pollner, pp. 319–29. New York: Holt, Rinehart and Winston.

Rosenthal, D. (1975) The concept of subschizophrenic disorders. In *Genetic Research in Psychiatry*, ed. R. R. Fieve, D. Rosenthal & H. Brill, pp. 199–208. Baltimore: Johns Hopkins University Press.

Rosenthal, D., Kety, S., eds. (1968) *The Transmission of Schizophrenia.* Oxford: Pergamon Press.

Rosenthal, T. T. & McGuinness, T. M. (1986) Dealing with delusional patients: discovering the distorted truth. *Issues in Mental Health Nursing*, **8**, 143–54.

Roth, J. A. (1963) *Timetables: Structuring the Passage of Time in Hospital Treatment and Other Careers.* Indianapolis: Bobbs-Merrill.

Roth, J. A. (1972) Some contingencies of the moral evaluation and control of clientele: the case of the hospital emergency service. *American Journal of Sociology*, **77** (5), 839–56.

Rothman, D. J. (1971) *The Discovery of the Asylum: Social Order and Disorder in the New Republic.* Boston: Little, Brown.

Rushing, W. A. (1964) *The Psychiatric Professions: Power, Conflict, and Adaption in a Psychiatric Hospital Staff.* Chapel Hill: University of North Carolina Press.

Russell, B. (1961) *History of Western Philosophy: And its Connection with Political and Social Circumstances from the Earliest Times to the Present Day.* London: George Allen and Unwin.

Ruzek, S. K. (1971) Making social work accountable. In *The Professions and Their Prospects*, ed. E. Freidson, pp. 217–43. Beverly Hills, CA: Sage Publications.

Sahlins, M. (1976) *The Use and Abuse of Biology: An Anthropological Critique of Sociobiology.* Ann Arbor: University of Michigan Press.

Sands, R. G., Stafford, J. & McClelland, M. (1990) 'I beg to differ': conflict in the interdisciplinary team. *Social Work in Health Care*, **14** (3), 55–72.

Scharfetter, C. (1975) The historical development of the concept of schizophrenia. *British Journal of Psychiatry*, Special Publication No. 10, 5–9.

Scheff, T. J. (1984) *Being Mentally Ill: A Sociological Theory.* Chicago: Aldine.

Scheper-Hughes, N. (1979) *Saints, Scholars and Schizophrenics.* Berkeley: University of California Press.

Schneider, K. (1974) Primary and secondary symptoms in schizophrenia. In *Themes and Variations in European Psychiatry*, ed. S. R. Hirsch, M. Shepherd & L. Kalinowsky, pp. 40–44. Charlottesville: University Press of Virginia.

Schreiber, F. R. (1975) *Sybil: The True Story of a Woman Possessed by Sixteen Separate Personalities.* Ringwood, Vic: Penguin.

Schutz, A. (1962) On multiple realities. In *Collected Papers 1: The Problem of Social Reality*, ed. M. Natanson, pp. 207–59. The Hague: Martinus Nijhoff.

Schutz, A. (1972) *The Phenomenology of the Social World.* London: Heinemann.

Schutz, A. & Luckman, T. (1973) *The Structures of the Life-World.* Evanston, IL: Northwestern University Press.

Scott, M. B. & Lyman, S. M. (1968) Accounts. *American Sociological Review*, **33** (1), 47–62.

Scull, A. (1979) *Museums of Madness: The Social Organization of Insanity in Nineteenth Century England.* London: Allen Lane.

Scull, A. (1984) Was insanity increasing? A response to Edward Hare. *British Journal of Psychiatry*, **144**, 432–6.

Seeman, P., Lee, T., Chau-Wong, M. & Wong, K. (1976). Antipsychotic drug doses and neuroleptic/dopamine receptors. *Nature*, **261**, 717–19.

Seeman, P., Ulpian, C., Bergeron, C., Riederer, P., Jellinger, K., Gabriel, E., Reynolds, G. P. & Tourtellotte, W. W. (1984) Bimodal distribution of dopamine receptor densities in brains of schizophrenics. *Science*, **225** (4663), 728–31.

Segal, H. (1973) *Introduction to the Work of Melanie Klein.* New York: Basic Books.

Shakespeare, W. (1951) Hamlet. In *William Shakespeare: The Complete Works*, ed. P. Alexander, pp. 1028–73. London: Collins.

Sham, P. C., O'Callaghan, E., Takei, N., Murray, G. K., Hare, E. H. & Murray, R. M. (1992) Schizophrenia following pre-natal exposure to influenza epidemics between 1939 and 1960. *British Journal of Psychiatry*, **160**, 461–6.

Sharrock, W. W. (1979) Symbolic interactionism as a perspective. In *Perspectives in Sociology*, ed. E. C. Cuff & G. C. F. Payne, pp. 89–120. London: George Allen and Unwin.

Sharrock, W. W. & Turner, R. (1978) On a conversational environment for equivocality. In *Studies in the Organization of Conversational Interaction*, ed. J. Schenkein, pp. 173–97. Orlando, FL: Academic Press.

Sherrington, R., Brynjolfsson, J., Pertusson, H., Potter, M., Dudleston, K., Barraclough, B., Wasmuth, J., Dobbs, M. & Gurling, H. (1988) Localization of a susceptibility locus for schizophrenia on chromosome 5. *Nature*, **336**, 164–7.

Silverman, D. (1975) Accounts of organizations: organizational 'structures' and the accounting process. In *Processing People: Cases in Organizational Behaviour*, ed. J. B. McKinley, pp. 269–302. London: Holt, Rinehart and Winston.

Singer, M. T. & Wynne, L. C. (1965) Thought disorder and family relations of schizophrenics. IV. Results and implications. *Archives of General Psychiatry*, **12**, 201–12.

Siporin, M. (1979) Essay review: practice theory for clinical social work. *Clinical Social Work Journal*, **7** (1), 75–89.

Smith, D. E. (1974) The social construction of documentary reality. *Sociological Inquiry*, **44** (4), 257–68.

Snyder, S. H. (1976) The dopamine hypothesis of schizophrenia: focus on the dopamine receptor. *American Journal of Psychiatry*, **133**, 197–202.

Snyder, S. H. (1982a) What is schizophrenia? *Schizophrenia Bulletin*, **8** (4), 595–7.

Snyder, S. H. (1982b) Schizophrenia. *Lancet*, **8305**, 970–4.

Spitzer, M. (1990) Kant on schizophrenia. In *Philosophy and Psychopathology*, ed. M. Spitzer & B. A. Maher, pp. 44–58. New York: Springer-Verlag.

Stanton, A. H. & Schwartz, M. S. (1954) *The Mental Hospital*. New York: Basic Books.

Stepan, N. (1985) Biological degeneration: races and proper places. In *Degeneration: The Dark Side of Progress*, ed. J. E. Chamberlin & S. L. Gilman, pp. 97–120. New York: Columbia University Press.

Stickey, S. K., Moir, G. & Gardner, E. R. (1981) Psychiatric nurse consultation: who calls and why? *Journal of Psychosocial Nursing and Mental Health Services*, **19** (10), 22–26.

Stoller, A. & Arson, K. W. (1955) *Report on Mental Health Facilities and Needs of Australia*. Canberra: A. J. Arthur at the Government Printing Office.

Strathern, M. (1981) Self-interest and the social good: some implications of Hagen gender imagery. In *Sexual Meanings: The Cultural Construction of Gender and Sexuality*, ed. S. B. Ortner & H. Whitehead, pp. 166–91. Cambridge: Cambridge University Press.

Strauss, A. L. (1978) *Negotiations: Varieties, Contexts, Processes and Social Order.* San Fransisco: Josey-Bass.

Strauss, A. L. (1982) Sentimental work in the technologized hospital. *Sociology of Health and Illness,* **4** (3), 255–78.

Strauss, A. L. & Bucher, R. (1975) Professions in process. In *Professions, Work and Careers,* ed. A. L. Strauss, pp. 9–23. New Brunswick: Transaction Books.

Strauss, A. L., Schatzman, L., Bucher, R., Ehrlich, D. & Sabshin, M. (1964) *Psychiatric Ideologies and Institutions.* New York: Free Press of Glencoe.

Strauss, J. S. (1969) Hallucinations and delusions as points on continua function. *Archives of General Psychiatry,* **21**, 581–6.

Strauss, J. S. & Carpenter, W. T. (1981) *Schizophrenia.* New York: Plenum.

Strong, P. M. (1979) *The Ceremonial Order of the Clinic: Parents, Doctors and Medical Bureaucracies.* London: Routledge and Kegan Paul.

Sudnow, D. (1965) Normal crimes: sociological features of the penal code. *Social Problems,* **12**, 255–64, 269–70.

Sullivan, H. S. (1962) Environmental factors and course under treatment of schizophrenia. In *Schizophrenia as a Human Process,* ed. H. S. Perry, pp. 246–55. New York: W. W. Norton.

Szasz, T. (1973) *The Manufacture of Madness: A Comparative Study of the Inquisition and the Mental Health Movement.* London: Granada/Paladin.

Szasz, T. (1976) Schizophrenia: the sacred symbol of psychiatry. *British Journal of Psychiatry,* **129**, 308–16.

Tagliavini, A. (1985) Aspects of the history of psychiatry in Italy in the second half of the nineteenth century. In *The Anatomy of Madness: Essays in the History of Psychiatry. Vol. II: Institutions and Society,* ed. W. F. Bynum, R. Porter & M. Shepherd, pp. 175–96. London: Tavistock.

Tamminga, C. A., Thaker, G. K., Buchanan, R., Kirkpatrick, B., Alphs, L. D., Chase, T. N. & Carpenter, W. T. (1992) Limbic system abnormalities identified in schizophrenia using positron emission tomography with fluorodeoxyglucose and neocortical alterations with deficit syndrome. *Archives of General Psychiatry,* **49**, 522–30.

Tannen, D. (1982) The oral/literate continuum in discourse. In *Spoken and Written Language: Exploring Orality and Literacy,* ed. D. Tannen, pp. 1–16. Norwood, NJ: Ablex.

Taussig, M.T. (1980) Reification and the consciousness of the patient. *Social Science and Medicine,* **14B**, 3–13.

Taylor, C. (1985) The person. In *The Category of the Person: Anthropology, Philosophy, History,* ed. M. Carrithers, S. Collins & S. Lukes, pp. 257–81. Cambridge: Cambridge University Press.

Thompson, E. H. & Doll, W. (1982) The burden of families coping with the mentally ill: an invisible crisis. *Family Relations*, **31**, 379–88.

Tiller, J., Schmidt, U. & Treasure, J. (1993) Compulsory treatment for anorexia nervosa: compassion or coercion? *British Journal of Psychiatry*, **162**, 679–80.

Torrey, E. F. (1988) Stalking the schizovirus. *Schizophrenia Bulletin*, **14** (2), 223–9.

Tsuang, M. T. (1993) Genotypes, phenotypes, and the brain: a search for connections in schizophrenia. *British Journal of Psychiatry*, **163**, 299–307.

Turkle, S. (1981) French anti-psychiatry. In *Critical Psychiatry: The Politics of Mental Health*, ed. D. Ingleby, pp. 150–83. Harmondsworth: Penguin Books.

Van den Berg, J. H. (1977) A metabletic-philosophical evaluation of mental health. In *Mental Health: Philosophical Perspectives*, ed. H. T. Engelhardt & S. F. Spicker, pp. 121–36. Dordrecht: Reidel.

Vaughn, C. E. & Leff, J. P. (1976) The influence of family and social factors on the course of psychiatric illness. *British Journal of Psychiatry*, **129**, 125–37.

Vaughn, C. E. & Leff, J. P. (1981) Patterns of emotional response in relatives of schizophrenic patients: a comparison of schizophrenic and depressed patients. *Schizophrenia Bulletin*, **7** (1), 43–44.

Verwey, G. (1985) *Psychiatry in Anthropological and Biomedical Context: Philosophical Presuppositions and Implications of German Psychiatry, 1820–1870*. Dordrecht: Reidel.

Waddington, J. L., O'Callaghan, E., Buckley, P., Larkin, C., Redmond, O., Stack, J. P., Ennis, J. T. & Kinsella, A. (1994) Are structural brain changes in schizophrenia solely of neurodevelopmental origin, or is there a neurodegenerative component? In *Abstracts of the Annual Meeting of the Royal College of Psychiatrists*, University College Cork, Republic of Ireland, pp. 39–40.

Walk, A. (1976) Medico-psychologists, Maudsley and The Maudsley. *British Journal of Psychiatry*, **128**, 19–30.

Wender, P. H. (1963) Dementia praecox: the development of the concept. *American Journal of Psychiatry*, **119** (12), 1143–51.

Westermeyer, J. (1991) Problems with managed psychiatric care without a psychiatrist-manager. *Hospital and Community Psychiatry*, **42** (12), 1221–4.

Wexler, B. (1980) Cerebral laterality and psychiatry: review of the literature. *American Journal of Psychiatry*, **137**, 279–91.

Wheeler, S. (1969) *On Record: Files and Dossiers in American Life*. New York: Russell Sage Foundation.

Wilkinson, G. (1987) Introduction to 'Dementia praecox' by E. Kraepelin. In *The Origins of Modern Psychiatry*, ed. C. Thompson, pp. 238–42. Chichester: Wiley.

Willis, E. (1989) *Medical Dominance: The Division of Labour in Australian Health Care*. Sydney: Allen and Unwin.

Wing, J. K. (1978a) The social context of schizophrenia. *American Journal of Psychiatry*, **135** (11), 1333–9.

Wing, J. K. (1978b) *Reasoning About Madness*. London: Oxford University Press.

Wing, J. K. (1980) Social psychiatry in the United Kingdom: the approach to schizophrenia. *Schizophrenia Bulletin*, **6** (4), 556–65.

Wong, D. F., Wagner, H. N., Tune, L. E., Dannals, R. F., Pearlson, G. D., Links, J. M., Tamminga, C. A., Broussolle, E. P., Ravert, H. T., Wilson, A. A., Toung, J. K. T., Malat, J., Williams, J. A., O'Tuama, L. A., Snyder, S. H., Kuhar, M. J. & Gjedde, A. (1986) Positron emission tomography reveals elevated D$_2$ dopamine receptors in drug-naive schizophrenics. *Science*, **234** (4783), 1558–63.

Wood, A. W. (1984) Kant's compatibilism. In *Self and Nature in Kant's Philosophy*, ed. A. W. Wood, pp. 73–101. Ithaca: Cornell University Press.

Woolf, V. (1933) *Orlando: A Biography*. London: Hogarth Press.

World Health Organization (1978) *International Classification of Diseases: Manual of the International Statistical Classification of Diseases, Injuries and Causes of Death*. Geneva: World Health Organization.

Wright, A. L. & Morgan, W. J. (1990) On the creation of 'problem' patients. *Social Science and Medicine*, **30** (9), 951–9.

Wyatt, R. J., Kirch, D. G. & DeLisi, L. E. (1989) Schizophrenia: biochemical, endocrine, and immunological studies. In *Comprehensive Textbook of Psychiatry*, ed. H. I. Kaplan & B. J. Sadock, pp. 717–32. Baltimore: Williams and Wilkins.

Young, J. M. (1992) Functions of thought and the synthesis of intuitions. In *The Cambridge Companion to Kant*, ed. P. Guyer, pp. 101–22. Cambridge: Cambridge University Press.

Young, R. M. (1985) *Darwin's Metaphor: Nature's Place in Victorian Culture*. Cambridge: Cambridge University Press.

Zerubavel, E. (1979) *Patterns of Time in Hospital Life*. Chicago: University of Chicago Press.

Zilboorg, G. A. (1941) *A History of Medical Psychology*. New York: Norton.

Index